Concepts and Practices of Healing

Glenn Molinari

Concepts and Practices of Healing

Soul Echoes and Metatron's Meditation Updated November 15, 2017

Glenn Molinari

P.O. Box 1534

Cornville, AZ 86325

Library of Congress

Copyright © 2017

Concepts and Practices of Healing / Glenn Molinari

Registration Number: TXu 2-024-247

Medical Advice Disclaimer

The information included in this book is not intended nor implied to be a substitute for professional medical advice. The reader should always consult his or her healthcare provider to determine the appropriateness of the information for their own situation or if they have any questions regarding a medical condition or treatment plan. The author assumes no responsibility or liability for how readers of this book choose to use the information contained within.

ISBN: 978-0-09854784-7-6

Table of Contents

Concepts and Practices of Healing

Preface

This book presents_information on the concepts of healing, and puts together a way to understand the connection between the body (physical), mind (mental and emotional), and spirit.

It also has practical and clear ways to implement what is presented.

As in any worthwhile undertaking the practices take effort, commitment and perseverance.

This will help guide you to ***your own way*** of understanding, healing and growing.

FREE downloadable and printable PDFs of the meditations, exercises and prayers in this book are available at http://www.twochoices.net/FREE_PDFs.html

They do not include the explanations and information in the book, so I suggest you read the book first.

Introduction

I gathered the information included here for myself and others beginning in the late 1980s. It is from various sources. I included the source information where I still have it. I strongly believe this information to be correct.

This book has information I have found valid and helpful for myself. I believe that connecting more closely to Great Spirit and LOVE also requires taking care of the physical body. I am still far from perfect in my eating habits and life style and yet I have noticed I am doing better as I continue my journey.

Like physical healing, when you do mental, emotional and Spiritual house clearing, your physical body can have reactions or go through detoxing symptoms. As with *any* type of healing, when you are detoxing, whether it be physical, mental, emotional or Spiritual you may have symptoms of the detox.

Great Spirit and Great Spirit's Helpers know what is best and what you can handle. Prior to healing you may ask Great Spirit and Great Spirit's Helpers as are best to make it gentle enough so you can continue your daily responsibilities.

You may have disorientation, vertigo, emotional release (unpleasant *feelings*/emotions, unpleasant dreams) while healing. This is often the case with any healing, including the use of such things as Flower Essences, Reiki, Shamanistic Practices, Soul Retrieval, Inner Child Healing, Prayer, Fasting and The Use of Antibiotics.

Allow the release and thank what is coming to the surface to be healed, erased, forgiven and loved (an emotion, *feeling*, thought, physical detox, etc).

You may get very tired for a few hours or for several days. If so, rest when your schedule permits.

NOTE: You may see immediate results or it may take a while before you see any changes in your life, awareness and health. Divinity knows what layers and what toxins need to be healed, erased, forgiven and loved. Divinity also knows the order in which to process them and the timing for each.

As you heal be careful as you reduce or even eliminate traditional therapies. If you are on prescription medicines consult with your doctor before discontinuing. As an example, blood pressure medicine can often be reduced or eliminated as you manage your weight, eat healthier and learn to reduce stress.

Glossary

Divinity/God/Great Spirit:
I prefer using the term Great Spirit to denote Divinity. Using the term that makes you most comfortable is best.

Aumakua: *(au·ma·ku·a)*
The Hawaiian name for what is sometimes called the super-conscious/connection with the divine. It is also defined as Hawaiian Ancestral Spirits.

Unihipili: *(u·hi·ni·pi·li)*
The Hawaiian name for what is sometimes called the subconscious /inner/emotional/intuitive mind. I use the name 'Unihipili' because there is nothing sub about the subconscious. It may need our LOVE and guidance; however, in many, and probably in most ways, it is much more powerful than the conscious mind.

Work
"Work", when doing healing 'work', includes healing, releasing, relinquishing, 'letting go', clearing and transmuting. It only includes 'curing' of physical symptoms and ailments if they are no longer needed for soul growth and spiritual development. If you are working on physical, emotional or mental symptoms make sure you remember the previous sentence. Keep enjoyment in the process.

Even though the Unihipili is much more powerful than the conscious mind, it is in many ways like a three or four year old child. It needs guidance and LOVE. It also likes to investigate. The Unihipili, or child within, will respond or react according to your "choice". The Unihipili, like children, dislikes work and likes to play; therefore I use the word carefully when doing any kind of healing, releasing and transmuting.

Uhane: *(u·ha·ne)*
The Hawaiian name for what is sometimes called the consciousness/waking/rational mind.

love: (lower case denotes human love as defined in the dictionary)
Is often defined as: feel affection for, adore, worship, be in love with, be devoted to, care for, find irresistible, be keen on and be fond of. This kind of love leaves room for judgment, anger, attachment, jealousy and other negative thoughts and feelings/emotions that are of a lower vibrational frequency.

Divine LOVE: (all upper case denotes Divine LOVE)
The word or phrase is basically indefinable, except to Know it leaves no room for anything that is out of harmony and attunement with God Source.

Violet Flame:
Some people have asked or wondered what the 'Violet Flame' is. Several definitions combined into one is that the Violet Flame is the essence of a unique Spiritual light, which has the qualities of mercy, forgiveness, freedom and transmutation.

Transmutation:

The dictionary definition is change/alteration/ transformation/metamorphosis.

As used in this book, transmutation is one of Divinity's tools for changing what is often referred to as dark/negative/evil into LOVE and LIGHT.

Healing, Transmuting, Releasing and Integrating:

Any time any form of the words *heal, clear* or *release* is used in a clearing or healing it includes the process of healing the energetic causes, transmuting any ‘negative’ into its ‘positive’ and Loving counterpart, releasing the unhealthy attachments and integrating the positive, life affirming and Loving aspects into yourself. If you have a pain, discomfort, injury or disease, treat it at the physical level with physical means. It is always a good idea to also treat the pain, discomfort, injury or disease by Healing, Transmuting, Releasing and Integrating at the spiritual, mental and emotional levels as well.

“As is best”:

Many of my prayers, the way I say them, are finished with “as is best”. This is my way of turning the prayer or request over to Great Spirit/God/Divinity without attachment to a desired outcome or an expectation. If you have another way of turning it over to Great Spirit use your way. Just make sure you turn it over. Also, remember you are responsible to do your part. If you sit on the couch and eat or drink all day and pray, “make me healthy” or “make me wealthy”, do you really expect to be made healthy or wealthy.

Feelings and Emotions:

There is such a fine line between the definitions of 'feeling' 'and emotion' that they can be easily confused. In many dictionaries one word is used to define the other. I understand feelings as held inside and often unexpressed, and emotions as expressed feelings, both literally and nonverbally. As an example, if you feel angry at someone **<u>but</u>** put on a happy face, that is a feeling. If you express the feeling outwardly that is an emotion. An emotion is the outward expression of a feeling. This is how I use the words in this book. Most places you will see 'feelings/emotions' rather than as separate words, since they are healed and released in the same way.

Co-Creation and Manifesting:

To me there is a difference between ‘co-creation’ with Great Spirit and ‘manifestation’. Co-creation is more at the spiritual and energetic level and Manifestation is more at the physical and human action level.

Entity:

Everything, everyone, every human, every non-human, every spirit, and each and every awareness, what we perceive and describe as Light and what we perceive and describe as Dark, is an entity. As an example, all of the following are entities: the earth, a rock, a grain of sand, a street sign, each hair on our heads, each molecule that makes up our hair, and each atom that makes up the molecule, each proton, electron and neutron. The energies that make up all of these things are entities. This can be expanded in all directions infinitely.

Judgment and Non-judgmental:

I use 'non-judgmental' as meaning **allowing** the other person or Being their own path, free will, truths and perceptions. A decision based on an objective observation is different than a 'judgment' and more like assessment. With objective assessment you can then take the appropriate action or inaction.

Accept, Accepting and Acceptance:

Rather than using the word non-judgmental it is more potent, more clear and more uplifting to say "unconditionally accepting" or "unconditional acceptance". This is at spiritual and energetic levels to allow others their own perceptions, choices and realities. It is appropriate and wise to protect yourself from any kind of abuse or mistreatment, whether verbal, physical or very subtle. If someone or an organization is abusing or mistreating you in anyway, distance yourself from them energetically **and** physically if you are able. If you are **temporarily** in a position where you are physically 'trapped', use a method to prevent taking on the energy as a personal belief. Acceptance is different than accepting negative people or circumstances into your life. It refers primarily to your feelings, as they are, relative to the negative people or circumstances. See yourself as safe.

Remember to unconditionally accept your self.

Compassion - As We Have Been Taught By Society and The Dictionary:

sorrow for the sufferings or trouble of another or others, with the urge to help; pity; deep sympathy; the feeling of empathy for others; emotion that we feel in response to the suffering of others that motivates a desire to help; suffering together with another; participation in suffering; requires walking with the other person and feeling with them their suffering; deep awareness of the suffering of another coupled with the wish to relieve it. This version of compassion defines someone as a victim and is thus a form of judgment.

Compassion - Higher Dimensional Version Of:

Deep awareness of the suffering of another without the need to relieve it, feeling total appreciation for its value; a state of unconditional acceptance and LOVE.

Accept that each person is choosing their problem(s) and have to connect with their own Higher SELF in order to heal;

We must shift our perspective of compassion and begin using a version that is beyond what we have been taught. We must move into the realm of unconditional acceptance, leaving pity and the need to 'fix' behind.

We must suspend all judgment of the actions of another. We must be aware of those actions, how painful they are and at the same time realize that they have a value and that this value pertains to the role they play in facilitating our spiritual growth as souls

Power - Dictionary Definition:

Authority, control, influence, supremacy, command, dominance, force.

Manipulation would be the key word; the power to manipulate situations and those around you.

Power - As Used In This Book:

Personal power comes from wisdom. Real personal power is a subtle quality of Beingness rather than a force.

Real power has nothing to do with control, especially the control of others. Conversely, real power is surrendering to the highest good.

Real power naturally settles within one's Beingness of its own accord as Wisdom and Love increase.

Wisdom - Dictionary Definition:

Understanding, knowledge, intelligence, accumulated learning, opinion widely held, accumulated philosophic or scientific learning, the judicious application of knowledge.

Wisdom - As Used In This Book

Wisdom has nothing to do with the level of one's attained knowledge, age, intelligence or I.Q. rating. Wisdom is born of LOVE arising from the heart. Wisdom becomes part of your Being.

Some aspects of wisdom: Acceptance, Patience and Perseverance, Attitude, Silence, Personal Responsibility, Gentleness and Serenity, Value and Priorities, and Respect

True Wisdom is beyond words and the intellect, and is only fully understood by the heart through Awareness.

To understand wisdom as clearly as possible with the intellect, the main aspects of wisdom also need to be understood. These are expanded on in my second book; *Awareness - A Path To Spiritual and Physical Health And Well-Being.*

"Amen" at the end of prayers

How many of us have said the word "Amen" at the end of a prayer without really giving it a second thought? Have you ever said "Amen", without thought, as a ratification of what is said? You may be saying, "May it be done as the speaker has prayed". Did you fully understand the prayer and did you fully agree with it?

As regards the etymology, which is the study of the origins of words, many believe "Amen" is a derivative from the Hebrew verb *aman* "to strengthen" or "confirm". Some believe the word was originally derived from a Sanskrit word "aum", meaning "to sound out loudly" and some believe it simply means "truly" or "so be it". Is it simply a form of affirmation or confirmation of the speaker's own thought?

In forms of worship a final amen, as now used, often sums up and confirms a prayer.

In many cases the word "Amen" is used as nothing more than a formula of conclusion — *finis,* indicating that the statement or prayer is ended and completed.

The seeming ambiguity of the word "Amen" is why I finish my prayers with "As is best" and "Thank you".

Stealing:

It is best never to steal. I'll leave it to you to decide if stealing a loaf of bread when one is literally starving is in Harmony with LOVE. It is best to ask for what one needs.

Breaking Promises:

It is best never to break a promise (unless it was made in anger or spite). If you do your best to keep your promise and a flat tire or true emergency interferes, explain and apologize.

Lying:

It is best never to lie. I'll leave it to you to decide if telling someone, "I forgot to buy your birthday present", is in Harmony with LOVE when you bought the present and want to surprise them.

Even though these are ‘my’ definitions, I hope they are thought-provoking for you. Think for yourself.

Personal Notes

Chapter 1

Philosophies and Concepts of Healing

Different Concepts Of The Cause Of Dis-ease

Traditional Western Concepts, Miasms (Homeopathy) and

Imprints On The Luminous Energy Field (Shamanism)

I hyphenated disease to emphasize that disease is something that is out of balance and is usually more than just physical. The disease can be caused by physical, emotional, mental or spiritual imbalances and toxins. Most, if not all, disease has components of more than one cause.

Concept As Practiced By Most Traditional Main Stream Doctors In The United States

Surgery and prescriptions without looking into the true underlying causes of disease.

More Complete Western Concepts

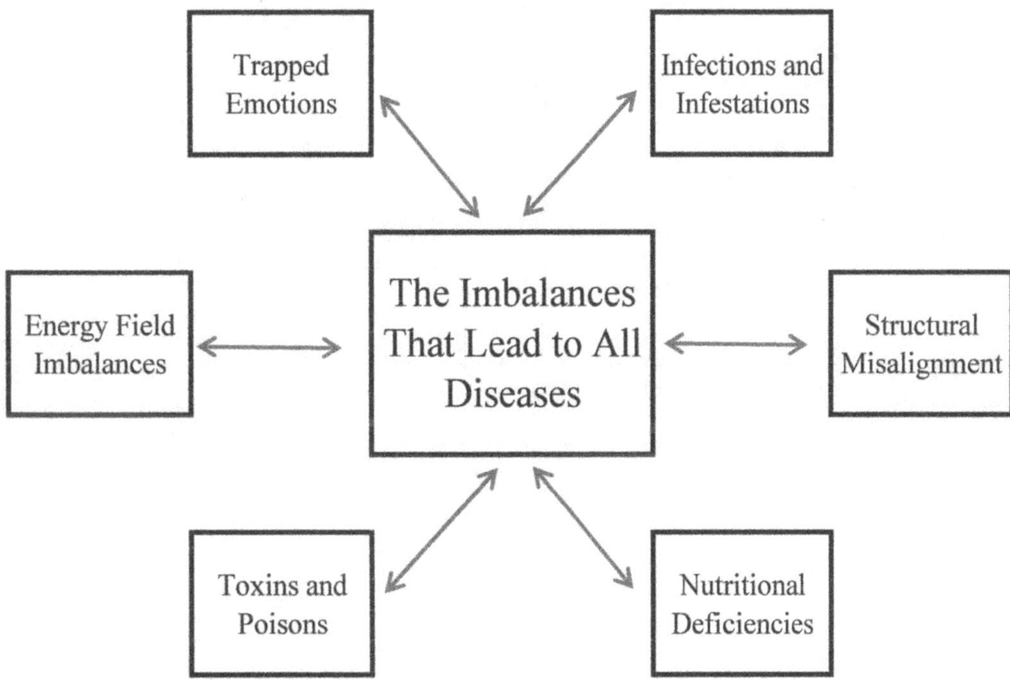

****

Below is adapted from http://www.klinghardtacademy.com>

The Five Levels Of Healing *By Dietrich Klinghardt, MD, PhD*

		Level Body / Sphere	Our Experience At This Level	Anatomical & Conceptual Designation	"Diagnostic" Method	Related Medical Treatment & Healing Techniques
		5th Level Spiritual Body	Oneness with God, Satori	Spirit, Higher Consciousness	Knowing & Awareness	Self Healing, Prayer, True Meditation, Chanting
	Soul is a composite of Levels 2 through 4	4th Level Intuitive Body	Intuition, Symbols, Trance, Meditative States, Dreams, Magic Curses, Spirit Possession, Out of body & near-death experiences	Collective Unconscious, "No Mind"	Intuition, systemic Family constellation, Sound & VoiceAnalysis, Radiesthesla, Dream Analysis, Syntonic Optometry, Art Therapy	Applied Psycho-Neurobiology (APN) II, Systemic Family Constellation, Color and Sound Therapies, Shamanism, Hypnotherapy, Jungian Psychotherapy, Radlonics, Rituals
Emotional Body is a composite of Levels 1 through 3		3rd Level Mental Body	Thoughts, Beliefs, Attitudes, Long distance healing, Consensus reality	Mind & Mental Field [conscious & Subconscious mind], Morphic field, The "Will"	AutonomiC Response Testing (ART) I & II, Applied Psycho-Neurobiology (APN) I & II, Psychological interview· (MMPI), Homeopathic Repertoirizing	Applied Psycho-Neurobiology (APN) I, Mental Field Therapy, Psychotherapy, TFT, EMDR, Homeopathy
		2nd Level Energy Body	Feelings - [anger, Joy, etc], Chi [qigong "energy"], 6th sense & other "energy" perceptions	Nervous system, Meridians, Chakras, Aura, Bio-Electric system, GAGS, Microtubules	Autonomic Response Testing (ART) I & II, Thermogram, EEG, EKG, EMG, VAS, EAV, KInesiOlogy, Chinese Pulses, Kirlian Photography, X-rays, MRI, CAT scan	Neural Therapy (A & B), Microcurrent Therapies, Acupuncture, BodyWork/Touch, Breath Therapy, Yoga, Qigong, Meditation, Radiation Therapy
		1st Level Physical Body	Sensations [touch, smell, etc], Action, Movement	Structure & Biochemistry	Direct Resonance - Autonomic Response Testing (ART) II, Physical Exam,Lab Tests, BDORT	Diet Therapy, Exercise, Osteopathy & Chiropractic, Surgery, Physical Therapy, Drugs & Herbs, Orthomolecular Medicine, Aromatherapy

Above is adapted from
http://www.klinghardtacademy.com/images/stories/5_levels_of_healing/Klinghardt_Article_5_Levels_of_Healing.pdf

Miasms As In Classical Homeopathy

When we ask someone, "What are miasms?", we usually get the answer, "Miasms are the fundamental cause of all diseases." or "Miasms are the factors which predispose us to diseases." But these answers tell us about the effect of miasms and not what they stand for.

Miasms are caused by a mis-integration (or dis-integration) of all of the parts of us. Particularly the disconnection of spiritual and physical. This misalignment creates a gap where susceptibility can reside and this is the miasm. That's why some of us suffer physically, some mentally, some emotionally, and some on a more spiritual level. When we can bridge the gap, reclaim our total selves and integrate them, the gap ceases to exist and so then does the susceptibility. This is what we need to do to heal.

The miasm is the cause, rather than the result, of this dis-ease or dis-integration'. This disconnectedness can occur on all levels, physical, spiritual, emotional, social, etc. Miasms can be inherited from your mother or father and you may notice that your siblings have it in one form or other, in lesser or greater degrees. Usually, when you see someone who has a miasm, you will find that their family members have it as well.

Imprints On The Luminous Energy Field

Luminous energy medicine has been used in different cultures for thousands of years.

Many Shamans and others who practice Luminous Energy Medicine believe our physical bodies are surrounded by a luminous energy field. Today many call this field our "aura," "halo" or "light body." This Luminous Energy Field has information on all our personal memories, early-life traumas and painful wounds as well as information from our ancestors and past lives.

These imprints also affect our physical bodies. While a physical mass can be removed by surgery, the blueprint (miasm or imprint) of the mass can still be in the Luminous Energy Field. When this occurs, it is only a matter of time before the mass returns unless the energy field's blueprint is healed. This is why many people are able to be healed of a serious physical condition, only to have it reappear years later down the road. The disease may have been cured. The cause was left unhealed. The cure can buy you time to heal the underlying energetic and Spiritual causes.

Many people believe the Luminous Energy Field has layers extending outward from the body.

A simple concept that is a good basis for understanding the Luminous Energy Field can be of layers as follows:

1. Causal (the Spirit)
2. Psychic (also known as etheric – the soul)
3. Mental-emotional (the mind)
4. Physical (the body)

The Luminous Energy Field contains an archive of all of our personal and ancestral memories, of all early-life trauma, and even of painful wounds from former lifetimes.

Are Misaims and 'Imprints On The Luminous Energy Field' The Same Thing?

It seems to me both are about the same thing, with different terminology and ways to heal the Miasm or imprint.

****

Healing On All Levels

Below is adapted from < http://www.katasee.com/2012/03/29/healing-on-all-levels/ from Kay Cordell Whitaker>

(web page no longer available)

Glenn's comment: This article talks about something called "Red Door Work". I have not looked into that. The basic information in this article feels right and makes sense.

In response to our post on "Healing with Energy and Spirit" William shared some great thoughts in the comments. He talked about how many of the alternative MD's are stressing the physical/emotional toxin load as well.

He also shared that he's worked with various physical level chelators and detoxers over the years and that his favorite right now is MCP (modified citrus pectin).

Here is our response to his comments.

There are slowly more and more MDs who are coming out with a similar perspective about the causes and treatment of disease.

In the Ka Ta See, Egyptian and radionics traditions we are always looking for the cause behind the cause behind the cause as well as the issues that appear circular in their influence on each other – sort of a chicken or the egg appearance.

An important factor which is often forgotten within the discussion of the role of emotional trauma within certain disorders and diseases are miasms.

Miasms are a huge focus in homeopathics.

This is too large a subject to go into in a blog post, but miasms are an hereditary, energetic, tendency for disease as well as an energetic condition that we can create in ourselves that leans us toward a particular type or group of disease conditions. We're not actually inheriting the disease, we're inheriting a tendency for acquiring it if our bodies get weakened; we are inheriting or building a weakness toward certain disorders.

They weaken our system so much that our inherent tendency for a particular disorder kicks in and we acquire a sickness that has been in our family before; or we become ill with disorders that we pass on to our own children in the same way.

One of the beauties about the Red Door work is that it can take miasms into account.

We have tracked physical toxins being drawn to certain organs because of emotional patterns being held there.

What we have observed consistently is that physical toxins as well as pathogens show up in areas, which are already weakened, whether by miasms, emotional traumas, previous injury or disorders, or malnutrition, where they have the most chance to thrive because they take the path of least resistance.

Poisons will also show up in any area and then proceed to severely weaken that tissue. And, of course, you can see where that could lead…the now weak tissue attracts more problems.

And that's where poisons come in. And by physical poisons I mean more than our man-made industrial and agricultural poisons. Emotional, mental and spiritual aspects that are out of harmony also attract more problems.

We need to look at the poisons in our diet that are legally labeled "food" or "edible" but are completely artificial, laced with toxins and over processed, such as white sugar, manufactured sugar chemicals, canola oil, soy oil, other newly invented monounsaturated and polyunsaturated oils, additives, monsters like Kool Whip, fast foods that no longer have a vitamin or mineral left, commercially raised animals. The list goes on for quite some length.

Unresolved negative emotions definitely play a role in weakening those systems, just like all other highly toxic poisons to the body.

It can be difficult to help people who keep shoveling in any of the various forms of poison.

Kay and I have been going through detox, specifically mercury and heavy metal detox for the past 5 years. About half way through we discovered MCP. It's amazing stuff.

What we have found in our work and in our own experience with detox is that it isn't so much about finding the latest and greatest chelator, which is a good thing, no doubt.

What is really crucial is to find the best combination of vitamins, minerals, supplements and diet where the nutrition and supplements support each other and the detoxing and the rebuilding processes in the best way possible.

All this has to be coordinated with every other supporting thing that's done such as the Red Door, lymph treatments, colon hydrotherapy and so on, in such a way that the chance for a healing crisis is kept to a minimum while the person gets rid of this enormous amount of poison the fastest way possible.

Kay cleared out her extremely high levels of mercury inside 2 years. That's been verified with lab tests. It's been rather remarkable.

The Red Door was invaluable in that process, but we also have been and still are using a list of ten different poison grabbers.

You probably could call them chelators, but we've come to refer to them as grabbers because not all fit the distinct definition for chelator.

Some of the most astounding things we sometimes observe are around the recommendations by practitioners as to what people should take and do to remove heavy metals from their body.

There are people who put essential oils on their feet and after they have done that for a short while the practitioner tells them that they are free of mercury. I challenge everybody doing that to take a DMSA challenge lab test to see where their mercury levels really are.

Another thing we run into quite a bit is that people come to us with certain symptoms and they have a list of supplements they are taking and in some cases we find their combination of supplement intake is part of the cause of their symptoms.

One simple example (but there are many more), we use Cholin (pure, by itself) with L-methionine and silimarin for liver cleaning and rebuilding.

Many practitioners recommend taking Choline with inositol, for other reasons, not as part of this combination.

So clients end up substituting the inositol mix for the pure choline that they then take with our mix. In our experience, inositol in the mix considerably lowers the liver cleansing effect of Choline and has some other strange side effects.

For us, and some of this is mentioned in the post, health, healing and especially detox is a combination of energy healing, the Red Door work, a supportive and highly effective combination of vitamins, minerals and supplements, together with lymph and colonics treatments and considerable attention on healthy food and emotional well being, being in Song and being happy which has helped us make such enormous progress in our own detox and healing.

We've met a friend recently whom we hadn't seen for almost ten years and his comment was, "you haven't aged, you look the same as you have ten years ago!"

As we always say, the proof for any work, but especially healing work, is in the pudding.

Thanks again for sharing.

Love and Song,

Helmut

Above is adapted from < http://www.katasee.com/2012/03/29/healing-on-all-levels/ from Kay Cordell Whitaker>

(web page no longer available)

****

Below is from: <http://www.mercola.com/forms/background.htm>

About Dr. Mercola

You are wise to question who you can trust when it comes to maintaining, enhancing, or rebuilding your health.

With all websites, newspapers, magazines, and other publications offering health advice important questions are.

1)What is their real motivation?

> Is the underlying motivation to make you as healthy as you can possibly be or is it whatever has the most profit potential and ego.

I fund this site, and therefore, am not handcuffed to any advertisers, silent partners, or corporate parents.

My motivation is to make you as healthy as you can possibly be. This involves:

1. Providing the most up-to-date natural health information and resources that will most benefit you and,
2. Exposing corporate, government, and mass media hype that diverts you away from what is truly best for your health and often to a path that leads straight into an early grave.

2)What are their qualifications?

My qualifications: first and foremost, I am an osteopathic physician, also known as a DO. DOs are licensed physicians who, similar to MDs, can prescribe medication and perform surgery in all 50 states. DOs and MDs have similar training requiring four years of study in the basic and clinical sciences, and the successful completion of licensing exams. But DOs bring something extra to the practice of medicine. Osteopathic physicians practice a "whole person" approach, treating the entire person rather than just symptoms. Focusing on preventive health care, DOs help patients develop attitudes and lifestyles that don't just fight illness, but help prevent it, too.

I am also board-certified in family medicine and served as the chairman of the family medicine department at St. Alexius Medical Center for five years. I am trained in both traditional and natural medicine.

My Education:

- University of Illinois at Chicago - UIC 1972-1976
- Chicago College of Osteopathic Medicine – Midwestern University 1978-1982
- Chicago Osteopathic Hospital 1982-1985 Family Practice Residency. Chief resident 1984-1985
- Board Certified American College Osteopathic General Practitioners July 1985

State of Illinois Licensed Physician and Surgeon

Above is from: <http://www.mercola.com/forms/background.htm>

****

Personal Notes

Chapter 2

Mind (Emotional and Mental)

****

Below is adapted from *Many Lives, Many Masters* by Brian L. Weiss, M.D.

Intellectual knowledge, easily acquired, must be transformed into 'emotional,' or subconscious, knowledge.

I recognized the influence of the messages from the Masters.

" ... Wisdom is achieved very slowly. This is because intellectual knowledge, easily acquired, must be transformed into 'emotional,' or subconscious, knowledge. Once transformed, the imprint is permanent. Behavioral practice is the necessary catalyst of this reaction. Without action, the concept will wither and fade. Theoretical knowledge without practical application is not enough."

"Balance and harmony are neglected today, yet they are the foundations of wisdom. Everything is done to excess. People are overweight because they eat excessively. Joggers neglect aspects of themselves and others because they run excessively. People seem excessively mean. They drink too much, smoke too much, carouse too much (or too little), talk too much without content, and worry too much. There is too much black-or-white thinking. All or none. This is not the way of nature."

"In nature there is balance. Beasts destroy in small amounts."

Ecological systems are not eliminated en masse. Plants are consumed and then grow. The sources of sustenance are dipped into and then replenished. The flower is enjoyed, the fruit eaten, the root preserved.

"Humankind has not learned about balance, let alone practiced it. It is guided by greed and ambition, steered by fear. In this way it will eventually destroy itself. But nature will survive; at least the plants will."

"Happiness is really rooted in simplicity. The tendency to excessiveness in thought and action diminishes happiness. Excesses cloud basic values. Religious people tell us that happiness comes from filling one's heart with love, from faith and hope, from practicing charity and dispensing kindness. They actually are right. Given those attitudes, balance and harmony usually follow. These are collectively a state of being. In these days, they are an altered state of consciousness. It is as if humankind were not in its natural state while on earth. It must reach an altered state in order to fill itself with love and charity and simplicity, to feel purity, to rid itself of its chronic fearfulness."

"How does one reach this altered state, this other value system? And once reached, how can it be sustained? The answer appears to be simple. It is the common denominator of all religions.

Humankind is immortal, and what we are doing now is learning our lessons. We are all in school. It is so simple if you can believe in immortality."

"If a part of humankind is eternal, and there is much evidence and history to think so, then why are we doing such bad things to ourselves? Why do we step on and over others for our personal 'gain' when actually we're flunking the lesson? We all seem to be going to the same place ultimately, albeit at different speeds. No one is greater than another."

"Consider the lessons. Intellectually the answers have always been there, but this need to actualize by experience, to make the subconscious imprint permanent by 'emotionalizing' and practicing the concept, is the key. Memorizing in Sunday School is not good enough. Lip service without the behavior has no value. It is easy to read about or to talk about love and charity and faith. But to *do* it, to *feel* it, almost requires an altered state of consciousness. Not the transient state induced by drugs, alcohol, or unexpected emotion. The permanent state is reached by knowledge and understanding. It is sustained by physical behavior, by act and deed, by practice. It is taking something nearly mystical and transforming it to everyday familiarity by practice, making it a habit."

"Understand that no one is greater than another. Feel it. Practice helping another. We are all rowing the same boat. If we don't pull together, our plants are going to be awfully lonely."

"How is it that you say "all are equal", yet the obvious contradictions smack us in the face...?"

On another' night, in a different dream I was asking a question. "How is it that you say 'all are equal', yet the obvious contradictions smack us in the face: inequalities in virtues, temperances, finances, rights, abilities and talents, intelligence, mathematical aptitude, ad infinitum?"

The answer was a metaphor. It is as if a large diamond were to be found inside each person. Picture a diamond a foot long. The diamond has a thousand facets, but the facets are covered with dirt and tar. It is the job of the soul to clean each facet until the surface is brilliant and can reflect a rainbow of colors.

"Now, some have cleaned many facets and gleam brightly. Others have only managed to clean a few; they do not sparkle so. Yet, underneath the dirt, each person possesses within his or her breast a brilliant diamond with a thousand gleaming facets. The diamond is perfect, not one flaw. The only differences among people are the number of facets cleaned. But each diamond is the same, and each is perfect."

"When all the facets are cleaned and shining forth in a spectrum of lights, the diamond returns to the pure energy that it was originally. The lights remain. It is as if the process that goes into making the diamond is reversed, all that pressure released. The pure energy exists in the rainbow of lights, and the lights possess consciousness and knowledge."

"And all of the diamonds are perfect."

Sometimes the questions are complicated and the answer is simple.

"What am I to do?" I was asking in a dream. "I know I can treat and heal people in pain. They come to me in numbers beyond what I can handle. I am so tired. Yet can I say no when they are so needy and I can help them? Is it right to say 'No, enough already?' "

"Your role is not to be a lifeguard" was the answer.

A message to other psychiatrists.

I awakened about six in the morning from a dream where I was giving a lecture, in this instance to a vast audience of psychiatrists.

"In the rush toward the medicalization of psychiatry, it is important that we do not abandon the traditional, albeit sometimes vague, teachings of our profession. We are the ones who still talk to our patients, patiently and with compassion. We still take the time to do this. We promote the conceptual understanding of illness, healing with understanding and the induced discovery of self-knowledge, rather than just with laser beams. We still use hope to heal."

"In this day and age, other branches of medicine are finding these traditional approaches to healing much too inefficient, time-consuming, and unsubstantiated. They prefer technology to talk, computer-generated blood chemistries to the personal physician-patient chemistry, which heals the patient and provides satisfaction to the doctor. Idealistic, ethical, personally gratifying approaches to medicine lose ground to economic, efficient, insulating, and satisfaction-destroying approaches. As a result, our colleagues feel increasingly isolated and depressed. The patients feel rushed and empty, uncared for."

"We should avoid being seduced by high technology."

Rather, we should be the role models for our colleagues. We should demonstrate how patience, understanding, and compassion help both patient *and* physician. Taking more time to talk, to teach, to awaken hope and the expectation of recovery - these half-forgotten qualities of the physician as healer - these we must always use ourselves and be an example to our fellow physicians.

"High technology is wonderful in research and to promote the understanding of human illness and disease. It can be an invaluable clinical tool, but it can never replace those inherently personal characteristics and methods of the true physician. Psychiatry can be the most dignified of the medical specialties. We are the teachers. We should not abandon this role for the sake of assimilation, especially not now."

Hearing what is said in the operating room while under anesthesia and how it can affect the outcome

Catherine the patient under hypnosis interrupts the therapist (Brian Weiss)

"Was more of a burden," she concluded. "Thoughts", she added, "thoughts. . . ."

"What thoughts?" I sensed she was in a new area. -

"About the anesthesia. When they give you anesthesia, can you hear? You *can* still hear!" She had answered her own question. She was whispering rapidly now, becoming excited. "Your mind is very much aware of what's going on. They were talking about my choking, about the possibility of me choking when they did the surgery on my throat."

I remembered Catherine's vocal cord surgery, which was performed just a few months before her first appointment with me. She had been anxious prior to the surgery, but she was absolutely terrified upon awakening in the recovery room. It had taken the nursing staff hours to calm her. Now it appeared that what was said by the surgeons during the operation, during the time she was under deep anesthesia, had precipitated her terror. My mind flipped back to medical school and my surgery rotation. I remembered the casual conversations during operations, while the patients were anesthetized. I remembered the jokes, the cursing, the arguments, and the surgeons' temper tantrums. What had the patients heard at a subconscious level? How much registered to affect their thoughts and emotions, their fears and anxieties, after they awakened? Was the postoperative course, the patient's very recovery from the surgery, influenced positively or negatively by the remarks made during the operation? Had anyone died because of negative expectations overheard during surgery? Had they, feeling hopeless, just given up?

"Do you remember what they were saying?" I asked.

"That they had to put a tube down. When they took the tube out, my throat might swell up. They didn't think I could hear."

"But you did."

"Yes. That's why I had all the problems." After today's session, Catherine no longer had any fear of swallowing or choking. It was as simple as that. "All the anxiety . . ." she continued, "I thought I would choke."

"Do you feel free?" I asked.

"Yes. You can reverse what they did."

"Can I?"

"Yes. You *are* .... They should be very careful of what they say. I remember it now. They put a tube in my throat. And then I couldn't talk afterward to tell them anything."

"Now you're free .... You did hear them."

"Yes, I heard them talk. ... "She fell silent for a minute or two, then began to turn her head from side to side. She seemed to be listening to something.

"You seem to be hearing messages. Do you know where that message came from?" I was hoping the Masters would appear."

"Someone told me" was her cryptic answer.

"Somebody was speaking to you?"

"But they're gone."

I tried to bring them back.

"See if you can bring back spirits with messages for us to help us out."

"They come only when they want *to,* not when I choose," she answered firmly.

"You don't have any control over it?"

"No."

"Okay," I conceded, "but the message about the anesthesia was very important for you. That was the source of your choking."

"It was important for you, not me," she retorted. Her answer reverberated through my mind. *She* would be cured of the terror of choking, yet this revelation was nevertheless more important for me than for her. I was the one doing the healing. Her simple answer contained many levels of meaning. I felt that if I truly understood these levels, these resonating octaves of meanings, I would advance a quantum leap into the understanding of human relationships. Perhaps the helping was more important than the cure.

"For me to help you?" I asked.

"Yes. You can undo what they did. You *have* been undoing what they did." *She* was resting. We had both learned a great lesson.

Above is adapted from *Many Lives, Many Masters* by Brian L. Weiss, M.D.

****

Below is adapted from http://www.slideshare.net/olivianightowl/habits-that-block-creativity and

http://http-server.carleton.ca/~gkardos/88403/CREAT/Block4.html (web page no longer available)

HABITS THAT BLOCK CREATIVITY

by Professor Geza Kardos (retired) Carleton University, Canada

Becoming more creative is not easy. Habits must be broken, perspectives changed, and thought patterns revised. Nevertheless, the results can be well worth the effort. Here are some reasons why it is difficult for most of us to be creative at all times.

It is a common myth that creativity declines with age beginning around the age of 11 or 12. It is also a myth that creativity also declines as education increases. These myths convey some idea that age and learning are obstacles to creative problem solving. This is not so it is just that as we gain experience and learning we develop more efficient tools for dealing with our daily activities.

The Known Vs. The New

The simplest definition of creativity is the ability to come up with new or unique ideas. Ideas do not have to be new to the world, just new to us. Because two or more people happen to make the same discovery or develop the same invention does not change the fact that each of them had to be creative to discover or invent the system independently.

Unfortunately, routine everyday decision-making works against searching for or accepting new ideas. In attempting to exercise good judgment and not make mistakes people usually base their decisions on the best, most complete, and most accurate information or experience available. These habits allow us to deal with most situations without difficulty or trauma. Unfortunately, such high-caliber information exists only about what is established, common, and known. The newer and more unique the solution required, the harder it is to get good and sufficient information. That is why the easiest solutions are not new and different. Creative solutions by their very nature must be new or different.

Obstacles To Creativity

The process of creating a new idea involves combining existing elements into original combinations. An example is Watson Watt's invention of Radar. All the elements, radio waves, amplifiers and oscilloscopes existed and were known to him. Nevertheless, he combined these elements into a new system and turned them into hardware. Once Watt succeeded, radar became just another of the "givens" from which newer systems and applications would be developed.

To unleash the creative process, much of what is usually known and taken for granted, must be looked at in a different way, for a new purpose. Here are some of the most basic obstacles that must be overcome:

Habits Restrict Awareness:

Habits are good in that they are efficient and conserve our mental energies for other tasks. However, habitual behavior can lead to a kind of blindness. One of the chief roadblocks to creativity stems from the physical, perceptual, and mental habits that we build up over time. Such habits tend to tune out those things and ideas around us that could be the basis for new insights.

Rigid Categories Prevent Insight:

We see the world selectively through a set of filters created by our experiences. These filters superimpose constraints on a problem that is not there. To find creative solutions we must discard our normal filtered perceptions and try a wholly new approach.

We begin life with essentially no experience or information. The solution to every problem is creative. We learn by interacting with our environment. This learning process fills our heads with raw data, which we organize into rules, mental pigeonholes. Each pigeonhole is the repository for a class of experience and/or information. Each pigeonhole is identified as good, if it leads to desirable results or bad if it does not. Soon our first instinct when faced with a situation is to try to fit it into an existing pigeonhole.

Wanting to fit new things into existing categories increases as we gain experience. Note the response of someone exposed to something new. They will probably start out saying, that it is the same as something they already know. If they are told it is not, they may take several tries at establishing identification based on similarity with something they know. If they are unable to do so, they may satisfy this need for mental equilibrium by saying: "Well, it is close enough." If they are open minded enough, they may accept it as totally new to them, and not fitting into a preexisting pigeonhole. They create a completely new category to reside beside the preexisting ones.

As we learn to cope with everyday living we learn to operate on automatic because we find it efficient and comfortable. We develop enough pigeonholes to get us through life, and we become reluctant to crowd in new ones. The net-effect is that even when exposed to something new, we try to treat it like something familiar, and immediately assume it belongs in an existing category.

There are several other creativity restraint mechanisms. For example, somewhere along the way we stop asking what we think are stupid questions. We somehow don't want to seem foolish and are afraid to show our ignorance. This tendency seems to increase as one's educational credentials increase. We are afraid to be laughed at or rebuffed.

Being different is difficult, to march to the beat of a different drummer. Our social instinct makes us want to belong to the group. Maintaining a view when those around you disagree with it is hard. Many psychological experiments have demonstrated that individuals may deny their own senses to make their judgments conform to what the overwhelming number of people in their group say or believe.

Most of these mechanisms are useful when it comes to getting us through life on a day-by-day basis. However, when the time comes to be creative, we must change the way we think and function. We must recognize these blocks to new ideas, for what they are and move beyond them.

Overcoming the Obstacles

The first step to becoming a more creative individual is to understand what conceptual blocks are and how they interfere with our ability to think about things in a new way. A conceptual block is a mind-set that prevents a person from seeing a problem or a solution in an unconventional way. The most frequently occurring conceptual blocks are perceptual blocks, emotional blocks, cultural blocks, environmental blocks and communication blocks.

- **Perceptual Blocks.** These are obstacles that prevent us from clearly perceiving the problem or the information needed to solve it. A few perceptual blocks are:
    - *Stereotyping:*- This assumes that once an item or idea is identified it can have no other use or function.
    - *Imaginary boundaries*:- We project boundaries on the problem and solution that need not exist in reality.
    - *Information overload:*- Trying to satisfy an excess of information and detail restricts the alternative that can be considered.
- **Emotional Blocks.** These blocks decrease your freedom to explore and manipulate ideas in a realm that makes you uncomfortable. They interfere with your ability to conceptualize fluently and flexibly. Emotional blocks prevent you from communicating your ideas to others. Some types of emotional blocks include:
    - *Fear of taking a Risk:*- Risk taking is always difficult, we start from childhood to be careful, not to fail, not to look foolish. These prohibitions are deeply ingrained in us by the time we become adults.
    - *Dislike for uncertainty:*- To be a good problem solver you must be prepared to deal with problems that are sometimes confusing. Some possible solutions must be explored when their relevance to the problem is not obvious or certain. Some best solutions may even seem contradictory.
    - *Judgmental attitude:*- This block comes from a negative attitude. Finding reasons why things won't work is easier than accepting a strange idea. Yet wild

ideas when explored further may lead to highly innovative solutions. A positive approach to strange ideas can overcome this block.

- *Not invented here:-* This block comes about when a new idea threatens a preferred idea or concept.
- *Lack of challenge:-* Sometimes problems or solutions seem too trivial or easy to waste our time on.
- *Inability to incubate:-* Attempting to rush a solution without taking time to mull it over can lock out additional and possibly better solutions.

- **Cultural Blocks.** These are blocks that we impose on ourselves due to the society, culture or group to which we belong. Cultural blocks refuse to accept that other societies or groups may see and desire things to be different. Some of these blocks are:
  - *Our way is right:-* This refuses to accept that there are other ways of doing things.
  - *We don't say or think that way:-* This is a reflection of the taboos we carry with us. But, sometimes good solutions must be approached by first considering the unacceptable and thinking the unthinkable.
- **Environmental Blocks.** These blocks are due to the distractions in our surroundings, real, imagined, or anticipated. Working in an atmosphere that is pleasing and supportive increases the generation of new ideas.
- **Intellectual Blocks.** These blocks occur because of insufficient knowledge of the kind needed to solve the problem being considered. Or because of a fixation on the specialty, with which we are comfortable, and denying the possibility that a better solution can be achieved using a different specialty.
- **Expressive Blocks.** This is the inability or willingness to express ideas clearly to others or oneself. Making models, sketches, drawings, or diagrams may clarify ideas and aid in communicating them.

Many of these perceptual Blocks reveal themselves by "killer phrases", phrases that stop consideration of any other solutions or of the problem itself. When these phrases surface, it is valuable to stop and think about the conceptual block that must be overcome. Some typical killer phrases are:

- **No!**
- **Guessing at the answer is wrong!**
- **Don't appear foolish!**
- **That's not my job (responsibility, concern)!**
- **I haven't been told what to do!**
- **I haven't been told how!**
- **I don't know how to start!**

- **I haven't been told exactly what is wanted!**
- **I don't understand!**
- **I don't want to be different!**
- **It looks too hard!**
- **It's too easy!**

Strategies for creative problem solving must include steps to overcome and avoid perceptual blocks. Some means of overcoming these blocks are:

- **Remove the fear of failure:-** Encourage wild ideas from all participants. Emphasize that all solutions belong to the group. Encourage humorous atmosphere. Have the ideas written down and passed around anonymously.
- **Adjust attitudes:-** Emphasize the positive aspects of the solution. Ensure that risks are worth taking. Encourage the acceptance of alternate solutions.
- **Change the rules:-** Temporarily suspend the rules and conditions for the problem and its solution. Especially where specific rules or conditions block progress.
- **Change the solution mode:-** If the problem is being explored verbally, try making a diagram or representing it mathematically. Use analogies. Assume a solution and see if it can be made to fit the problem.

Use provocative Questions:- Instead of dealing with the problem directly consider a question from beyond the perceived block. Then work backwards. Once the perceptual block becomes familiar, it ceases to exist. Ask "What if" questions. Use check lists.

Above is adapted from http://www.slideshare.net/olivianightowl/habits-that-block-creativity and

http://http-server.carleton.ca/~gkardos/88403/CREAT/Block4.html (web page no longer available)

****

Below is adapted from chapters 4 and 5 of *Are You Really Too Sensitive* by Marcy Calhoun

Are You Really Too Sensitive

Telepathy is mentally receiving/sending information from one being to another being. This is the most common kind of information received and sent by the communication center, and is experienced by all three kinds of ultra-sensitives.

Psychometry is the ability to pick up information by touching a person, place, or thing.

Empathy is feeling/ experiencing/ knowing/ seeing what other people are experiencing/ knowing/ seeing/ feeling on the physical, mental, emotional and spiritual levels.

Physical empathy is the ultra-sensitive picking up physical pain from another person or animal living in present time or living in past memory or living in pure precognitive experience.

Mental empathy is the ultra-sensitive picking up attitude or judgment from another person, movie, book, dream, social or cultural belief, childhood attitude/memory, or group opinion about someone, then followed by "emotional empathy."

Emotional empathy is the ultra-sensitive picking up the feelings of others: people who are thinking about them, people they are thinking about, people they have seen in their daily life, friends, relatives, coworkers, immediate family, loved ones at a distance, people the ultra-sensitive is in conflict with, people that have died and have left the physical plane of existence, people remembered from the present lifes past (such as childhood memory), past life connections that cannot be logically connected to anything of the present. These are often accompanied by physical sensations from others. Receptors almost always believe it is theirs because it is so real and strong.

Visions: A vision is a visual experience of something that is about to happen, has happened, or is happening. Some visions are literal and some are symbolic.

A vision is an experience that you have when you are physically awake but your mind/emotions are in a drifting or floating state. To have a vision you must be in an "altered state." Altered states occur more often than most people believe. The first altered state of a vision is the state a person is in when s/he is daydreaming. The second stage of a vision is a feeling of disconnectedness with the sense of the physical-world reality.

Sometimes you can experience a vision physically by feeling it with your physical body sensations as if it were actually happening to the physical-body-you, and not just a mirror image actually happening to someone else. Many times visions can be experienced by feeling what the person is experiencing in your vision. Many times you can bring back the physical sensations as well as the emotional sensations with your will.

Mediumship is the awareness that someone or something outside yourself is wanting to communicate with you through you.

Channeling is spontaneously receiving information without any personal interpretation, often without even an awareness of information coming through until the thought/concept is complete. It can happen at times when there is no awareness at all of being a channel for someone else-for instance, in a meeting.

How to Handle Your Sensitivity

I would like to replace the word "psychic" with the word "ultra-sensitive." Being ultra-sensitive means deeply and lovingly caring about the world we live in and the people in that world. An ultra-sensitive is in tune. In tune means that there is an awareness of the world, which includes taking care of the people, animals, plants, earth ... but not always themselves. Ultra-sensitives know, feel, or see that they are an integral part of all things of the earth.

As an ultra-sensitive you need to create a filtering system to help you survive in the world. A filtering system would consist of methods or techniques that filter out most of the negativity or emotional bombardment that you deal with in life until you strengthen yourself to the point where you need no protection at all.

Once you need no filters you will be living in the state of unconditional love. Unconditional love is a state of being that has no judgment, no need to see things as bad" or "good," no need to change people into being happy, no need to change people into your idea of what you think would make them happy.

This filtering system is called "intuitive self defense." When you use this protection you are not defended against the world. You are filtering out the energies that are destructive to you at the moment, while at the same time you are building your strength to more than just survive.

Glenn's note: The main filtering systems I have used:

1) Running around in circles as a five to seven year old. My parents put a throw rug in our living room so to keep me from wearing the out good carpet.

2) Playing sandlot football and basketball when running in circles was no longer age appropriate. I was good enough to almost always find a game and played many hours until I broke my ankle badly in eleventh grade.

3)When I could no longer 'filter' using extreme physical activity I began smoking. I still smoke as I am writing this. How much I am filtering/blocking, how much is habit and how much is addiction is unclear. It is all three to some extent and someday I will let go of the perceived need to smoke.

If somebody gets hurt, ultra-sensitives also experience the pain unless they protect themselves. If they are protected they can be clear and focused and can send energy that is available to them in order to help the people they want to help. Being "protected, means that you can be loving, caring, nourishing, healing and effective. One of my deepest goals in life is to be EFFECTIVE because in the past I have been ineffective when I have felt the hurt as deeply as other people have felt it. Now I can live my life being loving, open, caring, and sensitive without taking on other people's pain.

I can love people exactly where they are, whether they approve of me or not. For the moment I can feel their hurt and pain, then my being adjusts to understanding what it is without suppressing myself in any way - just by understanding that they need to be where they are until they choose to change. The moment they choose to change I will be available to help them in any constructive way I can.

Recognition/Naming of What is Happening

About eighteen years ago I awakened in the middle of the night not able to get my breath, trying to figure out what was going on. I was gasping for breath, frightened and not understanding what was happening to me. Then I lapsed into a comatose state, not wanting to respond to anyone or anything. Then - after many hours - instantly I felt full of energy. I found out later that I was experiencing a heart attack that a friend was having. At that point I did not understand what was happening to me. I was "stuck" in the experience until' my friend died. I thought it was me. I heard one day after my experience that he had died. When I was told what happened to him, I realized that I had my picking up experience at the same time he was having the heart attack. I experienced his distress even to the point of having a total lack of energy and no response to my husband, children, or life, while my friend was in a coma.

I experienced the very same things he was experiencing. At the moment of his death I was filled immediately with knowledge of myself, my life, and my loved ones, and I was once again filled with the energy of a young woman, rather than that of a man in his sixties who was ill and weak.

Now when I experience anything similar, I know what is happening to me. These are the techniques that I use, which you can also use, when you are in rapport or connected in empathy to anyone:

Ask these questions of yourself:

> Where is this coming from? Who is it?
>
> Listen to your thoughts. Listen by seeing/hearing who is on your mind or who keeps coming into your mind.
>
> Then make this statement out loud:
>
> THIS IS NOT MINE. I AM WHOLE, HEALTHY, AND HEALED. I AM (YOUR NAME). Say your name over and over until the feeling/ experience has stopped.
>
> Say your name with INTENT AND FEELING.
>
> Mean it. In this exercise you are using your name as a powerful mantra.

Uses of Your Name

Your name is the most powerful mantra you have. Everyone else uses your name with their belief of who you are. When they say your name, you become for a moment what they believe you to be, unless your belief in yourself is stronger than theirs.

I have also found that at the very time you need to say your name the most, in order to gather yourself back to yourself, you will experience resistance in doing so. The resistance comes because the person or persons connected to you unconsciously (and sometimes consciously) will not want to let go. Use your will and strong intent in saying your name. Your need to be yourself must be stronger than their need to be connected to you.

1. When saying your name, say it as if you were slipping into your body - as though you were putting on a pair of gloves.

2. Say your name and really believe what you are saying is true.

3. If you do not like your name, find another name that feels good to you and use that name as a clearing and centering tool.

   Glenn's note: You may also want to clear on your birth name and any nicknames if there is a negative emotion or memory attached.

The "Name Mantra" for Clearing and Protection

I am (your name). I am only (your name). There is no one within or connected to me that is not (your name). I am totally and completely (your name): body, mind and spirit. I own my own universe and fill it with being (your name).

In ancient mystery schools people would be given new names. You were told not to give others your sacred name or to allow others to know it. Your name was sacred. If you told someone else your name, then you gave them control over your life. Giving someone your sacred name meant giving them your energy. In this lifetime it is still important to honor your name and understand that it is the name of your body, your world, your universe, your life. Your name is powerful for you whether you feel powerful yet or not. It is a tool you may have not gained the full use of yet.

Protection

Glenn's note: I let go of the word 'protection'. If you are standing in and surrounded by Divine LOVE and LIGHT anything that is of "anything Else" will automatically stay away from you. When you are ready you can simply ask:

"Great Spirit and Great Spirit Helpers as are best, keep me fully surrounded and standing in your pure LOVE, LIGHT and VIOLET FLAME. Thank you."

The "Three Jewel" Protection

Visualize an emerald - hard, solid, and a beautiful rich green - deep inside your body, at the level of the solar plexus. Let it expand, still solid, until it has own to a radius of two feet in all directions around your body. In other words, you are surrounded by a hard, green, emerald, four feet in diameter, anchored at your solar plexus. Visualize bringing bright sunlight with all the colors of the rainbow into the emerald, charging it with light and protective energy.

Next visualize a deep blue sapphire, faceted in all directions, hard, solid, inside your solar plexus center 'and expanding out until it has grown to a radius of two ;feet in all directions, pushing the emerald out two more feet. You are now surrounded by an emerald four feet in diameter and a sapphire two feet in diameter, both anchored securely at your solar plexus center.

Finally, visualize a hard, brilliant diamond inside our body at the solar plexus. Do not use a crystal at this point for your protection. Use a diamond when you need strong protection inside the sapphire and emerald. Start the diamond as a solid, hard, multi-faceted jewel that has all the colors of the rainbow playing within it, always moving and never still.

It has a life of its own coming from your creative force designed to protect you. Let the diamond expand until it has grown to a radius of two feet in all directions, pushing the sapphire and emerald out further.

Now you are surrounded by an emerald six feet in diameter, a sapphire four feet in diameter, and a diamond two feet in diameter, all anchored solidly deep inside your body at the solar plexus center.

Now for the final part of your protection, place in your heart's golden center an unconditional loving child that is the purest form of you to radiate out all your unconditional loving energy, to remind you to be unconditional in all your connections with all people including yourself. Now charge all your gems with more sunlight to give them life. I suggest that you use this exercise daily and on some days reinforce it as many times per day as is necessary to keep you a clear, loving, open, person that shows forth your light to the world.

Above is adapted from chapters 4 and 5 of *Are You Really Too Sensitive* by Marcy Calhoun

****

Below is adapted from http://kundalini-teacher.com/guidance/discern.php

Discernment

The essence of discernment is really listening to your body, and especially to your heart. Most people who do not get to hear the heart voice, at least get a sense of warmth that is a non verbal affirmation. The body has a built in lie detector, and the signals of it can be unique. The most common signals:

> A sense of opening, expansion, warmth and/or joy in the heart chakra communicates a "yes".
>
> A sinking feeling in the stomach is a negative answer.
>
> Goosebumps and shivers is a positive answer.

This guidance from your body comes through most clearly, if you are grounded and clear of entities. If you are not grounded, then you may get responses from your ego fears or your mind. If you have entities, then they may want to put their two cents worth in. Especially entities occupying the heart and power chakra.

Here is a series of statements: Get grounded, then read them as truth and see how your body responds! Your signals may be unique to you and you will usually find that there is some consistent reaction in your body to statements that are true, and a different reaction to statements that are false. The signals are often subtle, however you can ask for them to be made clearer.

Remember!!! This is about **feeling**, not **thinking**. Do not think about the answers; feel for the responses of your body. You already know what you think. Thinking takes you out of your body and intuitive knowing and into your head. You want to know the truth of the body mind, and it speaks in feelings and sensations, not words.

> I am male.
> I am 250 years old.
> My name is Horace.
> I breathe.
> Your name is Ferdinand.
> I am alive.
> I am female.
> I have blue eyes.
> I am infinite.
> I have black hair.
> I have two arms.
> I am an asshole.

I like to drink beer.

The sky is blue.

I am married.

My dog's name is Bill.

My car is red.

I work hard.

I am ugly.

Great Spirit loves me unconditionally.

Once you have had some practice hearing the signals of these obvious true/false statements, check out these ideas, using the resonance of the heart chakra for a lie detector. It only works if you are grounded. I find that when I do this the Heart will also fill in the blanks with additional information that is not in words. Reading the words, and listening to the heart both at once, you will find that your heart provides a subtle commentary to your life experience. Hopefully your Heart will elaborate on these spiritual concepts for you.

The logical mind is producing limitation after limitation. Because it must, that is its job. It is for 3D navigation.

It can only work with what it knows, and it can know very little, in the overall scheme of things.

Einstein used imagination to discover E=mc2, imagining himself to be a photon, and traveling an imaginary trip in his mind... or was it an out of body experience?

He said: **"Imagination is more important than knowledge."**

It is normal to try to fall back on logic for safety when the enormity of everything gets scary, however in the end it is usually of little use. We must discard logic and reach for faith and imagination.

Know that logic can come up with Reasons and limitations endlessly.

That's what it is good at.   Keeping you stuck in 3D.

It always comes down to choosing to ignore logic and focus on faith and desire. Leaps of faith are often illogical, expect for the previous experience that shows they work. You may not be an engineer to understand electricity; however you can still use a toaster. Faith is not built on reasons that are a logical understanding of how Great Spirit works.

Joseph Campbell said "Follow your Bliss."

That means, chase after what makes your heart feel warm and joyful; the things you love and get passionate about. It is said, that if you do the work you love, you will never work a day in your life. It is not that you will be unemployed, however that your work will feel like play.

Space and time do not exist, and we are All One.

Love transcends space and time, because it is the E that =mc2, the very fabric of the universe of 3D we perceive; it is All.

The key to the unified field theory.

The energy that is limitless, that transcends Newton's physics.

LOVE.

Matter and energy are one, and energy is LOVE.

As Darkness is the absence of light, so fear is the absence of LOVE.

Expectations are a way of creating limitations on our experience. If you have an expectation that (______________), you also close yourself off to the possibilities of (_____________) anywhere, with anything. This is also known as "if-then" thinking. The mind takes you out of the moment, into imaginary fears or desires of the future, and you make choices based on expectations grown from the fantasy, not from what Is.

The choice of how you perceive resides with you. It is your world.

If you have expectations that you are vulnerable to the negative energy of others, then you will be. If you have expectations that life is hard then you die, then those are the thought-prayers that shape your experience of life.

Richard Bach said, **"Argue for your limitations, and you get to keep them."**

I mean that kindly.

We know way more than we think we know. To access it we have to give up what we think we know.

We are exactly as limited as we believe we are.

Releasing the fear/separation beliefs is the process of enlightenment.

The words you are reading are a partial communication of idea and intention. The total of the communication we are actually exchanging goes far, far beyond these words, and is not dependent on any mechanical or physical system.

Do not underestimate the power of your imagination. It is the most powerful tool we have. Close your eyes for a moment and feel the energy resonating from this idea, and ask yourself (heart chakra) if what I say is true.

You might get an emotional response, you might get an internal explanation, you might get anything.

Release expectations and listen.

It takes some practice to stay grounded and observe yourself without letting your thoughts run away with you. Give yourself the patience you would give to a small child learning to walk. It is your inner child, after all, that has the imagination power to make this real. And the determination.

A child falls down a hundred times, yet you do not see any adults who are crawlers. Learning to do this is written in the plan of your DNA, just as walking is.

We all get it eventually. We fall down over and over, forgive ourselves and cry, and get on our feet again to try to take that first step.

We learn to walk, then run, then we learn to forget all that and give up the limitations so we can levitate...

Above is adapted from http://kundalini-teacher.com/guidance/discern.php

****

Below is adapted about 2007 from < http://types-of-dreams.info>

Web page no longer available as of June 2016

What Is A Dream

What Is A Dream?

What exactly is a dream? According to some, a dream is a trip into the subconscious mind. Others believe a dream is just a person's imagination being allowed to break free. Perhaps it is a little bit of both. Is it totally symbolic or somewhat literal?

Types of Dreams

LUCID DREAMS

When we are awake, we associate this with being who we are. It is the part of us in charge of all the decision making we do in the day. It is who think we are as an awake human. In a dream state, our waking consciousness is normally turned off, so all the important faculties such as analytical abilities, logic and questioning tend to be dormant. In a lucid dream, you literally walk a door from physical reality into one of pure mental existence. Your thoughts effortlessly paint the dreamscape and you have full mental faculties as you would if you were awake. Lucid dreaming is probably one of the best forms of dreaming that I can think of. You extend your conscious existence into a realm where you are the creator. Your abilities to imagine are increased to quantum levels where the very thought of a building can create architecture unlike anything imagined in our physical world. This is a place where you discover just how real and unlimited your imagination can be. The level or quality of the dream is yours to command. The rules of conduct are yours to decide. Anything imaginable can be expressed in fluid graceful motion in this dreamscape. It also opens up a great avenue for your curiosity.

PRECOGNITIVE DREAMS

This is where time and space no longer seem to fit any rational logical meaning. These dreams will put the twist on any logical thinker. Precognition is an ability to know and experience a future event before it ever occurs. Not everybody has had a precognitive dream that they remember, but many do. And déjà vu is the shadow of such colossal events in human consciousness. A part of you just skipped the time/space continuum to check out what it will be doing in some later date. Seldom controlled, these dreams are spontaneous, faint and ghost like. You may wake up having full memory of them, which usually quickly fades. And in the thoughts that a dream might be precognitive, such clear memory tends not to hold any precognitive value. These in my opinion are the hardest, and most stealthy of the dreams for our consciousness to behold. And probably for a good reason, as we probably aren't ready for that knowledge until something in us decides that we are. If you have ever observed your waking state, you'll notice that your body with all of its senses records your reality and stores this recording into memory as time progresses.

Occasionally for a precognitive dreamer, it is like a record has just skipped and you are playing the same verse over again. If you remember the dream, and have a clear memory, the accuracy can scare you. These dreams can hold an eerie 100% accuracy down to the finest of details. Even to the details we think are totally spontaneous like our own inner contemplation and emotions. For example imagine that in a dream you are standing in a park that you have never been to before. An old man wearing a blue jacket with a brown furry collar and yellow-grey pants walks up to you and asks you if you have the time. You check your watch and your thoughts remark on the man's jacket. You check the watch and tell the man it is 12:15 pm. He thanks you and walks off. You wake up, remember this clearly and let it slip back into the sub-conscious memory banks.

Months later, you are on vacation at some city. You go for a walk in a park to absorb the natural beauty that the city presents. The very man in your dream walks up as if in perfect timing, and he asks you the time, you respond and tell him it's 12:15 pm, but this time you suddenly have a flash of déjà vu. Something is really familiar about that man, the park, the time. You struggle with how you could know this and with some luck, you remember the dream. It was so clear at the time and both the memory of the dream and the physical event map over each other like a perfect glove.

For many, this kind of small excerpt is common. A very brief one or two minute reminder that something more is going on than what you consciously know. Yet, not something that is totally hidden or alien to your consciousness. It's something we all naturally do, just some remember better than others.

Precognitive dreams can come once in a life time, or in an assault of unrelenting waves. The fact is, some people have them and remember them whether they want to or not. You may be one of these people. And they are part of the tip of the iceberg for a much deeper spiritual you. If you have them, that's normal and actually there is nothing to be frightened of. I find that a lot of people tend to be intimidated by powerful precognitive dreams.

NIGHTMARES

Actually, I like them, you may not. Nightmares can scare the *you know what* out of any of us. These dreams hold the paralyzing fears we have stored layer after layer in our jumbled consciousness. To me, they are nothing more than some crazy horror show gone haywire. It's the realm of demons, monsters, goblins, aliens, freak shows, murder, insanity, darkness. It's the realm of our deepest human fears struggling with our moral mind as to why we think what we think.

Nightmares force us to fight, flee or LOVE. They are patterned after our survival instinct, and contain a warped Hollywood style to them when our hellish imagination gets the better of us. When I have a nightmare, I just change them to something more desirable. And if they get the better of me, I usually laugh right in them because I know that it's just a silly dream and I can change it at will. For my personal investigation into myself, my nightmares reflected only what I truly feared. When I realized that I could exist in such a state as myself untouched by it all, the nightmare was harmless. Like a painter who got scared of the picture he painted. We still have control.

I like nightmares for one basic fundamental. They let us know we dream in a very loud and clear way. We may not like them, and it may detour the timid from expanding forward with conscious exploration of the dream state. If you are not easily frightened or intimidated, you can have some real fun with nightmares. I tend to mimic some of my earlier role models such as Bugs Bunny's ability to stylishly deal with his vile villains. And like a villain, a nightmare can be turned into some really funny solution for problem solving. Nothing can hurt you if you don't let it. Self-control and discipline in dreaming is like achieving a black belt in karate. You will now have effective tools to deal with anything you don't want to dream about should you willfully desire to control it.

DAYDREAMS

Daydreaming is often overlooked as a proper dream, and regarded instead as wandering thoughts. However, the meanings to your nightly dream symbols are also applicable to your daydreams. The content in your daydreams are helpful in understanding your true feelings and will help you in achieving your goals.

Daydreaming is the spontaneous imagining or recalling of various images or experiences in the past or the future. When you daydream, you are accessing your right brain, which is the creative and feminine side of your personality. Worrying about something creates visual images in your brain of the worst outcome that you are imagining and is a form of daydreaming. By repeating these negative images in your mind, you are more likely to make them happen. So the next time you start worrying, try to think of a positive outcome. Positive daydreaming is very healthy and acts as a temporary escape from the demands of reality. It is also a good way to release built up frustrations without physically acting them out.

What Causes Dreams

Dreams serve a purpose. They serve a specific function for our bodies and mind. While many dream analysts at the turn of the century focused on dream interpretations, dream experts of today focus on the scientific approach of what causes dreams. Usually we define a dream as an experience remembered upon awakening that comes through nonphysical channels. Basically, it is an altered experience we have when we are sleeping and that we remember when we wake. However, there are lots of other variations on the definition. Some people define dreams as life goals and wishes for the future. This is another way we use the word. Many different theories, nothing for sure.

According to the Freudian school, dreams are the result of subconscious thoughts and desires. The other extreme attributes dreams to random "noise" in the neurons without special meaning.

My own understanding is that dreams are made of many small parts, from memory and imagination. These are united to generate images of dream. It is a process which operates from the subconscious.

There is definitely value behind dreams; nevertheless nobody knows precisely, what causes them. The general theory is that they occur from subconscious thoughts from our daily thoughts and actions.

5 Different Types of Dreams

They often blend and merge with one another.

1) Revelatory
This category speaks of things to come in a form of revelation and prophecy. It may involve words of knowledge about a condition or situation you or a friend may be in. We wake up with the knowledge that "decisions" we thought were made artfully and wisely on our own, are actually due to our childhood, our upbringing, the war zone nursery.

2) Directional
It is as its name implies, directional in nature, specifically for the dreamer. It may make you aware of conditions or blind spots in your life. This would also include warnings of danger in choices made or show 'calling' in one's life. This category also includes inventions and ideas that God may be communicating to you.

3) Cleansing
This type of dream is a way of Spirit to clean you from negative things you have been exposed to visually, chemically or spiritually. The dreamer can receive disposal and healing through this type of dream.

4) Spiritual Warfare
Dreams can be a spiritual field of fight. The things won in dreams are often won in life. These dreams of struggle can also mean that you petition for yourself or for others.

5) Dark dreams
Are false dreams coming from negative spiritual forces? False dreams or sometimes nightmares usually come in black and white or sepia coloring. These dreams are meant to intimidate you or bring fear into your life.

3 Types of Dreams

1) **Recurring dreams**

They repeat themselves with little variation in story. They may be positive but often, they're nightmarish in content. Dreams may recur as a conflict in the dream still needs to be resolved. Once you have found a solution to it, your recurring dreams will stop.

Other dreams may have a message for you but you tend to forget it. With recurring dreams, the message might be so strong that it just will not go away.

These dreams are so frequent, that they force you to notice. They are desperately trying to tell you something. These dreams are often extended and could be caused by a situation or problem in your life. They can come back often, with little change to history. They usually point to a personal weakness or fear in your life, be it the past or the present

2) Epic dreams

They're so compelling and vivid that it's hard to ignore them. The details of such dreams remain with you for years as if you dreamt it last night. When you wake up from such a dream, you feel like you have discovered something amazing about yourself or the world. It'll feel like a life changing experience.

3) Healing dreams

Many experts believe that dreams can help to avoid potential problems of health and to help to begin to live. Dreams of this nature could speak to us to go to the dentist, go to the doctor or go on a spiritual journey. They serve as messages in relations to our health and well-being

Dream Symbols

Dream symbols often vary from dream to dream and from dreamer to dreamer. This makes it difficult to try to interpret your dream from a symbol book purchased in a bookstore. A skilled dream interpreter will interpret symbols based on the context of the dream and the dreamer.

The "shadow" of our personalities is that portion that we repress or refuse to acknowledge - even the most kind-hearted nun has emotions and urges that are not confessed. Each of us has access to mythological, cultural and historical symbols that we somehow genetically inherited from our ancestors. This knowledge can be thought of as the "collective unconscious". It is my personal belief that we have access to this knowledge and symbolism as a result of our previous lives - we remember everything, but can (usually) only access it in our dreams.

Common Dreams

Common Dreams are a communication of body, mind and spirit in a symbolic communicative environmental state of being. That's it!

Above is adapted about 2007 from < http://types-of-dreams.info>

Web page no longer available as of June 2016

****

Below is adapted from a web site around 2007. I can't find it as of 2016.

Consciousness

Beyond Matter

Perceived by the human senses, matter is a thing or substance that has shape and form, yet upon electroscopic investigation (according to Quantum physicists) it is made up of individual molecules with even smaller sub-atomic particles. Relatively speaking (according to Astrophysicists) there is about as much space between the planets and stars as there are between the atoms that make up matter. Apparently, our tangible reality is more vacuous than we thought. Still, even though matter itself makes up a miniscule portion of our universe (like the tip of an iceberg) this is the part that we are most conscious of - especially while we are living under its spell ("Maya"). Yet, if we take away all this matter that we objectively and subjectively experience... what's left? What is residing within this "empty space"? If we go below the surface of our perceived reality, what will we find? If it is not matter, then is it energy, vibration, sound, light or some other intangible like consciousness... or is it God?

Consciousness

Let's just say that we find ourselves floating in the vacuum of empty space. The light from our sun and the stars shine forth to us unimpeded (unless we close our eyes). We could say that this outer light brings us "consciousness" or "awareness" of the physical universe... for when one turns on the light, one is "awakened" from sleep (and ignorance) and becomes "conscious" or "aware" of things (thus increasing our intelligence).

Yet, independent of the outer light, there is an inner light that also shines - the "light behind the light" so to speak. This is the "spiritual light" - when you remove the physical, this spiritual light is shining, subtly, but it's still there. When we are asleep and dreaming, our eyes are closed, yet we are aware - we see light and images (and hear sounds too) all independent of the outer light (and outer sound). It logically follows that when the body dies, the light of our spirit would still be alive.

If there was no separation between inner and outer, there would be a state of oneness, union, bliss. Yet, between the seeing and the seen, between the subject and the object, between our minds eye and the light, there is often something in between. This something separates the two – to various stages of distinction.

Let's say that we (the subject) are looking at the universe (the object) through a camera with a pristine sparkling clear lens. If we looked out of that camera, we would see the images of life just the way it is. But if the lens collected some dust, or someone added on a red colored lens (called a filter) or another lens with scratches on it... when we next looked out of our camera... we would see life – not as it is, but tainted with this red color (it would be a bit cloudy from the dust, and scratchy too). So too is our inner consciousness affected by all the "stuff" we collect inside. All the filters we start adding on to our lens, these would be all those things that our egos get attached too - the identifications and belief systems and thoughts and feelings that are enmeshed within the material phenomena and reality.

For example, if one dusted upon that clear lens... images (or thoughts) of material possessions, then when you would look out through the lens of your camera, what you would see would be images (or thoughts) of your things... and one would say you are "materially conscious". Wherever you go, that's what you will see overlaid on top of all your perceptions. And if one has angry red feelings filtered over that clear lens, then when you would look out of your camera, what you would see (or feel) would be a red glow (these angry feelings). It's like wearing rose colored glasses - everything is perceived rosy, but that's not its true objective reality. In other words, our conscious personal experience of reality is defined by that which overlays it – this is what our ego-minds hang its hat on. If we have dark over our lens, then our consciousness identity and awareness is darkness, and so on.... we may even have subtle shades of colored filters, pink, gold, violet, and so on, yet they are still filters... still not a direct pure unadulterated perception of what is.

Levels of Consciousness

But where do these other filters covering our minds come from?

Within all of Creation, there are many mansions, many dimensions, many universes... of different lights (and sounds). Just like there is a vast spectrum of visible light, so too are there different spectrums of consciousness... ones that reach from the more dense solid colors to the subtler pastel colors of the light spectrum... way beyond the invisible. Whatever dimensions our soul and our spirit have ever traveled on, even ones where we existed as incorporeal beings... we accumulated (as part of our karmic repertoire) a variety of consciousness filters - some very fine and subtle, others very dark and intense. All these filters overlay our current life experience. Imagine if you will, a person who has accumulated so many of these filters, that their vision becomes so dark, all they can see is in shades of black - this is a possibility (in this case, they would be virtually blind).

Not only is each one of these filters (of consciousness) covering our vision, but each one clouds our body, emotions and mind. These are the layers of stuff that must be peeled off (like the onion analogy) within your healing. This can be a lot of stuff, and could take a long time. It is your stuff and it has to go if you want to experience pure reality).

Glenn's Comment: It can be instantaneous when healed with LOVE and GRACE instead of working through Karma

Depending upon your past experiences in these various dimensions of consciousness, one band or filter of consciousness can hold a whole different set of memories and feelings – some positive, some negative. In other words, each one of these layers and their stuff may be sensed somewhat differently by you than another. Again, some may be very subtle and fine (almost imperceptible) others dark and intense (and overbearing). All are affecting (clouding) your experience of reality. In order to ascend through the limitations of these consciousnesses, one has to clear out these filters – this does take time and a lot of patience and faith.

Many people live exclusively within the awareness and energy of one consciousness over another. Telling them that they are stuck in one is a hard idea for them to swallow. The existence to us of different consciousnesses (just like the existence of God) must be taken with a great deal of faith... considering that "consciousness" is like the air (or gas) we breathe – we can't see it, but we somehow sense its presence within and all around. And like gas, there are subtleties in it – like carbon monoxide, some have toxic qualities that cannot be sensed until it's too late.

The Pure at Heart

The more clear and pure the inner screen of our consciousness (or if you will - mind) the more we can perceive the true nature of reality. When all our internal filters are removed - when our lens is polished and clean - we can see things as they are, not what we have made them to be.

The state of having this blank and neutral lens is what is sometimes referred to as "Pure Consciousness", "Enlightened Consciousness", "Pure Awareness", "Beginners Mind" or simply just "Being". Nothing is added or subtracted from reality – it just "is".

Above is adapted from a web site around 2007. I can't find it as of 2016.

****

Below is adapted from Robert Burney
http://www.woundedsouls.com/index.php/emotional-incest;

http://www.suite101.com/article.cfm/codependency_recovery/50739
Oct 18, 2000 (Web page is no longer available as of June 2016);

http://www.healyourinnerchild.com/Book-Content/inner-child-healing-how-to-begin

http://www.woundedsouls.com/index.php/emotional-incest

Inner Child Healing

Unintentional, Damaging, Emotional Programming

"Consider a scenario where a mother is crying in her bedroom and her three year old toddles into the room. To the child it looks as if mom is dying. The child is terrified and says, "I love you mommy!" Mom looks at her child. Her eyes fill with love, and her face breaks into a smile. She says, "Oh honey, I love you so much. You are my wonderful little boy/girl. Come here and give mommy a hug. You make mommy feel so good."

A touching scene? No. Emotional abuse! The child has just received the message that he/she has the power to save mommy's life. That the child has power over, and therefore responsibility for, mommy's feelings. This is emotional abuse, and sets up an emotionally incestuous relationship in which the child feels responsible for the parent's emotional needs.

A healthy parent would explain to the child that it is all right for mommy to cry, that it is healthy and good for people to cry when they feel sad or hurt. An emotionally healthy parent would "role model" for the child that it is okay to have the full range of emotions, all the feelings - sadness and hurt, anger and fear, Joy and happiness, etc."

I witnessed a scene a few years back that was graphic proof that the best thing any of us can do for our loved ones is to focus on our own healing. At a CoDA meeting one day a little four year old boy, who had been going to twelve-step meetings with his mother for two years, was sitting on a man's lap only six feet away from where his mother was sharing and crying. He didn't even bother to look up when his mother started crying. The man, who was more concerned than the little boy, said to him, "Your mommy's crying because she feels sad." The little boy looked up, glanced over at his mother and said, "Yea, she's getting better," and went back to playing. He knew that it was okay for mom to cry and that it was not his job to fix her. That little boy, at four years old, already had healthier boundaries than most adults - because his mother was in recovery working on getting healthier herself.

There are several facets of that scene that are remarkable because of their rarity in our society. One was that the adult had a safe place to share and express her feelings. The second was much rarer, a child with some semblance of healthy boundaries between self and parent.

One of the most pervasive, traumatic, and damaging dynamics that occurs in families in this dysfunctional, emotionally dishonest society is emotional incest. It is rampant in our society but there is still very little written or discussed about it.

Emotional incest occurs when a child feels responsible for a parent's emotional well-being. This happens because the parents do not know how to have healthy boundaries. It can occur with one or both parents, same sex or opposite sex. It occurs because the parents are emotionally dishonest with themselves and cannot get their emotional needs met by their spouse or other adults. Some people in the field refer to this dynamic as a parent making the child their "surrogate spouse."

This type of abuse can happen in a variety of ways. On one end of the spectrum the parent emotionally "dumps" on the child. This occurs when a parent talks about adult issues and feelings to a child as if they were a peer. Sometimes both parents will dump on a child in a way that puts the child in the middle of disagreements between the parents - with each complaining about the other.

On the other end of the spectrum is the family where no one talks about their feelings. In this case, though no one is talking about feelings, there are still emotional undercurrents present in the family which the child senses and feels some responsibility for - even if they haven't got a clue as to what the tension, anger, fear, or hurt are all about. The child feels responsible for it because they suffer the consequences - whether it is through outbursts from the parents or being shut out emotionally by the parents.

Often a parent who has a passive, traditionally codependent defense system will be married to a parent that has an aggressive, counter-dependent defense system. As I say in my book, traditionally in this society men were taught to be John Wayne and women to be self sacrificing. That is a generality; it is entirely possible that your mother was the John Wayne aggressive type while your father was the passive one.

What happens in this dynamic - a very common one - is that the passive parent allows the aggressive one to abuse him/her and the children in some way (verbal, emotional, mental, and/or physical.) And then that parent turns around and makes excuses to the children for allowing that behavior. A child that grows up hearing abuse being excused with rationalization and justification, is going to become an adult that will swing between the extremes of tolerating an abusive relationship or avoiding relationships altogether.

I came from a traditionally dysfunctional family, in that my father was the emotionally unavailable angry person while my mother was the martyr with no boundaries. I so hated how my father behaved that I became a martyr like my mother. I was a martyr because I did not speak my Truth or set boundaries, avoided confrontations, tried to please the other person to keep her liking me.

In my first relationship in my codependence recovery, I realized that for me, setting boundaries in a romantic relationship felt to my inner child like I was being abusive. The very thing I had sworn to myself I would never be - like my father. I had to constantly be alert to that child's feelings and let that wounded part of me know that it was not only OK to set boundaries and say no - but that it was not Loving to do otherwise.

I discovered that there was a 4 or 5 year old age of my inner child who felt overwhelming shame that I could not protect my mother from my father. I thought that was my job. To make my mother happy.

I thought that I was not worthy of Love because I had been unable to do my job. So, in my adult life I was attracted to emotionally unavailable women who were verbally abusive. To my disease, it was better to be in relationship with someone like my father, than to fail to do my job in a relationship with someone who was available emotionally.

I had a relationship phobia that for the most part kept me from getting into relationships because I felt I was defective in my ability to be responsible for another person's happiness.

Until we do some healing of our childhood wounds, it is impossible to really understand our adult patterns. If we have never experienced ourselves as independent emotional beings separate from our parents, we cannot truly be present for a relationship in our adult lives.

Emotional incest is a violation and invasion of our emotional boundaries. It is not sexual abuse, nor is it sexual in nature - although sexual incest is often accompanied by emotional incest. It can however cause great damage to our relationship with our own gender and sexuality. Emotional incest, along with religions that teach that sexuality is shameful and societal beliefs that one gender is superior to the other fall into a category that I call sexuality abuse - because they directly impact our relationship with our own sexuality and gender.

Our parents were our role models. We learned how to be emotional beings from their behavior and attitudes. We learned what a man is, what a woman is, from their example. We cannot undo that programming without being willing to heal those emotional wounds. We cannot know who we truly are without separating ourselves on the emotional energetic level from our parents.

Inner Child Healing - How to begin

"Recovery involves bringing to consciousness those beliefs and attitudes in our subconscious that are causing our dysfunctional reactions so that we can reprogram our ego defenses to allow us to live a healthy, fulfilling life instead of just surviving. So that we can own our power to make choices for ourselves about our beliefs and values instead of unconsciously reacting to the old tapes. Recovery is consciousness raising. It is en-light-en-ment - bringing the dysfunctional attitudes and beliefs out of the darkness of our subconscious into the Light of consciousness.

On an emotional level the dance of Recovery is owning and honoring the emotional wounds so that we can release the grief energy - the pain, rage, terror, and shame that is driving us.

That shame is toxic and is not ours - it never was! We did nothing to be ashamed of - we were just little kids. Just as our parents were little kids when they were wounded and shamed, and their parents before them, etc., etc. This is shame about being human that has been passed down from generation to generation.

There is no blame here, there are no bad guys, only wounded souls and broken hearts and scrambled minds."

Inner child work is in one way detective work. We have a mystery to solve. Why have I been attracted to the type of people that I have been in relationship with in my life? Why do I react in certain ways in certain situations? Where did my behavior patterns come from? Why do I sometimes feel so: helpless; lonely; desperate; scared; angry; suicidal; etc.

Just starting to ask these types of questions, is the first step in the healing process. It is healthy to start wondering about the cause and effect dynamics in our life.

In our codependence, we reacted to life out of a black and white, right and wrong, belief paradigm that taught us that it is shameful and bad to be wrong, to make mistakes, to be imperfect - to be human. We formed our core relationship with our self and with life in early childhood based on the messages we got, the emotional trauma we suffered, and the role modeling of the adults around us. As we grew up, we built our relationship with self, other people, and life on the foundation we formed in early childhood.

When we were 5, we were already reacting to life out of the emotional trauma of earlier ages. We adapted defenses to try to protect ourselves and to get our survival needs met. The defenses adapted at 5 due to the trauma suffered at earlier ages led to further trauma when we were 7 that then caused us to adjust our defenses, that led to wounding at 9, etc., etc., etc.

Toxic shame is the belief that there is something inherently wrong with who we are, with our being. Guilt is "I made a mistake, I did something wrong." Toxic shame is: "I am a mistake. There is something wrong with me."

It is very important to start awakening to the Truth that there is nothing inherently wrong with our being - it is our relationship with our self and with life that is dysfunctional. And that relationship was formed in early childhood.

The way that one begins inner child healing is simply to become aware.

To become aware that the governing principle in life is cause and effect.

To become aware that our relationship with our self has been dysfunctional.

To become aware that we have the power to change our relationship with our self.

To become aware that we were programmed with false beliefs about the purpose and nature of life in early childhood - and that we can change that programming.

To become aware that we have emotional wounds from childhood that it is possible to get in touch with and heal enough to stop them from dictating how we are living our life today.

That is the purpose of inner child healing - to stop letting our experiences of the past dictate how we respond to life today. It cannot be done without revisiting our childhood.

We need to become aware, to raise our consciousness. To create a new level of consciousness for ourselves that allows us to observe ourselves.

It is vitally important to start observing ourselves - our reactions, our feelings, our thoughts - from a detached witness place that is not shaming.

We all have an inner critic, a critical parent voice, that beats us up with shame, judgment, and fear until we heal it. The critical parent voice developed to try to control our emotions and our behaviors because we got the message there was something wrong with us and that our survival would be threatened if we did, said, or felt the "wrong" things.

It is vital to start learning how to not give power to that critical shaming voice. We need to start observing ourselves with compassion. This is almost impossible at the beginning of the inner child healing process. Having compassion for our self, being Loving to our self, is the hardest thing for us to do.

So, we need to start observing ourselves from at least a more neutral perspective. Become a scientific observer, a detective - the Sherlock Holmes of your own inner process as it were.

We need to start being that detective, observing ourselves and asking ourselves where that reaction / thought / feeling is coming from. Why am I feeling this way? What does this remind me of from my past? How old do I feel right now? How old did I act when that happened?

One of the amazing things about this process, is that as one starts to become more aware of our own reactions, we also start to become more aware of others. We start seeing when the people in our lives are reacting like a little kid, or adolescent, or teenager, or whatever. The more we become aware of their reactions, the easier it becomes to stop taking their behavior personally - which then makes it easier to detach from our own reactions and observe ourselves.

It is an amazing, miraculous process, that can help us to change our relationship with our self, with other people, and with life. Becoming more aware, becoming conscious of a new way of looking at ourselves and life is the beginning of a process of learning to forgive and Love our self.

A detective always looks at cause and effect. By becoming a detective, solving the mystery of why we have lived our lives as we have, we can start to free ourselves from our past. By doing the inner child healing, we can start to learn how to really be alive instead of just surviving and enduring.

Inner Child Healing - Why do it?

"We are set up to be emotionally dysfunctional by our role models, both parental and societal. We are taught to repress and distort our own emotional process. While we are children we are trained to be emotionally dishonest.

This emotional repression and dishonesty causes society to be emotionally dysfunctional. Additionally, urban based civilization has completely disregarded natural laws and natural cycles such as the human developmental process. There is no integration into our culture of the natural human developmental process.

As just one blatant example of this, consider how most so called primitive or aboriginal societies react to the onset of puberty. When a girl starts menstruating, ceremonies are held to celebrate her womanhood - to honor her coming into her power, to honor her miraculous gift of being able to conceive. Boys go through training and initiation rites to help them make the transition from boyhood to manhood. Look at what we have in our society: junior high school - a bunch of scared, insecure kids who torture each other out of their confusion and fear, and join gangs to try to find an identity.

This lack of integration of the natural human growth process causes trauma. At each stage of the developmental process we were traumatized because of the emotionally repressive, Spiritually hostile environment into which we were born. We went into the next stage incomplete and then were retraumatized, were wounded again.

For all of the so called progress of our modern societies, we still are far behind most aboriginal cultures in terms of respect for individual rights and dignity in some kind of balance with the good of the whole. (I am speaking here of tribal aboriginal societies - not urbanized ones.) Nowhere is this more evident in terms of our relationship to our children.

Modern civilizations - both Eastern and Western - are no more than a generation or two removed from the belief that children were property. This, of course, goes hand in hand with the belief that women were property. The idea that children have rights, individuality, and dignity is relatively new in modern society. The predominant and underlying belief, as it has been manifested in the treatment of children, has been that children are extensions of, and tools to be used by, their parents.

A very telling insight into the basic beliefs underlying Western attitudes towards children is shared by inner child pioneer Alice Miller in her book *The Drama of The Gifted Child.* She shares how the 19th Century German Philosophers who laid the groundwork for modern psychology, emphasized the importance of stamping out a child's "exuberance." In other words, a child's spirit must be crushed in order to control them.

Children are to be seen and not heard. Spare the rod and spoil the child.

It is only in very recent history, that our society has even recognized child abuse as a crime instead of an inherent right of the parent. The concept of healthy parenting as a skill to be learned is very new in modern society.

Any society that does not respect and honor individual human dignity, is going to be a society that does not meet the essential needs of its members. Patriarchal societies, that demean and degrade women and children, are dysfunctional in their essence.

We form our core relationship with our self and with life - and of course with other people - in early childhood in reaction to the messages we get from the way we are treated and the role modeling of the other people in our lives. We then have no training or initiation ceremonies, no culturally approved grieving process, to help us let go of the old programming and learn a different relationship with our self and life. So, we build upon the foundation laid in early childhood.

As adults, we react to the programming of our childhood. To contend that our childhood emotional wounds have not affected our adult lives is ridiculous. To think that our early programming has not influenced the way we have lived is to be in denial to an extreme.

Because societies standards for what constitutes success are dysfunctional, many people can be pointed out who "have risen above" their past to be a success. It is those people, who are supposedly successful, that are running the world. How good a job do you think they are doing?

It is our world leaders, reacting out of the fear and insecurity of their inner children, and the dysfunctional belief systems underlying civilization, who give us war and poverty, billionaires and homelessness.

My book, Codependence: The Dance of Wounded Souls, evolved out of a talk that I first did in 1991. In the talk, I stated that I would like to one day make up a bumper sticker that said "Work for World Peace, Heal Your Inner Child." I did have these bumper stickers printed when I published my book. It is, I believe, an essential Truth. We will never have world peace, or a civilized society which is based upon respect and dignity - to say nothing of Love - unless we can heal our relationships with ourselves enough to learn to Love and respect our self.

We cannot Love our neighbor as our self, as long as we are judging and comparing our self to them in order to feel good about our self. We cannot have a society that meets the essential emotional and spiritual needs of its members as long as we are reacting to life in alignment with rules of interaction that we learned in junior high school.

We are all connected - not separate. We all have worth and deserved to be treated with dignity and respect - instead of earning societies version of worth by stepping on and over our fellow humans, to say nothing of destroying the planet we live on.

It is through healing our inner child wounds that we can learn to respect and Love our self so that we can know how to treat others with respect and Love. It is through healing our inner children that we can save our planet and evolve into a society that does meet the essential needs of its members.

Inner child healing is not some fad or pop psychology. Inner child healing is the only way to empower ourselves to stop living life in reaction to the past. We have been ignoring history and repeating it for centuries. If we are going to have a chance to reverse the self destructive patterns of human kind, it is going to come from individuals healing self. By healing our inner child wounds, we can change the world.

Learning to Love our self

Codependence is an emotional and behavioral defense system which was adopted by our egos in order to meet our need to survive as a child. Because we had no tools for reprogramming our egos and healing our emotional wounds (culturally approved grieving, training and initiation rites, healthy role models, etc.), the effect is that as an adult we keep reacting to the programming of our childhood and do not get our needs met - our emotional, mental, Spiritual, or physical needs. Codependence allows us to survive physically but causes us to feel empty and dead inside. Codependence is a defense system that causes us to wound ourselves.

We need to take the shame and judgment out of the process on a personal level. It is vitally important to stop listening and giving power to that critical place within us that tells us that we are bad and wrong and shameful.

That "critical parent" voice in our head is the disease lying to us. . . . This healing is a long gradual process - the goal is progress, not perfection. What we are learning about is unconditional Love. Unconditional Love means no judgment, no shame.

We need to start observing ourselves and stop judging ourselves. Any time we judge and shame ourselves, we are feeding back into the disease, we are jumping back into the squirrel cage.

Codependence is a dysfunctional defense system that was built in reaction to feeling unlovable and unworthy - because our parents were wounded codependents who didn't know how to love themselves. We grew up in environments that were emotionally dishonest, Spiritually hostile, and shame based. Our relationship with ourselves (and all the different parts of our self: emotions, gender, spirit, etc.) got twisted and distorted in order to survive in our particular dysfunctional environment.

We got to an age where we were supposed to be an adult and we started acting like we knew what we were doing. We went around pretending to be adult at the same time we were reacting to the programming that we got growing up. We tried to do everything "right" or rebelled and went against what we had been taught was "right." Either way we weren't living our life through choice, we were living it in reaction.

In order to start being loving to ourselves we need to change our relationship with our self - and with all the wounded parts of our self. The way which I have found works the best in starting to love ourselves is through having internal boundaries.

Learning to have internal boundaries is a dynamic process that involves three distinctly different, but intimately interconnected, spheres of work.

These three spheres are:

1. Detachment
2. Inner Child Healing
3. Grieving

The purpose of the work is to change our ego-programming - to change our relationship with ourselves by changing our emotional/behavioral defense system into something that works to open us up to receive love, instead of sabotaging ourselves because of our deep belief that we don't deserve love.

I need to make the point here that Codependence and recovery are both multi-leveled, multi-dimensional phenomena. What we are trying to achieve is integration and balance on different levels.

In regard to our relationship with ourselves this involves two major dimensions:

They are the horizontal and the vertical. In this context:

The horizontal is about being human and relating to other humans and our environment.

The vertical is Spiritual, about our relationship to a Higher Power, to the Universal Source.

If we cannot conceive of a God/Goddess Force that loves us then it makes it virtually impossible to be loving to ourselves. So a Spiritual Awakening is absolutely vital to the process in my opinion.

Changing our relationship with ourselves on the horizontal (being human) level is a necessary element and is made possible by working on and integrating Spiritual Truth into our inner process.

Because Codependence is a reactive phenomena it is vital to start being able to detach from our own process in order to have some choice in changing our reactions. We need to start **observing** our selves from the **witness** perspective instead of from the perspective of the **judge**.

We all observe ourselves - have a place of watching ourselves as if from outside, or perched somewhere inside, observing our own behavior. Because of our childhoods we learned to judge ourselves from that witness perspective, the "critical parent" voice.

The emotionally dishonest environments we were raised in taught us that it was not ok to feel our emotions, or that only certain emotions were ok. So we had to learn ways to control our emotions in order to survive. We adapted the same tools that were used on us - guilt, shame, and fear (and saw in the role modeling of our parents how they reacted to life from shame and fear.) This is where the critical parent gets born. It's purpose is to try to keep our emotions and behavior under some sort of control so that we can get our survival needs met.

So the first boundary that we need to start setting internally is with the wounded / dysfunctionally programmed part of our own mind. We need to start saying no to the inner voices that are shaming and judgmental. The disease comes from a black and white, right and wrong, perspective. It speaks in absolutes: "You always screw up!" "You will never be a success!" - these are lies. We don't always screw up. We may never be a success according to our parents or societies dysfunctional definition of success - but that is because our heart and soul do not resonate with those definitions, so that kind of success would be a betrayal of ourselves. We need to consciously change our definitions so that we can stop judging ourselves against someone else's screwed up value system.

We learned to relate to ourselves (and all the parts of our self - emotions, sexuality, etc.) and life from a critical place of believing that something was wrong with us - and in fear that we would be punished if we didn't do life "right." Whatever we are doing or not doing, the disease can always find something to beat us up with. I have 10 things on my "to do list" today, I get 9 of them done, the disease does not want me to give myself credit for what I have done but instead beats me up for the one I didn't get done. Whenever life gets too good we get uncomfortable and the disease jumps right in with fear and shame messages. The critical parent voice keeps us from relaxing and enjoying life, and from loving our self.

We need to own that we have the power to choose where to focus our mind. We can consciously start viewing ourselves from the "witness" perspective. It is time to fire the judge - our critical parent - and choose to replace that judge with our Higher Self, who is a loving parent. We can then **intervene** in our own process to protect ourselves from the **perpetrator within** - the critical parent/disease voice.

It is almost impossible to go from critical parent to compassionate loving parent in one step - so the first step often is to try to observe ourselves from a neutral position or a "scientific observer" perspective.

This is what enlightenment and consciousness raising are all about. Owning our power to be a co-creator of our lives by changing our relationship with ourselves. We can change the way we think. We can change the way we respond to our own emotions. We need to detach from our wounded self in order to allow our Spiritual Self to guide us. We are Unconditionally Loved. **The Spirit does not speak to us from judgment and shame**.

To me, the process of recovery is about reprogramming my ego-defenses so I know that it is ok to feel the feelings. That feeling and releasing the emotions is not only ok it is what will work best in allowing me to have my needs fulfilled.

We need to change our relationship with ourselves and our own emotions in order to stop being at war with ourselves. The first step to doing that is to detach from ourselves enough to start protecting ourselves from the perpetrator that lives within us.

Loving the Wounded Child Within

It is through having the courage and willingness to revisit the emotional "dark night of the soul" that was our childhood, that we can start to understand on a gut level why we have lived our lives as we have.

It is when we start understanding the cause and effect relationship between what happened to the child that we were, and the effect it had on the adult we became, that we can Truly start to forgive ourselves. It is only when we start understanding on an emotional level, on a gut level, that we were powerless to do anything any differently than we did that we can Truly start to Love ourselves.

The hardest thing for any of us to do is to have compassion for ourselves. As children we felt responsible for the things that happened to us. We blamed ourselves for the things that were done to us and for the deprivations we suffered. There is nothing more powerful in this transformational process than being able to go back to that child who still exists within us and say, "It wasn't your fault. You didn't do anything wrong, you were just a little kid."

As long as we are judging and shaming ourselves we are giving power to the disease. We are feeding the monster that is devouring us.

We need to take responsibility without taking the blame. We need to own and honor the feelings without being a victim of them.

We need to rescue and nurture and Love our inner children - and STOP them from controlling our lives. STOP them from driving the bus! Children are not supposed to drive, they are not supposed to be in control.

And they are not supposed to be abused and abandoned. We have been doing it backwards. We abandoned and abused our inner children. Locked them in a dark place within us. And at the same time let the children drive the bus - let the children's wounds dictate our lives.

When we were 3 or 4 we couldn't look around us and say, "Well, Dad's a drunk and Mom is real depressed and scared - that is why it feels so awful here. I think I'll go get my own apartment."

Our parents were our higher powers. We were not capable of understanding that they might have problems that had nothing to do with us. So it felt like it was our fault.

We formed our relationship with ourselves and life in early childhood. We learned about love from people who were not capable of loving in a healthy way because of their unhealed childhood wounds. Our core / earliest relationship with our self was formed from the feeling that something is wrong and it must be me. At the core of our being is a little kid who believes that he/she is unworthy and unlovable. That was the foundation that we built our concept of "self" on.

Children are master manipulators. That is their job - to survive in whatever way works. So we adapted defense systems to protect our broken hearts and wounded spirits. The 4 year old learned to throw tantrums, or be real quiet, or help clean the house, or protect the younger siblings, or be cute and funny, etc. Then we got to be 7 or 8 and started being able to understand cause and effect and use reason and logic - and we changed our defense systems to fit the circumstances. Then we reach puberty and didn't have a clue what was happening to us, and no healthy adults to help us understand, so we adapted our defense systems to protect our vulnerability. And then we were teenagers and our job was to start becoming independent and prepare ourselves to be adults so we changed our defense systems once again.

It is not only dysfunctional, it is ridiculous to maintain that what happened in our childhood did not affect our adult life. We have layer upon layer of denial, emotional dishonesty, buried trauma, unfulfilled needs, etc., etc. Our hearts were broken, our spirit's wounded, our minds programmed dysfunctionally. The choices we have made as adults were made in reaction to our childhood wounds / programming - our lives have been dictated by our wounded inner children.

History, politics, "success" or lack of "success," in our dysfunctional society/civilizations can always be made clearer by looking at the childhoods of the individuals involved. History has been, and is being, made by immature, scared, angry, hurt individuals who were/are reacting to their childhood wounds and programming - reacting to the little child inside who feels unworthy and unlovable.

It is very important to realize that we are not an integrated whole being - to ourselves. Our self concept is fractured into a multitude of pieces. In some instances we feel powerful and strong, in others weak and helpless - that is because different parts of us are reacting to different stimuli (different "buttons" are being pushed.) The parts of us that feel weak, helpless, needy, etc. are not bad or wrong - what is being felt is perfect for the reality that was experienced by the part of our self that is reacting (**perfect for then** - but it has very little to do with what is happening in the now). It is very important to start having compassion for that wounded part of ourselves.

It is by owning our wounds that we can start taking the power away from the wounded part of us. When we suppress the feelings, feel ashamed about our reactions, do not own that part of our being, then we give it power. It is the feelings that we are hiding from that dictate our behavior, that fuel obsession and compulsion.

Codependence is a disease of extremes.

Those of us who were horrified and deeply wounded by a perpetrator in childhood - and were never going to be like that parent - adapted a more passive defense system to avoid confrontation and "hurting others." The more passive type of codependent defense system leads to a dominant pattern of being the victim.

Those of us who were disgusted by, and ashamed of, the victim parent in childhood and vowed never to be like that role model, adapted a more aggressive defense system. So we go charging through life being the bull in the china shop - being the perpetrator who blames other people for not allowing us to be in control. The perpetrator that feels like a victim of other people not doing things "right" - which is what forces us to bulldoze our way through life.

And, of course, some of us go first one way and then the other. We all have our own personal spectrum of extremes that we swing between - sometimes being the victim, sometimes being the perpetrator. Being a passive victim is perpetrating on those around us.

The only way we can be whole is to own all of the parts of ourselves. By owning all the parts we can then have choices about how we respond to life. By denying, hiding, and suppressing parts of ourselves we doom ourselves to live life in reaction.

A technique I have found very valuable in this healing process is to relate to the different wounded parts of our self as different ages of the inner child. These different ages of the child may be literally tied to an event that happened at that age - i.e. when I was 7 I tried to commit suicide. Or the age of the child might be a symbolic designator for a pattern of abuse/deprivation that occurred throughout our childhood - i.e. the 9 year old within me feels completely emotionally isolated and desperately needy/lonely, a condition which was true for most of my childhood and not tied to any specific incident (that I know of) that happened when I was 9.

By searching out, getting acquainted with, owning the feelings of, and building a relationship with, these different emotional wounds/ages of the inner child, we can start being a loving parent to ourselves instead of an abusive one. We can have boundaries with ourselves that allow us to: take responsibility for being a co-creator of our life; protect our inner children from the critical parent within; stop letting our childhood wounds control our life; and own the Truth of who we really are as Spiritual Beings. This way we can open up and receive the Love and Joy that is ours to have.

It is impossible to Truly love the adult that we are without owning the child that we were. In order to do that we need to detach from our inner process so that we can have some objectivity and discernment that will allow us to have compassion for our own childhood wounds. Then we need to grieve those wounds and own our right to be angry about what happened to us in childhood - so that we can Truly know in our gut that it wasn't our fault - we **were** just innocent little kids. Then we can de-energize the anger with unconditional LOVE.

Feeling the Feelings

Attempting to suppress emotions is dysfunctional; it does not work. Emotions are energy: E-motion = energy in motion. It is supposed to be in motion, it was meant to flow.

Emotions have a purpose, a very good reason to be - even those emotions that feel uncomfortable. Fear is a warning, anger is for protection, tears are for cleansing and releasing. These are not negative emotional responses! We were taught to react negatively to them. It is our reaction that is dysfunctional and negative, not the emotion.

The way to stop reacting out of our inner children is to release the stored emotional energy from our childhoods by doing the grief work that will heal our wounds. The only effective, long term way to clear our emotional process - to clear the inner channel to Truth which exists in all of us - is to grieve the wounds which we suffered as children. The most important single tool, the tool which is vital to changing behavior patterns and attitudes in this healing transformation, is the grief process. The process of grieving.

Until we are fully healed we all carry around repressed pain, terror, shame, and rage energy from our childhoods, whether it was twenty years ago or fifty years ago.

> Glenn's note: This energy can be from what we perceive as past lifetimes and may even be inherited from our ancestors.

We have this grief energy within us even if we came from a relatively healthy family, because this society is emotionally dishonest and dysfunctional.

Emotions are energy that is manifested in our bodies. They exist below the neck. They are not thoughts (although attitudes set up our emotional reactions.) In order to do the emotional healing it is vital to start paying attention to where energy is manifesting in our bodies. Where is there tension, tightness? Could that "indigestion" really be some feelings? Are those "butterflies" in my stomach telling me something emotionally?

When I am working with someone and they start having some feelings coming up, the first thing I have to tell them is to keep breathing. Most of us have learned a variety of ways to control our emotions and one of them is to stop breathing and close our throats. That is because grief in the form of sadness accumulates in our upper chest and breathing into it helps some of it to escape - so we learned to stop breathing at those moments when we start getting emotional, when our voice starts breaking.

Western civilization has for many years been way out of balance towards the left brain way of thinking - concrete, rational, what you see is all there is (this was in reaction to earlier times of being out of balance the other way, towards superstition and ignorance.) Because emotional energy cannot be seen or measured or weighed ("The x-ray shows you've got 5 pounds of grief in there.") emotions were discounted and devalued. This has started to change somewhat in recent years but most of us grew up in a society that taught us that being too emotional was a bad thing that we should avoid. (Certain cultures / subcultures give more permission for emotions but those are usually out of balance to the other extreme of allowing the emotions to rule - the goal is balance: between mental and emotional, between intuitive and rational.)

Emotions are a vital part of our being for several reasons.

1. Because it is energy and energy cannot just disappear. The emotional energy generated by the circumstances of our childhood and early life does not go away just because we were forced to deny it. It is still trapped in our body - in a pressurized, explosive state, as a result of being suppressed. If we don't learn how to release it in a healthy way it will explode outward or implode back in on us. Eventually it will transform into some other form - such as cancer.

2. As long as we have pockets of pressurized emotional energy that we have to avoid dealing with - those emotional wounds will run our lives. We use food, cigarettes, alcohol and drugs, work, religion, exercise, meditation, television, etc., to help us keep suppressing that energy. To help us keep ourselves focused on something else, anything else, besides the emotional wounds that terrify us. The emotional wounds are what cause obsession and compulsion, are what the "critical parent" voice works so hard to keep us from dealing with.

3. Our emotions tell us who we are - our Soul communicates with us through emotional energy vibrations. Truth is an emotional energy vibrational communication from our Soul on the Spiritual Plane to our being/spirit/soul on this physical plane - it is something that we feel in our heart/our gut, something that resonates within us.

Our problem has been that because of our unhealed childhood wounds it has been very difficult to tell the difference between an intuitive emotional **Truth** and the **emotional truth** that comes from our childhood wounds. When one of our buttons is pushed and we react out of the insecure, scared little kid inside of us (or the angry/rage filled kid, or the powerless/helpless kid, etc.) then we are reacting to what our emotional truth was when we were 5 or 9 or 14 - not to what is happening now. Since we have been doing that all of our lives, we learned not to trust our emotional reactions (and got the message not to trust them in a variety of ways when we were kids.)

4. We are attracted to people that **feel familiar on an energetic level** - which means (until we start clearing our emotional process) people that emotionally / vibrationally feel like our parents did when we were very little kids. At a certain point in my process I realized that if I met a woman who **felt** like my soul mate, that the chances were pretty huge that she was one more unavailable woman that fit my pattern of being attracted to someone who would reinforce the message that I wasn't good enough, that I was unlovable. Until we start releasing the hurt, sadness, rage, shame, terror - the emotional grief energy - from our childhoods we will keep having dysfunctional relationships.

I became willing to do the emotional healing in the summer of 1987 when I set myself up to be abandoned on my birthday one more time. I called a counselor that I had been told was good with the emotional work. It turned out that he was in the middle of moving to Hawaii and wasn't doing counseling anymore. But he said I could come over and talk to him as he packed.

I don't remember anything that he said to me that day - what I do remember is that as I sat in his house watching him pack I had a feeling, and a visual image, that I had just opened Pandora's Box - the monsters were loose now and I would never be able shut that box again.

Doing the grief work can be absolutely terrifying. The word I came up with to describe how I felt was terrifying. It felt like if I ever really owned the pain, I would end up crying in a rubber room for the rest of my life. That if I ever really owned the rage, I would just go up and down the street shooting people. That is not what happened. The Spirit guided me through the process and gave me the resources I needed to release great quantities of that pent up, pressurized emotional energy. To release enough to start learning who I really am, to start seeing my path more clearly, and to start forgiving myself and learning about love.

I still need to do the grieving/energy release work from time to time. There is still a hole in my soul - a seemingly bottomless abyss of wish-to-die-pain, shame, and unbearable suffering. But it is a much smaller hole and I don't have to visit it very often.

The wounds don't automatically go away. They have less power to dictate my life as I heal. I needed to own that wounded part of me in order to start getting to know, and have compassion for, me. I also needed to learn to have a balance because we can't live in those feelings. We need to own them and honor them in order to own and honor ourselves - but then we need to learn to have internal boundaries that will allow us to find some balance in our life, allow us to trust the process and our Higher Power.

We are on a Spiritual journey - and the Force is with us. It will help and guide us as we face the terror of owning how painful our human experience has been. The more we are able to feel and release the feelings / emotional energy, the more clearly we can tune into the emotional energy that is Truth - and Love, Light, Joy, Beauty - coming from The Source Energy.

Above is adapted from Robert Burney (http://www.woundedsouls.com/index.php/emotional-incest;)
http://www.suite101.com/article.cfm/codependency_recovery/50739
Oct 18, 2000 (Web page is no longer available as of June 2016);
http://www.healyourinnerchild.com/Book-Content/inner-child-healing-how-to-begin
http://www.woundedsouls.com/index.php/emotional-incest

Below is adapted from http://www.creativegrowth.com/teresa.htm

Growing Towards Wholeness Through Grief:

The Journey of the Wounded Child Within

by Teresa M. Kaplan

Note: The following article was originally written by Teresa Kaplan as part of her Master's-level graduate work in psychology. It is a moving blend of valuable information about what inner child therapy is - and how it is conducted with therapy clients - interwoven with her heartfelt account of her own personal journey of growth and healing. When she shared this written work with us, we asked if we could post it on our Center's website, knowing that it was an informative and inspiring piece. We are very happy to share her most excellent article with you, in the hopes that you, too, will find it useful in your own path of growth and healing. (The names of her therapy clients, referred to later in the article, have, of course, been changed to preserve confidentiality.)

"We shall not cease from exploration

And the end of all our exploring

Will be to arrive where we started

And know the place for the first time."

T.S. Eliot

I am six years old. It is sunny outside, it must be spring or summer. We are just getting home from our day. My father, my nine year old brother and I are walking up the steps to our rented house on Regency Drive. As my brother walks inside, my father turns to me and says, "Mom and I got a divorce, and she is living in New York now." I tell him it is okay. Both my brother and I state that we are not sad, and in fact, I truly remember not feeling sad in that moment. And that was that. Never again in my 18 years of living at home did my family discuss my mother. We simply went on and "forgot" that she existed.

Twenty one years later, I am in my studio apartment, living on my own for the first time. The phone rings and I expectantly pick it up, imagining it might be my older brother. "Holli just gave birth to a baby girl," he says, with the pride of a husband and new father. I begin to tear as I congratulate him, moved by this emotional moment. Yet as we hang up the telephone, I realize that my tears are not that of an excited and touched new Aunt, but are tears of immense pain. My tears turn to sobs, my heart experiencing a depth of pain that I have never known before. I don't know why I feel this, I just know it hurts. The pain is unbearable. It feels intolerable. I feel as if I am experiencing the pain of the entire world in my one little body. There are no words, no thoughts. I am only feeling, feeling so much I can't stand it. I question if I can make it through the night like this.

I did make it through that night, and have survived other nights of almost similar intensity. I even welcome them now. I sometimes encourage them. This notion may sound strange, as our culture, our families, even our own natural protective instincts encourage us to avoid our painful feelings. The goal of life is to feel good and be happy! Thus we find ways to avoid, deny, distract, repress, dissociate, forget. And yet ultimately these defenses are not helpful, bringing us pain anyway. I truly believe, then, that we must go through the darkness, not around it, in order to get to the light. And thus, I present here the grief work that I so strongly understand as a path to healing. I will take you on my own journey last year as my child self began to mourn the loss of my mother, I will share the works of authors in the field of the "inner child" and grief work, and I will present the beginning journey's of my clients and case examples of clinical interventions and the framework I hold in therapy. With my personal experience, witnessing my clients, and reading outside materials, I feel strongly at this point that one of the most powerful ways of healing is through tapping into the grief of our child self. This is how we reconnect with who we really are. This is how we grow towards Wholeness.

It wasn't until over one year later that I began to understand the deep pain that was triggered in me on the night that my beautiful niece was born. The pain is still difficult to name with words. Her birth, the first birth of the next generation in my family, the birth of a baby girl, brought with it a glimpse of the reality that I had always denied; the disconnection of the mother-daughter relationship, and the emotional understanding that my baby self was essentially born and raised "motherless," that even before her physical departure when I was six, she had departed mentally through "schizophrenia" when I was an infant. One year later, after over 27 years of repressing my child pain, I was finally ready to accept and to feel that at a very early age my child self was abandoned and wounded deeply. I was determined now to know this in my body, my mind, my heart. Thus I decided to take an inward journey, to heal my past in the present.

The journey I took last year began with a strong desire to know, to feel, to heal. Soon after this intention was declared, my "journey" took on a life of its own. The next several months included extreme hard work through individual therapy, Mendell's Process work, dreamwork, expressive arts modalities, psychodrama, journaling, poetry, energy work, and a written integration of it all through a 65 page personal process paper. Before this, beginning since I was 11 years old, poetry had been the one tool I used in order to express myself and my feelings in relation to my mother. I begin that paper with a poem I wrote after speaking with family and learning more about my infancy. It seems fitting for this paper as well, and so I share it here:

She left, before I even came out of her.
And when I lay in my crib, new born and vulnerable
voices screamed at her
"Kill your child" they said.
And I had left, an exhausted mother
fighting to keep us both alive.
I did survive that childhood
where brothers teased and fathers were always right.
I put on my happy face
and with love and light inside to anchor me,
I hid myself from the pain that always comes with truth.
Oh sure, it came out in poems,
and once a year visits to a coughing woman

but that memory of fear sat deep inside
covered, with layers. . . so that I might not feel a thing.
Now here I am at 27, with a flood of emotion at my feet.
More vulnerable, more fragile than my child self.
You don't go backwards silly.
I want to shake me and scream,
"Listen up and remember, you are a woman and you are strong."
But can a child, that has needs and no mother,
become a woman, whole and strong?
I am too tired now, to ponder that question.
I just want to find some peace.

I then write in the introduction of that paper, "In some ways, this deep inner work has felt like an awakening. I have experienced pain, fear, excitement, pleasure, loss, anger, power, sadness, clarity, understanding, love. I have felt young, fragile, wounded, wise, brave, strong, proud. I have tapped into buried emotions and connections, years of denial and confusion now leading into insight and clarity."

I go on to write, "I continued to flow with the process, inquiring inside, reflecting, digging, searching, feeling, writing, reading, expressing, allowing. I gave myself permission to explore and be in it, to push myself to the growing edge while giving myself assurance that I am safe and able to hold what was to come up. I have thus been able to feel my young child's pain and loss, while my woman self has held her hand with comfort and soothing knowledge of healing. I have learned I am big enough now, to dive into the darkness. The work I have been doing - the young trauma - includes mother loss, emotional caretaking, sacrifice of self, unmet needs, double messages, confusion, emotional repression, denial, disempowerment, . . . all weaving together to encompass the core of my wounding. The 'factual' puzzle pieces I may never 'know,' but through the process of opening up to my core issues, the puzzle pieces of my self and my psyche have begun to fit together to present glimpses of the Whole."

Jung understood my desire to journey and the significance of our inner child. "In the adult there lurks a child-an eternal child, something that is always becoming, is never completed, and that calls for increasing care, attention, education. This is the part of the human personality that wishes to develop and become whole" (cited in Abrams, 1990, p. 203). And I am drawn to the healing powers of grief work, especially grieving the losses of our childhood and our child selves, because I have personally experienced the immense transformation that occurs when we open up to it. During this time, I cried and screamed and went mad. But I believe the permission I gave to myself to do this, to dive to the depths of places that I had never allowed myself to go before, allowed for a strength and fullness to emerge. Through our grief, we can feel the incredible bittersweet beauty that comes with life lived in depth. Through my own grief, I experienced this profoundly. Ironically, through tapping into my loss, I now experience a fuller sense of completeness inside of me. I have always been fortunate to experience self-love, but through my deep pain an even deeper more expansive self-love and self-compassion were tapped into. Connection to the Divine became more solid than I have ever known. And in grieving my child wounds, my authentic voice became louder, clearer, more solid, unafraid of the whole Teresa Kaplan who is here on this earth to be who she is.

Although my own experience involves actual loss of my mother through mental illness, I believe we all experience the trauma of loss in some form during childhood, and I have seen that my experience includes childhood wounds that are similar to many other's experiences. I remember sharing my experience of loss during an in-depth presentation in class one time, and was surprised to see tears on so many faces that could relate to my story in their own way. But most of us do experience loss and "abandonment" as a child, whether it be more subtle or more dramatic. Often our adult selves are not aware or conscious of these losses, as they may be less tangible and more invisible because they are gradual, partial, or even symbolic (Whitfield, 1987, p. 89). Most of us experience a loss of the part of our beautiful innocent selves that was unacceptable to our particular family. Even when we were loved, we were not fully seen or acknowledged or appreciated as our whole selves. Or worse yet, we were judged or criticized for it. All of us at one point felt hurt, rejection, neglect, unfairness. And especially, all of us had unmet needs. "People seek psychotherapeutic help largely because of the pain, despair, rage and unfulfilled needs of the neglected inner child" (Stein cited in Abrams, 1990, p. 264). Thus all of us can benefit from grieving these experiences.

When we are young, we are at our greatest time of need. This time is crucial for the development of our sense of self. Our needs are simple, yet essential. Charles Whitfield (1987) describes many of the needs that when left unmet, may stifle the child self. They include a sense of safety, physical touching, attention, mirroring, guidance, listening, acceptance, freedom to be our self, tolerance of our feelings, validation, respect, support, trust, nurturing, and unconditional love (pp. 17-22). And in order to become our true self, we actually require most of these needs. And yet this is often not possible. Whitfield (1987) points out that rarely does one have a mother or other figure who is even capable of providing or helping us to meet all of our needs. "There is usually no such person available. . . Thus, in our recovery, we grieve over not having had all our needs met as infants. . ." (p. 22).

It seems the greatest and most crucial need a child has in order to develop fully is to receive "mirroring." When we are young we need to have our true feelings-our true self- mirrored, in order to help us develop trust in our own experiences. I have witnessed the wounds and pain and "holes" in myself, as well as my clients, due to this lack of mirroring. It is clear this is an essential aspect in facilitating the continuation of our authentic development. In Winnicott's terms, when we receive empathic attunement (mirroring), this nurturing environment allows the blossoming of the "true self" of the child (cited in Firman & Russell, 1994, p. 10). In Psychosyntheses, this true self can be called "authentic personality." It is seen in a similar way, with the understanding of mirroring being a crucial factor. "If at each stage of life we receive this mirroring, we are able to recognize, accept, and include the unfolding aspects of ourselves at that stage . . . Through this mirroring we can actualize all the richness of our unfolding human potential . . . " (Firman & Russell, 1994, p. 11). And thus when we are young, instances of major failures in mirroring can cause deep wounding to our sense of identity.

I agree with John Bradshaw (1990) in the belief that we are all born with a sense of wholeness and completeness, even though we are not fully developed yet. We are valuable and special as no one is exactly like us. "The story of every man's and every woman's fall is how a wonderful, valuable, special, precious child lost its sense of 'I am who I am'" (p. 39). As most of us are not completely accepted or unconditionally loved exactly for who we are, we may disconnect from our full sense of self. During the time of our infant and child development, this connection to our Self appears-and essentially is-less important than the real or imagined emotional abandonment that may occur if we retain the parts of our selves that are unacceptable. “To the child, abandonment by its parents is the equivalent of death” (Peck cited in Abrams, 1990, p. 106). Thus the choice we have then appears, and often is, conflicting. This means choosing to identify with the “false” self in order for survival. (Abrams, 1990, p. 118).

Our false self is the part of us that emerges for our protection. When our parents have not worked through their own childhood wounds, they continue to have unconscious needs. Our child selves then intuitively sacrifice our own self-realization in order to gratify them and thus maintain connection. Often, rather than the adult parents meeting unconditionally the needs of their children, it is the children who unconditionally meet the needs of their parents. It is understandable then that a pattern thus unfolds throughout the generations . . . until courageous members begin to face their grief and thus begin to break the cycle. Until then, we see the tragedy of the loss of our beautiful complete authentic Selves.

As Jung says, “If parents because of their own insecurity cannot accept sufficiently the basic nature of the child, then its personality becomes damaged. If it is beyond the normal bruising of life the child becomes estranged from his center of being and feels forced to abandon his natural pattern of unfoldment” (cited in Abrams, 1990, p. 202). Thus the goal of our adult selves is to reclaim that natural path of unfoldment, to travel to and remain in the “center” of our being. It is possible to reconnect with who we really are-the complete authentic self we were born as that may still be hidden underground. And this is the transformation that occurs through our child’s grief. Alice Miller strongly affirms this when she says, "The true self has been in 'a state of noncommunication,' as Winnicott said, because it had to be protected. The patient never needs to hide anything else so thoroughly, so deeply, and for so long a time as he has hidden his true self. Thus it is like a miracle each time to see how much individuality has survived behind such dissimulation, denial, and self-alienation, and can reappear as soon as the work of mourning brings freedom from the interjects." (cited in Abrams, 1990, p. 136) The painful difficult work this entails is worth it. I can validate the experience.

Thus, I feel fortunate that when my dam broke I had the courage to continue swimming in the waters of darkness. For many of us, including myself for 27 years, the fear of drowning, of the currents, of the imagined engulfing never-ending river of our emotions is too great to allow us to do more than splash with our toe and run back to the “safety” of land to dry off. Others of us, are still unaware of the water. We remain disconnected or dismiss our childhood experiences through minimizing their impact. This is how I lived for many years. This is how many live, denying their inner child’s wounded experience and thus continuing, maybe unknowingly, to suffer. We do this because most of us believe what we intuitively knew in childhood-that we cannot handle our pain. Although now as adults we can learn to efficiently hold our pain, we still imagine, “. . .that we will die, or go crazy, or that the pain or discomfort will be unending, or that we are wrong or weak for having those feelings. So we try to protect ourselves. We ignore, deny, or discount our feelings; and in so doing, we abandon our Inner Child” (Paul, 1992, p. 56). And we unconsciously imagine that somehow by continuing to disconnect from the pain of our child self, we will not experience pain.

And yet as Carl Jung says, "Whatever is denied conscious access continues to influence the individual anyhow-but via unconscious processes" (cited in Walker, 1995, p. 19). When we do not explore our feelings, these "unconscious processes" can have a significant impact on our sense of self, our adult relationships, and our lives. Although we can deny or discount our emotions, this does not make them magically disappear. They remain hidden, or turn against the self, or project outwards effecting others with whom we are in relationship. Some of the difficulties that I have witnessed when we remain unconscious of our child's pain, are; co-dependence, feelings of emptiness, trust issues, difficulties with intimacy, depression, hostile self-criticism, low self-esteem, irritability (due to holding in anger), anxiety, fear, and excessive need of approval or attention. I imagine this list describes just a few of the possible consequences that may occur when we do not really listen to our child inside and work through our inner pain. "...The pressure from such hidden wounds can and does eventually wreak havoc in our lives and in the world" (Firman & Russell, 1994, p. 19).

Much of our unnecessary emotional pain is due to the pressure that comes from not releasing stored up energy that has accumulated throughout our lives. I believe, further, that without the release that comes through our grief work, we may be holding so much deep inside that it can affect us emotionally, physically, mentally and spiritually. As our bodies, hearts, minds, and spirit are interconnected, when we experience wounding, it is a wounding to our entire being. And as I myself have physically experienced, our emotional trauma is stored up as energy in our bodies. When not processed, this can have a great effect on us. As Whitfield (1987) says, "When we are not allowed to remember, to express our feelings and to grieve or mourn our losses or trauma, whether real or threatened, through the free expression of our Child Within, we become ill" (p. 58). I believe this "illness" can and does take on many forms.

And not only do we possibly suffer when we do not allow our grief, we also simply may not experience the full depth of our experiences. By repressing or ignoring our childhood experiences and our still living inner child, "we are limiting our consciousness and our ability to experience life" (Short cited in Abrams, 1990, p .203). Through our grief work we can begin to live in a more full, rich, deep way. It has been claimed that when we repress one emotional aspect of ourselves, we then dim all of the others. If we are afraid to dive into our pain, we may not be allowing ourselves to experience the full intensity of our joy. As Walker (1995) shares,

Along with love and peace and beauty, God made pain and loss and suffering. Our ability to fully appreciate life depends on our willingness to sometimes feel sad and angry about our own and others' misfortunes and difficulties. The tools of grieving are gifts from God that enable us to integrate and grow from life's inexorable hardships, and then to return to gratitude for its wonders. (p. 203) Thus it is clear that the ungrieved pain of our child self can affect our adult lives in deep ways. I believe that much of our adult suffering stems from our ungrieved past. Many of our issues stem from the core of our inner child's wounding and the still neglected pain that silently, somewhere, yearns to be felt.

Before my journey last year, I myself was stuck in denial for many years, minimizing the effects of the difficulties of my childhood, completely disconnected from my inner child's pain. I remember a few years ago an acquaintance asked me over dinner one night about my mother. I said in an almost amused tone, "She is schizophrenic, she thinks she works for the CIA, has won the Nobel Peace Prize, and talks to me about the special powers she has. It is interesting." He looked at me with shock and almost disdain, "That is one of the saddest things I've ever heard." I felt a little embarrassed, but his words did not penetrate into my heart. And yet I did not imagine I was in denial, for I was aware and acknowledging of the situation. But although I knew the information, I did not "know" the feelings of it. It appears this is a common phenomena. "Minimization is a subset of denial; it is acknowledging, but making light of, childhood losses. Many survivors minimize hurtful childhood memories by transmuting their pain into jocularity. . ." (Walker, 1995, p. 71). For years I could tell my story to anyone who inquired, yet it never felt real to me. And yet my unconscious wounds came through in my adult life. I see now how these behaviors and emotions were my traumatized child self screaming out, crying gently, angry and sad and attempting to be nurtured.

So how do we get from this place of minimization and denial to a place of acceptance and feeling and then healing. As John Bradshaw (1990) says, "In order for grief to be resolved several factors must be present. The first factor is validation. Our childhood abandonment trauma must be validated as real or it cannot be resolved" (p. 228). I know this was very true for me. As I sat in lost silence, I felt my childhood a puzzle in which many of the pieces were missing. And then last year I realized I needed to build that puzzle, filling in the pieces in whatever way I could. My desire for growth and health outweighed any fear or defense. So I read the book, "Motherless Daughters; the legacy of loss" by Hope Edelman, which by validating my experience for the first time, began to finally help lift my protections. Rather than numbly thinking about it feeling as if it were the life story of someone else, I finally began to realize-to feel-that this was in fact, sadly, my life story. Now I was ready to meet her, my vulnerable hurt little girl.

The experience of validation allowed me to begin to do this. I write about the significance of this in my process paper. Mother loss is a significant event for boys as well as girls. Reading letters and studies of women who have lost their mothers (due to death or mental illness) shows me that I can be allowed to feel. This may sound strange but the message I have received in my life is to minimize my loss-it is not significant, nothing to mourn. Thus I have never felt the permission to really feel, for fear that I am simply being overly dramatic. Finding my own truth in this book-not just in the significance of loss but also the ways of my family's denial and dynamics-I am beginning to trust myself. I want to fight now for what I am entitled to, embracing the reality of my experience with eyes and heart open. Wow, a mother is often the most significant figure that a child has in his or her life and the mothers influence continues throughout life as the child grows into adult-hood..

Once we begin to understand that our experiences and emotions are important and valid , we then seem to allow ourselves the permission to acknowledge and feel them. I have seen with my clients that as I mirror their experience and continue to validate them, and especially take their experience seriously on a feeling level, their true emotions begin to awaken. Once the tragedy of my situation was named and acknowledged from outside sources, I began to open up to the reality of the experience of my child within. And for me I noticed that once I made this conscious choice to accept her, she began to come to me. After feeling the validation that I needed through reading as well as finally speaking with family members, my pain awakened for the first time through a dream.

I wrote the experience in my journal. "I am at my old elementary school, the school in which I now work. It is a beautiful sunny day. I look down the steps, and I see my mother. She is young, and so incredibly beautiful. She is happy and light and radiant. She is real. I walk over to her and she looks into my eyes. We connect deeply. I am overwhelmed with love and joy to be with this amazing woman, to have a mother whom I admire in so many ways. I can't believe how beautiful she is. . .how lucky I am. . . I awake alone in my studio apartment. My unconscious has just given me the gift this night of tapping into the connection-and thus the loss of connection-that I have experienced in my life in relation to my mother. As I shift from dream state to waking life, my emotions do not leave me. I awake with intense sadness, and release tears that I really have access to for maybe the first time. A flood of tears emerge, coming from a deep, deep place inside...the core of my being. I do not feel like 27 year old Teresa Kaplan in this room, I feel transported to another time/place . . . I feel like an infant, helpless and small. My heart feels broken, as if I have lost a part of myself, or the closest thing to me. It hurts . . . I feel sad defeat . . . very deep and alone . . . The denial has lifted-I lost my mother. And this is very, very sad. On this night I am now feeling the emotions of this sadness."

Intuitively, I knew the healing power that feeling my feelings could bring me. I thus called to my little girl self, encouraging my wounded child to come out from hiding after these many years. I needed to remind her of her experience in order to help her into her feelings. I write in my journal to myself: "Oh my incredible strong and beautiful Teresa. You are amazing. . . and you have such young wounds. Imagine neglected baby T. Helpless. Needy. Uncomfortable. In pain. Scared. Hungry for attention and nourishment. And you had to sit with that. Your mother was not present. She wasn't able to care for you, fulfill your needs. She was self absorbed. She was in her own world. You were abandoned at your time of greatest need. And your father was no help. He was in denial. He was away, working three jobs and writing his dissertation. Now in intimate relationship in adult life you have feared abandonment. You have been hurt when you were not paid attention to. You experienced narcissistic rage when your needs couldn't be fulfilled. You have felt devastated. This is your helpless infant crying out. These are your baby wounds hurting, wishing to heal. It is time now to express them to and from their real source. Let the abused infant be seen and felt. Let it be clear. Then let her be taken care of. Take care of her! Let her know she deserved attention and nourishment. And remind her that she probably did not receive it. Let her be angry, devastated-this will not drown her. Gently and sadly remind her that she will never get what she lost out on then. No one can be there for her now the way a mother is there for her infant. You cannot expect that sweety. Mourn this loss. Accept it. Know that pain. And then you will begin to heal. Slowly, it will take time. You may still get hurt. You may still feel disappointed and get angry. But it will be cleaner. And the wound won't go so deep. It will not be so big. You will not be so small. You will continue into health. I love you amazing T."

My child within listened to these words, and trusted enough to come out from hiding. Her pain continued to come up through my dreams, during experiential exercises with my psychodrama groups, in therapy, in my journal writings, when I called to her as I lay alone in my studio at night, in the safety of the arms of my partner in bed, and spontaneously and uncontrollably in various situations that triggered the old pain of abandonment and loss. I became aware of every mother daughter pair walking together down the street. Situations, interactions and words that at one time went unnoticed, now became painful reminders of the immense wounded child whose painful feelings were now so accessible inside. I was integrating her, and her grief was a part of my common experience now. I write to myself in my journal at this time, “You are integrating . . . able to hold the deep connection and love of mother and daughter, and at the same time the tremendous painful loss and absence. Both are true. Both are real. Both can give you power.”

During this work, most of my grief was experienced as painful sadness and expressed through tears. This is an extremely important aspect of grief work. Our emotional pain is stored up energetically in our bodies. Through the act of crying we can finally begin to release this stored up energy. When we are able to let go and open up to our pain and cry-not just silent tears but deep bodily sobs-we are naturally healing ourselves. When we give ourselves the space to sit in the pain and allow it to move through us physically via unrestrained tears, we are being there for our child self (Walker, 1995, p. 79). We can surrender to our bodies and allow them to do the work, shaking and releasing “primal” sounds from deep down, carrying the hurt out of our body. We can let ourselves sob and shake, knowing this is the body’s way of letting go of the pain it has been holding for many years. It is extremely therapeutic to surrender to this trembling as it marks the release of the deepest levels of pain” (Walker, 1995, p. 80). And yet most of us are not familiar with this deep core crying. Most of us are afraid to let go of “control” and trust enough to allow our bodies to experience deeply. But when we open ourselves to the experience, the healing that takes place through this grieving process is truly transformational.

This of course takes much strength and courage. Sometimes during a “grief session” I am amazed that I-that one person-could be holding so much pain. The reservoir that I tap into has seemed bottomless at times, yet I dive in anyway, certain in the healing aspects that come with the experience. A few months ago, after my inner work last year, again my child self was triggered one night. This session was the most powerful I have experienced. Having my partner with me, who is comfortable, safe and supportive, who is big and unafraid, further encouraged my hurt girl to feel her feelings in their fullest. For over three hours I cried, sobbed, and released primal sounds that came from deep within my center. My body shook, trembled, contracted and released. My emotional pain and physical pain seemed to merge, I was unable to differentiate them. I could physically feel the energy releasing out through my mouth via sounds, and course through my body eventually releasing out of my feet and hands. This healing work is profound and powerful, yet simple: we need not “do” anything . . . just allow ourselves to be open to the experience and be with it. Hold the hand of our hurt little child and let her deeply cry.

In the process of grieving, experiencing and expressing our child’s anger is just as important as releasing our sadness through tears. “We are learning that in healing our Child Within it is appropriate and healthy to become aware of and to express our anger” (Whitfield, 1987, p. 104). Many of us are not aware of this. As we move through our grief process, we may experience blocks at any phase, and I see this is especially true for the experience of anger. I know this was true for me. During my own process, I knew somewhere inside I must be angry, yet I had a difficult time touching into those feelings. As it has always been my mother whom I see as the victim, and as I witness her innocent childlike self full of love and vulnerability I couldn’t imagine how I could be angry with her. But intuitively, I also understood that intentions are not relevant in this work, what is relevant is what I actually experienced. As John Bradshaw (1990) explains, “It’s okay to be angry, even if what was done to you was unintentional. In fact, you have to be angry if you want to heal your wounded inner child. . ." (pp. 78-79). Thus I did open to the experience of my anger. I did get in touch with a lot of anger towards my father during this time. And eventually I was able to experience anger for the experience of being abandoned and the unfairness of not having a mother. For me, this was just as healing.

Allowing and experiencing our anger during grief work is necessary in many ways. As with allowing our tears of sadness, feeling and expressing our anger helps us to release the stored up emotions that have accumulated inside due to our childhood experiences. This process is extremely important. Otherwise, in our adult lives we may continue to hurt ourselves or others with our unconscious behaviors that come from old unresolved anger. When we work through our past anger, we are less likely to carry anger in our adult lives. When we attempt to deny it we then allow it to come up unconsciously and this is when it turns against us-becoming rage, suicidal depression, creating violence in the world. I agree with Walker (1995) that most of us fear our anger and hide from it, as we are afraid of this energy and of its seeming power to damage us. Ironically, it is truly damaging only when we do not embrace it. And thus we see the necessity of allowing our anger to manifest during our grief work.

But not only is our experiencing of anger necessary, it can also be extremely beneficial. Many possibilities for transformation occur when we embrace our anger and work with it. As Walker (1995) says, "Angering unlocks our joy. When we finally end our lifelong repression of our anger, we often feel exuberant relief" (p. 87). Anger empowers us. It releases our fear so that we can more fully embody ourselves and feel more free to express who we are. It allows us to hold boundaries. It gives us assertive strength, without the need for aggression. It builds confidence. Interestingly, it may even create more peace within us. Our relationships and interactions may also shift. Walker (1995) found that his anger actually helped him to feel safe enough to risk being vulnerable with others, and says, "Truly intimate relationships finally began to flower in my life" (p. 69).

And during grief work we need not fear our anger as there are many healthy nonviolent ways to explore and express it. It is important to understand that almost always the least helpful way to express our anger is actually releasing it directly towards others, even the person we our angry with. Some other more helpful techniques, most of which I myself actively participated in, include psychodrama, art, writing letters (not to be sent), role-plays, sharing with others, yelling, voicing primal noises, journaling, pounding, dancing to "angry" music, expressing with self out loud or silently. Through using our feelings therapeutically in this way, experiencing our anger frees us from our fear of it, and we come to learn that our expression of anger is not always dangerous—it can be safe and healing. And as Walker (1995) says, "What a wonderful paradox that the safe letting go of control actually insures us that control will not be lost destructively! Safe angering insures this won't occur because it prevents rage from becoming an explosive pressure cooker without a release valve" (1995, p. 150).

Within this discussion of experiencing our anger, I feel it is important here to discuss blame, and the idea of "blaming" our parents during this grief work. What seems most common to me as I witness my clients struggle, is their fear of blame. Many of us are afraid of blame because as children we were "abandoned" for challenging our parents. We may thus unknowingly carry an unconscious fear of rejection. Although we are not technically still needy children of our parents, our lives no longer threatened by their abandonment, the emotional dynamic is deep within us from childhood. Also, as I shared earlier, because I have so much love and compassion for my mother, I have a "block" to blaming her. How could I blame her, with her large innocent heart and vulnerability and illness, her incredible poetry and depth. How could I do anything but love her. I have seen my clients, when attempting to share their childhood pain, experience much hesitation, as they imagine that by doing this they are being unloving to their parents. They imagine that if they present their pain, they are blaming harshly and then discounting all of the positive aspects of their parental figures. We may feel guilt or shame. We may feel, as I myself did at various points, that by feeling our anger and blaming, we are "bad." We may find it easier to blame indirectly and feel anger towards the unfairness of the experience, as I have-rather than the direct person. In cases of unintentional hurt (death, illness), I believe this may be just as helpful. Yet also, I remind my clients, as I did myself, that acknowledging the difficulty, does not have to take away our appreciation. We can hold both. Our pain falls within the experience of our love.

Further, it is now clear to me that experiencing our anger around childhood and expressing our "blame," is ultimately a more loving act towards ourselves and towards our parents. Through our grief-the blame and anger and sadness we experience around our childhood issues-we are finally truly able to forgive our parents. Walker (1995) shares an intense experience of feeling anger towards his mother. He then says, "On the other side of one particularly intense role-play of catharting blame at my mother, I felt my heart open with more love for her than I had ever felt before. This feeling of love then expanded into compassion for her and finally culminated in an authentic feeling of forgiveness" (p. 157). Our stored up pain is released and the energy of the emotions has moved through us, and thus real acceptance and love can be available. Yet if we "forgive" before we feel our blame, we may carry our child's hurt and anger around forever (Walker, 1995, p. 148). Not until we fully experience our anger, do our resentments begin to fall away. Not until we fully express our blame, do we release it and open our hearts to truly seeing, accepting, and loving. And we naturally begin to hold our parents with compassion as we see their innocent wounded child selves. We then have the opportunity, if we choose, to create a less defensive more honest and meaningful relationship.

For me this happened naturally as I went through my grief. At one point in my process, my anger towards my father manifested. I felt too hurt and angry to continue in our relationship, and thus took a "break" from it. Through taking my space, feeling my feelings and creating temporary distance, my internal relationship with him was transformed, and thus our external relationship was shifted when we reconnected. My idealization of him had melted, finally allowing me to project less and see more clearly. My sensitivity and intensity of emotion around my father dissipated. My boundaries strengthened. I believe we both experience now a clearer easier connection. I love him deeply and also see and accept him in his humanness. As I went through the darkness, not around it, I authentically moved towards the light. One year ago, I could not speak to him. Now one of my very favorite weekly experiences is having Friday night dinners at my dad's house.

I have noticed a great shift in my relationship with my mother as well. The other morning I telephoned her. She began to share her usual "delusional" news. In the past I have listened, feigned response, and felt completely disconnected from her not knowing how to be "real" or relate because her reality is so different than mine. For the first time the other morning, I felt sincerely emotionally connected to her throughout our entire conversation, and it was effortless. She asked me if I had heard anything about her winning the Nobel Peace Prize or Pulitzer Prize. I told her I had not, but that she certainly deserved all of that. And I felt this; I see what she goes through, how hard she must work inside, and feel that she certainly deserves recognition. She told me about the beautiful new houses she owns, and how she would like to spend her time painting and growing roses. I told her what a wonderful plan that was; it felt beautiful to me. She told me about her lover who she is wishing to be with but cannot because he has a spell cast on him that makes him invisible. She shared that she is very thin ("103 pounds!") but she appears 200 pounds because her old teacher is "throwing bulk" on her. Listening to her, sensing her feelings behind her story, I told her how frustrating this all sounded. She told me that she is in charge of a courthouse and gave me a telephone number of the judge who would be there for me if I ever needed help. I felt her intention of protection, and told her what a wonderful mother she is. I felt this in my heart. She replied back to me, "And you are a wonderful daughter." I felt her feeling this, but more importantly I felt it myself. The entire feeling and ease of this conversation was a great shift. In the past I have heard her delusional words and thus instantly felt distant. I have had to "force" a feeling of connection. But this conversation felt clean and clear and easy. My unconscious guilt, shame, fear, judgment, hurt, discomfort, defenses (denial, dissociation), emptiness and yearning melted and transformed into a natural openness, acceptance, joy, energy, true authenticity. I saw clearly her Narcissistic wound, her child-like regression, her fantasy and wishes and I naturally and intuitively responded to that. What was incredible to me, is that her different sense of reality did not threaten my sense of connection to her, for I could hear what she was feeling and understand her and respond from that place. In my past I would have never imagined this. I am aware that this transformation occurred through my grief and anger. Thus when I see my clients begin to approach the anger phase of their childhood grief, I am aware that their feelings and blame are a part of the larger process of unfolding love.

I would not be able to enjoy these conversations with my mother so much without my grief work and experiencing my anger. I feel fortunate that I was able to do this. During my journey the universe set me up with the perfect "gift" one night to facilitate my own anger for the first time. I was triggered spontaneously. I write in my journal, "For the first time in my life, I DON'T WANT COMFORTING. I don't want to be held and soothed. I want to be alone in my anger. I walk outside and allow myself to scream. It is so fucking unfair. Why can't you be here. It is so, so unfair. Although this is a painful experience, it feels right. . . I cannot speak, but I want to release. From deep within the noises come. Noises of anguish. Noises of frustration . . . pain . . . sorrow . . . noises of deep, deep . . . anguish. I am O.K. in this, I feel strong enough and I feel safe. . ."

I was beginning to get in touch with the anguish-the pain and anger-of my experience of abandonment. When I was young, at the age of the actual experience, my little child self could not have tolerated this pain. I thus held it, stored it, waiting until a time when I became "big" enough to be able to sit with it, live through it and survive. Bradshaw (1990) speaks of this when he says, "The natural response to emotional abandonment is a deep-seated toxic shame that engenders both primal rage and a deep-seated sense of hurt. There is no way you could grieve this in infancy. You had no ally who could be there for you and validate your pain, no one to hold you while you cried your eyes out or raged at the injustice of it all. In order to survive, your primary ego defenses kicked in and your emotional energy was left frozen and unresolved." (p. 88). Years later when we are ready, we may then begin to work towards resolution.

And now I did have someone there to validate my pain, to hold me while I felt this grief. I had my intimate friends, and my incredibly supportive partner. But most importantly, I had myself. "We also discover that there is only one person that can assure that we get the nurturing we need, and that one person is us . . . . We are our own nurturer . . . . We may at times get others to help us get what we need, but basically we are the only one that can attend to our needs" (Whitfield, 1987, p. 130). My nurturing mother self was there for me and with me in an unconditional way that was profound. She was big and strong, validating, encouraging and full of love. She can love me and fulfill my needs like no other separate human being can. I/she journals to myself after the night my anger was triggered: "My incredibly strong girl. How painful it is that you didn't get to experience what almost all other women experience throughout their lifetime. The joy and love and support and strength-you missed out on. The little girl in you feels how unfair this is and is angry that her mother was taken away. Let her feel this and know it is okay, in fact appropriate, justified and necessary. You are so strong now that you are able to hold this deep hurt and know you are all right. You can be in it and not get lost. You can be in it because you are so strong. The fear is gone. And know that even your mother supports you in this anger and pain. She knows it doesn't mean you don't love her, she knows in fact it means you are more connected to her. I am so incredibly proud of you my beautiful strong girl. You are big and you are safe in yourself now. You are large enough to contain yourself. You did not have that strong container-a mother-to hold you when you were young, and for many years understandably you were unable to hold yourself. But you have grown solid and powerful, and I admire the incredible depth of your journey." My Higher self, or mother self, nurtured me through writings like this, as I tapped into a large well of self-compassion.

I believe the most beautiful aspect that occurs through our grief work is the awakening of true self-compassion. This seems to occur naturally as we awaken to our pain. Stephen Levine says, "We seldom let go of our judgment and make room in our heart for ourselves. How can we so lack compassion for this being we feel suffering in our heart? If we fully acknowledge our pain, it would be difficult not to be swept with a care and compassion for our own well-being" (cited in Walker, 1995, p .57). As we begin to contact our inner child, we can separate her painful wounds from other aspects of ourselves. In doing this, what was once the shame we have taken in from identifying with our young experiences and our external environment, transforms into a new perception of our innocent self. This holding of our child naturally elicits a loving self-compassion within us which then may replace self blame and criticism. Our relationship to our self shifts. We can learn to contact our nurturing parent inside, and begin to reparent ourselves by giving and receiving the complete acceptance that we couldn't possible get from another yet so much deserve. We begin to find True Love. We begin to truly heal.

"When we have compassion, pain dissolves into love" (Stephen Levine cited in Walker, 1995, p .57). I remember experiencing this self-love profoundly one day during a therapy visit. I write about it in my paper: "At the end of this session...I really see myself and feel myself. I feel so much love for myself that I begin to cry. I tenderly share how proud I am of myself, that I feel that I am an amazing person . . . I feel so much appreciation towards myself, as one would feel towards another person. I have always had so much love inside, and a lot of love to myself that I express (usually through poetry or writings from Higher Self), but somehow healing with my mother. . . has transformed it a little. Love exchange can go on inside me now - and is a part of me TK. I can give it to myself and receive it from myself. Before I just felt this love inside...saw it just as a beautiful yet stagnant emotion. Today it is a most touching sweet exchange."

Going through my grief and nurturing my child self allowed me to tap into and experience this intense self-love. The power of self-love and compassion is one of the greatest I can imagine. This self-compassion and self-love is what leads us towards our authentic, whole spiritual Selves. We gain acceptance and love for who we are, we thus become more fully Who We Are. We gain access to the Divine within us. As contacting and grieving our child self can awaken our connection with the Divine, some call this self the "eternal" child. Metzer says, "Out of the turmoil and darkness of dying come the sparkling vitality of the newborn self. This new self is connected to the eternal source of all life, that source from which we all derive, the divine essence within. It is therefore aptly named the 'eternal child'" (cited in Abrams, 1990, p. 16). In Psycho synthesis, the term "inner child" represents this transpersonal openness as well. Firman and Russell (1994) state, "If we were continuously aware of this connection. . . . we would be walking the path of Self-realization, living with ongoing communion with Self" (pp. 5-6). When we contact our inner child and gain self-compassion, it seems we open up more fully to the larger realms of Love and Spirit.

For Walker (1995), "Grieving has also moved me to notice the spiritual beauty of many other human beings" (p. 204). I would say the same is true for me. And thus when we hold love and compassion for ourselves inside, we are then able to hold it more fully for others. As is said throughout all of the inner child literature that I have encountered, the way we treat our outer child is a reflection of the way we treat our inner child. I believe it is true that the more loving we are towards ourselves, the more loving we naturally are towards others. We also become more clear. We are more conscious of our defenses, of when we are coming from our still somewhat wounded child, and when this contaminates our adult interactions. We are able to react less, to be more honest, to take responsibility and own our own feelings. We no longer blindly project or easily blame others. Inner child grief work creates the self-compassion that allows us to then love others on deeper levels than before. "In reclaiming and championing your wounded inner child, you give him the positive, unconditional acceptance that he craves. That will release him to recognize and love others for who they are" (Bradshaw, 1990, p. 40).With this connection and self compassion, we no longer feel like a victim, for we are healing ourselves inside. With self love, we are more loving and empowered. We are big. We are grown.

I felt this empowerment through the work of my own journey. Through my grief I discovered a sense of my own self, of my own "power." I write in my journal one day after therapy, "The feeling I have-standing there in front of another in my own power space-is that I am finally reclaiming my self . . . after a long, long time . . .before I leave the session Lane tells me he truly felt he was in the presence of a woman." In the past I had always judged and feared this, having learned what most of us learn in childhood-that being in myself completely, authentically, was not okay. Through my grief I realized I was always, unconsciously, "giving away" my power, having associated being "powerful" with being "unloving." Through my grief work I began to let go of that fear and judgment. In the last page of my personal process paper I write, "Lately, I have simply felt completely full in myself, big. Nothing is wrong or hurtful about this my dear. This is true beauty. Today Lane left me with Nelson Mandela's inaugural speech, a powerful assurance of this message:

"Our deepest fear is not that we are inadequate.
Our deepest fear is that we are powerful beyond measure.
It is our light, not our darkness, that most frightens us.
We ask ourselves, who am I to be brilliant, gorgeous, talented and fabulous?
Actually, who are you NOT to be? You are a child of God.
Your playing small doesn't serve the world.
There is nothing enlightened about shrinking
so that other people won't feel insecure around you.
We are born to make manifest the glory of God that is within us.
It's not just in some of us; it's in everyone.
As we let our own light shine, we unconsciously give other people permission to do the same.
As we are liberated from our own fear, our presence automatically liberates others."

When I remember this, that being in my self and my power is actually coming from a loving intention, which it always is, then I realize it is not only okay but 'good' and even necessary." This is how I grew through grief, becoming my own full self.

Although I have much grief from my childhood, and experienced abandonment from my ill mother, I have also been extremely fortunate as the expression of love emotionally was great in my family, both from my mother and especially my father. Even through her altered state my mom exudes a profound amount of loving energy. And my father, even during my difficult days in adolescence, came into my room at least once a day to tell me just how much he loved me. Love was the central most accepted and thus expressed emotion in my household growing up. Thus for me, feeling self-love has come rather easily. There are many situations for others though, as I have witnessed with my clients, that access to love is much more difficult as it is, sadly, unfamiliar. And as Marion Woodman says, "Children who are not loved in their very beingness do not know how to love themselves. As adults, they have to learn to nourish, to mother their own lost child" (cited in Bradshaw, 1990, p. 205). Thus in the field of psychology and inner child work there are many techniques and exercises that facilitate one to contact the inner child, experience our grief, and build "reparenting" skills to encourage self-love and compassion.

These skills are essential for our healing, as "The more disconnected your Adult and Inner Child are, the greater your pain" (Paul, 1992, p. 27). We can learn how to connect and nourish the relationship between these parts of ourselves. But first we must simply contact our child within, as she has probably been hidden for many years. We have built defenses to protect her. She has been hurt and may be frightened to come out. I agree with Firman and Russell (1994) that, contacting our inner child is a matter of mirroring, of empathic attunement. "It was a disruption in mirroring which caused the splitting off of the inner child, and it is only mirroring which can heal the break with our inner child" (p. 23). We need to be patient and gentle. We need to create or seek a safe environment.

One simple yet powerful way we can then gain more emotional awareness of our child is by sharing with others. "Telling our story is a powerful act in discovering and healing our child within" (Whitfield, 1987, p. 96). And as we share, within the context of a safe mirroring environment, we become a witness to our own story. We get to hear our own story, and the more we do so the more we begin to contact the character of this story, our inner child. We then begin to separate slightly from our identification with our wounded child self, and allowing some "distance," we can begin to conceptualize the hurt child inside of us. Doing this, "disidentifying" from this aspect of ourselves and labeling her, seems to create deeper feelings of safety and allow the pain (pained child) to emerge further.

One of the most powerful ways to awaken our child self and begin to nurture her is through meditation and visualization techniques. Most authors share their own version of guided meditations for the inner child. Bradshaw (1990) for example, has created various exercises for our different phases of development, including infancy, toddlerhood, preschool and school-age years. "You need to go back to those (threatening) scenes and let your championing adult give your wounded inner child some new words that are nurturing and soothing" (p. 217). He has a list of affirmations, scenes and specific meditations. Many others give the example of "playing our childhood movies" which can bring old memories into consciousness. Bry for example, explains that we are to watch the movie, unhappy or scary as it is, and feel whatever feelings it brings up, knowing they will pass (cited in Abrams, 1990, p. 255). Sinor (1993) instructs us to watch the movie and then recreate those scenes and recreate our emotional experiences (p. 159). Sheldon Kramer (1994), in his brilliant book "Transforming the inner and outer family," gives meditation exercises and imagery for contacting our inner child, as well as accessing our "intragenerational family" (inner parents, siblings, grandparents, etc.) in order to heal our internal images and those inner aspects of ourselves that have been in pain. Throughout his book he gives healing meditation techniques (as well as specific techniques for the therapist to use with clients). Others emphasize the power of simple imagery such as that of our adult selves holding our child, gently being with her, stroking her, showing acceptance, compassion and respect. Branden shows the power of this imagery when he quotes a client saying, "All of these years I've tried to be an adult by denying the child I once was. I was so ashamed and hurt and angry. But I truly felt like an adult for the first time when I took her into my arms and accepted her as a part of me" (cited in Abrams, p. 247).

These are a few ways of gaining contact with our child self. The most important step then in caring for this inner child is to recognize her presence and to develop an awareness of her feelings and needs. There are techniques to help facilitate this as well. We can work with our wounded child and develop her presence more fully through expressive arts and psychodrama. Ritual can be extremely powerful. We can use various forms of journaling as well. We can write about various childhood events, including milestones and traumas that we experienced during our developing years. We can continue to do this through various exercises such as "sentence completion," in which we finish various sentences such as "When I was five years old, One of the things I had to do as a child to survive was . . ., When my child self tries to talk to me . . ., When I recall how my body felt when I was very young . . . " (Paul, 1992, p. 245). Reflecting and allowing ourselves to complete these sentences, to sink into the experience, is one simple way for our child to present herself and for us to become more aware.

Another helpful way of contacting and nurturing our child is through internal dialogue. "The first dialogue with the vulnerable child may simply involve sitting quietly and encouraging it to come forth. It is often preverbal and may sit quietly or cry" (Stone & Winkelman cited in Abrams, 1990, p. 178). As we continue to work this way, our child's verbal feelings and words may begin to come through. We can dialogue silently inside, verbally aloud, or with a facilitator in therapy. One of the most popular modes of dialoguing with our child self is through writing. The most common writing technique used in dialogue is for our adult self to write with our familiar hand, and our child self to share by writing with our non-dominant hand. We can ask our child questions, such as "What are you feeling, How can I help, Am I shaming you, What do you need from me . . . " and give reassurances such as, "It's okay to cry, I'm here for you, You are not alone . . . " (Paul, 1992).

These dialogue techniques can be especially helpful in allowing our true hurt and uninhibited child self to speak up. It is extremely important to remember that our full and complete acceptance is essential in facilitating this. "And without a non-judgmental, empathic, mirroring atmosphere, our inner child simply will not emerge" (Firman & Russell, 1994, p. 24). And with it, our true child self feels she can begin to safely speak after these many years, encouraged through dialogue. We may wish to ask for our inner child's forgiveness for neglecting her for so many years. We listen to our child selves, respond from a loving place, dialogue, and take action to meet both our inner child and inner adult's needs. Through dialogue work, we can hear the child's voice and gradually begin to love our child self and take over the responsibility of "child-rearing," reparenting our selves in the unconditional way we so desire.

And thus we begin to take over child-rearing and take care of our inner child. Walker (1995) believes, "The most essential task of self-mothering is restoring the individual to a deeply felt sense that he is lovable and deserves to be loved. Self-mothering is the practice of actively and passively loving the inner child in all his mental, emotional, and energetic states" (p. 211). We give understanding, compassion, and guidance. We can write letters to our child selves, or have our child selves write a letter to us (again with the non-dominant hand) to express what she wants or needs. As discussed earlier, we can meditate with her, visualizing her vulnerable self and give her solid attention and love. We can facilitate this further through positive healing affirmations such as, "You are a gift to the world, You are exactly perfect the way you are, I am very proud of you" (Walker, 1995). To cultivate deep love we can also journal from our mother or Higher Self in a similar way that I shared in my own process earlier. We may also need to learn how to discipline her/him in a loving way. And we give her/him new permissions. It is important to create the time and space for her/him. Many authors emphasize the importance of "taking time" for our child, making inner parenting a priority. This means living with her/him, listening to her/him, attempting to meet her/him needs appropriately, even making agreements with her/him if necessary. And in return, as Barbara Sinor (1993) emphasizes in her book, we may receive many gifts from this contact with our inner child. And once we contact her/him, we now continue this relationship throughout our lifetime.

There will always be our child self inside of us. She/he may always remember the pain and hurt she/he has experienced. This may not change. What we may shift is the relationship we have to her/him, how we hold her/him-this is the healing that is in our power. I appreciate how Firman and Russell (1994) state, "'healing the inner child,' is misleading, while 'healing my relationship with the inner child' is more accurate" (p. 24). We are the responsible adults now, and it is a choice we make that allows us to shift from discounting, criticizing and shaming to the healing nurturing we may give. And being this loving adult means shifting the way we see ourselves-we begin to see ourselves through the eyes of gentle acceptance, as we would our own actual child. Thus it appears the most essential aspect of inner child work is learning to "reparent" our inner selves and to give the love that they so much yearn for. As discussed earlier, the process of grieving seems to naturally trigger the beginnings of this self love for our child. And as we continue to nurture her/him, she/he comes to trust us, knowing finally that we will not abandon her/him. Then, "to be our self requires no work or effort. There is nothing to do" (Bradshaw, 1990, p. 256). And by reparenting our inner child, we can release and heal the pain from the past. "This healing through reparenting is the way to bring freedom and joy into the present" (Paul, 1992, p. 81). It is a way to bring love.

"The power of inner bonding is the power of love as the force that heals, love from Inner Adult to Inner Child. Other's love can help support this process-love from mate to mate, from friend to friend, from therapist to client; but it is only when the Inner Adult loves the Inner Child that true healing and joy occur" (Paul, 1992, p. 6). This is what I attempt to help facilitate during my work with clients. I do strongly believe in the power of the therapist's love and acceptance. When a person is given mirroring, acceptance and love, he or she begins to heal her or his wounded self. We can be helped to gain self-love through internalizing the love of others, and self-acceptance through internalizing the acceptance of the therapist. And yet of course, another's love alone, and as a therapist my love alone, will not automatically bring about transformation. But, "If the defenses of the self are worked through and the individual receives the appropriate reflection, the Self will reconstellate. Proper reflection means that the divine child is being accepted by another and so eventually by oneself" (Satinover cited in Abrams, 1990, p. 155). Although, ultimately, it is the act of inner love from self to self that truly heals the wounded child within, also it may be in the therapy room that one first learns how to cultivate this act.

Throughout my two years of seeing clients, I have been a witness to this healing work. I have sat with clients, holding the space for them to get in touch with their childhood grief. I have guided them through inner child/adult self dialogues, allowing self-compassion to manifest. I have seen clients begin to disown the internalized projections from their parents, dissolving self-criticism and blame. I have felt shame begin to release as acceptance from myself and then their own self is honored. I have witnessed pain, tears, anger, laughter, self-love, and hard, hard work. I thank my clients for touching me and allowing me in to their deepest exploration. I thank them for the sharing that has aroused my interest and created my passion for the topic of grief and the wounded child. I will share here some glimpses into our experience in the therapy room.

Mark is a male in his mid-fifties, who came in for therapy as an adjunct to his spiritual work. During this session he began discussing the difficulties he has when attempting to communicate with his mother. We begin to talk about his relationship with her when he was younger. The session continues as follows:

Mark: I guess just little things (pause) I mean I don't know how important things are to talk about my childhood. There are things that I experienced that were really traumatic for me that involved her.

Therapist: It sounds like it's really important.

Mark: One thing was (pause) it was the first day of the first grade (begins to tear). And during the middle of the day I peed in my pants sitting at my desk because I was too shy to ask the teacher to go to the bathroom. So I was sitting there during recess. I did not get up and leave my desk I was so petrified at such a (pause) blowing it so hard. So after school I waited until everyone else left. Then I got up to leave. I was supposed to walk home with my sister who was in kindergarten. I was so miserable I didn't want to walk with my sister because I didn't want her to find out what I had done. So I ended up throwing rocks at her to keep her away from me (sad laugh) so she would walk farther away. I was like "leave me alone leave me alone I don't want to talk to you." She starts crying, gets upset. She goes in and tells my mother that I was throwing rocks at her. So I come home and my mother is just raging mad (crying).

Therapist: Mmm...

Mark: And just shrieking and yelling, just really freaked out and just really, I just remember her being incredibly angry even when I told her what had happened. She was so mad at me that I had done that in the first place.

Therapist: You were trying to protect yourself.

Mark: Yeah (crying). (pause) So I don't know that was a really heavy experience.

Therapist: I'm also really struck by the sense of shame that you felt and it wasn't okay that you went to the bathroom

Mark: No exactly, it was like just guilt, shame, just feeling like this is really (pause) not cool.

Therapist: What was the message that you were given?

Mark: That I was a bad person. That good people don't do those kind of things. So that's what I carried with me for a long time

Therapist: Yeah

Mark: I've never forgotten that. There's just a lot of real intense guilt and shame around all of that kind of stuff, anything that had to do with your body.

Therapist: Let me ask you how you see that first grader now?

Mark: Pretty sad. Not very happy. And definitely not able to understand how to make friends very well.

Therapist: And if you were to tell him something about that incident, about his going to the bathroom in his pants because he was shy. What would you tell him now?

Mark: (cry). Whew. (very emotional) (pause) (cry) I would have to tell him he is okay.

Therapist: (softly) Yeah. Yeah.

Mark: That that's no big deal (cry).

Therapist: (again softly) Yeah.

(towards end of session)

Therapist: It feels like you're beginning to find compassion for that boy

Mark: Yeah, I'd like to. I'd like to find that. I'd like to let that boy know that it is all right (cry). He's not a bad kid.

Therapist: It is painful when you hear other things.

Mark: Yeah. Just this little bit today, I can tell I can be more aware of my feelings and how I was feeling then. It is so painful to go there but I know that's the direction to go in.

Mark has begun to get in touch with his sadness around his child's experience to cry for him. He can also then begin to hold him and heal. I look forward to our continuing work.

Another client of mine, a 23 year old female, has been getting in touch with much of her shock and anger as her denial is beginning to disappear. She comes from a physically and emotionally abusive father and an alcoholic and neglectful mother, who divorced when she was young. During this session she is feeling the upset of the reality of her past. She is feeling her anger and now wishing for the first time she could tell her parents and get validation from them. I attempt to give it to her in the session. The session continues as follows:

Sarah: I have been thinking about it a lot. I mean am I ever going to get my chance to say what I want to say. What is it, "You hurt me," is all I really need to say. And then you blamed me for doing the things that I did to survive that, which was like sex or food or whatever. I hated my dad because he was so scary, but my mom, she was just drunk all the time, all the time. By the time I was in high school it didn't bother me anymore. But no one intervened, I can't believe my dad didn't do anything about it. And if they only knew what I did, snuck out all the time, shoplifted.

Therapist: So let's just stay with that, what you just said. You as a child were left with a mother who was drunk and negligent of you, and no one intervened.

Sarah: Right. Why didn't they? I was just so unsupported. It was like no one cared.

Therapist: Can you feel that?

Sarah: Yeah, it makes me really angry

Therapist: Yeah.

Sarah: Everything I did in high school, I was valedictorian, I started all these clubs, all on my own, I had no help from them. They never once helped me with my homework. I never felt like they helped me. It astounds me now.

Therapist: And I hear it makes you really angry.

Sarah: It does. I'm angry because I was not acknowledged. The world from my eyes was just written out of the family consciousness.

Therapist: So you really did not have anyone understanding from your perspective.

Sarah: And I guess one of my goals now is to be able to just tell them. But I can't count on them.

Therapist: I know that would feel and be really healing for you; to be able to share with them and have them respond to you and I also know that it might be too difficult for them to be able to hear. I imagine what you're wanting is validation from them, it could be painful for you then. I do strongly believe that it is possible to work through that hurt and anger without having to do that.

Sarah: Okay.

Therapist: And I'm not saying "Don't do that." I imagine, you are 23 years old, I imagine there may be a time when you can talk with them.

Sarah: So where do you think we should go from here?

Therapist: It can be helpful to get in touch with that hurt and that younger hurt can be seen by you and I.

Sarah: (large sigh). (pause).

Therapist: And we can validate the anger. There is anger around not being seen and heard and being neglected. That is very understandable. If 8 year old Sarah was here, getting in touch with feeling how she felt, what would you say to her?

Sarah: (sigh) God (crying)

Therapist: What can you imagine 8 year old Sarah wanted to hear?

Sarah: (sobbing) I can't believe you have to be here (long pause). There are other places in the world. There are other places for you, I promise. (long pause) (crying).

Therapist: How do you feel about yourself right now?

Sarah: I feel pretty strong.

Therapist: I want to tell you what I see over here. I see you are very strong and you are getting in touch with your pain, and also beginning to get in touch with a nurturing part of yourself.

Sarah: (crying).

Sarah is continuing to work with her anger, as well as her hurt, and is realizing that her harsh inner critic is a false voice that she internalized from her father. Rather than continuing to accept it as "truth," she is now attempting to grieve through her painful experiences and is beginning to feel that she is more than she has believed. Currently she feels as if she is going through a transformation, and I have seen a tremendous shift in her feelings of self-worth. I admire her incredible courage.

Another client of mine, a 22 year old female, Becky, has been attempting to penetrate through her feelings of shame and self-hate. She continues to slowly share more with me, including an eating disorder she struggles with. I have seen a shift in her communication with me, although it can still be somewhat difficult for her. Because she has difficulty sharing verbally she has brought in many journal entries and poems for me to read. She believes her self-hate comes from incidents when she was younger with other kids in school. She feels deeply wounded by other children teasing her. Most of her writings are focused around this pain. The beginning lines from one poem she shared expresses her experience well:

"I took in your words as my own. Your voices tell me I am...worthless...undeserving... unlovable...unworthy...bad...I tried to understand why you would say such things. Then 13 year old me understood...I deserved that cruel treatment because I am me."

I feel honored that Becky has felt safe enough to let me in. I have seen a lot shift in her, and yet she is still unable to make much room for any other feeling towards herself besides self-critical blame and shame. As she says she is unable to imagine any positive feelings towards herself, including her child self, I decided one session to "bring in a third party" to begin with. (Some authors suggest the metaphor of 'adopting a child' to start with). I took her through a visualization in which she left therapy that day and was walking home through a park. There she came upon a group of children and witnessed them teasing a little girl. How does she see this little girl. What would she do. With this exercise, Becky was able to get in touch with care and concern and empathy for this imagined girl. Seeing this little girl as "other" and not a part of her self, she was able to have the distance that elicited compassionate feelings for her. Although she is not projecting this towards herself, I believe it is a small helpful step. Becky came in the following session and handed me a writing. I read it out loud to her so she could really hear it. This writing had a tone unlike any other I had heard from her before:

"If I were at a park and saw other kids picking on her, what would I want to say to her?

I would kneel in front of her and sit on my heels. I would gently hold her close, stroking her hair and back. I would talk to her calmly as she cries. "It's okay. You are all right. They told you lies. Those kids said those cruel things to make themselves feel better about themselves, and to feel powerful. They actually could be hurting inside, too, and this is all they know to do in order to deal with their own pain. I'm sorry they felt they needed to take their insecurities and pain out on you. You are not bad. You've done no wrong" . . . "You don't deserve to be hurt. What they tell you hurts a lot, though. It's okay to do well. You don't deserve the pain and hate they give you. Send it back to them in your heart. Don't take it in. You don't deserve to hurt."

Becky says she still believes she deserves to hurt. Although she works hard and has accomplished a lot since she began, she still believes her core is ultimately and undoubtedly "bad." But when I read this writing I was amazed, just to hear her write these nurturing words. Although when I read them to her she said she was unable to really feel that message towards her self, I believe the act of writing it was helpful. Somewhere, unconsciously, it may have a slight chance to sink in. As she herself once said, "It has to be when I'm not looking, and then it (positive self-expression) can slip in." I feel so proud of her for her effort and work. I hope one day she can know her beauty, and see in herself all that I see as I sit across from her. I hope she can allow the above writing to be directed towards herself.

The last client that I will share, Tina, a 30 year old lesbian female, seems to effortlessly take in her experiences in therapy and then continues to apply her learning to her life. After some visualizations, she easily contacted both her inner child and soothing mother self (her own mother was an alcoholic and Tina left home at age 16), and she actively now utilizes this process. She has begun to build a relationship between her pained child self and her knowing adult. During one session she shares with me that when feeling nervous and fearful during a situation recently, she was able to help herself through it using self-talk. She goes on to share this experience:

Tina: I said to myself, "It's okay. Stay calm, stay in your body, it is not a big deal." I just brought it down, "Okay, bring it (her energetic boundary) in."

Therapist: What I'm hearing from that is that you have, looking at parts of self, your mother was there.

Tina: Yes. The mother part that we have talked about has really helped. I just say now, "Okay Mother Tina, come out and take care of me right now." It has also helped me at times when I have felt abandoned. I use it sometimes when I need to be strong and I use it at other times when I feel, "Oh I'm sad right now, I'm feeling abandoned."
When I feel that unhealthy part of me begin to come out, I try to get in touch with the Mother Self, just talking myself down from things that can seem really scary.

Therapist: Mmm. When there is the younger part of you feeling abandoned, what happens during those times?

Tina: I do a lot of putting it into perspective. "Okay, right now you are feeling kind of sad and you are parting with somebody but there are going to be these new exciting things you are going to do with your day instead." It's always about putting it in reality because for me sometimes I can get so crazy making in my head that I go to this land that doesn't make any sense and I'm like "oh my God" so a lot of times it is just self talk around that.

Therapist: Yeah. The part that is so able to go into those places is that younger wounded part and it sounds like you are having a pretty good relationship between the two right now, where you can use your adult mother self for reality checks.

Tina: Yeah.

She is able now for the first time to soothe and ground herself. The session prior to this one further illustrates some of this process:

Tina: (has been discussing a party she went to) It was so much fun. It was the first time I felt comfortable with my girlfriend's friends too. I wasn't jealous of them or feel threatened by them and my girlfriend's relationship.

Therapist: What was it that allowed you to be experiencing in the moment the joy rather than having some difficult feelings?

Tina: I noticed some difficult feelings coming in at times and I would just sit with them and talk with myself about them. It was interesting, I really would just feel them and be like, "Okay, let's just reframe how you are looking at this right now," and just start telling myself, "okay Kelli (her girlfriend) is still here, everything is fine, she's not flirting with anybody like all your past girlfriends, we're just having fun and these are great people." And I (the other part of her) was like, "Oh this is great!" Then I would just be in a moment of having fun again.

Therapist: You were doing an internal reality check with your wise parental part of you.

Tina: Right.

Therapist: That's great.

Tina: It was really fun.

Therapist: And that's new.

Tina: Very new. Instead of just being like "I want to go home" and being a cranky person and feeling scary feelings of like my mom talking to boys at parties and men at parties and feeling like she's going to run off with some guy and never...ya know, that fear of abandonment that sometimes comes up at social situations.

Therapist: Right.

Tina: And just really nurturing myself and not going into that, "Well I'm going to leave." That was fun.

Therapist: So that more observing part that is able to help you out at times, that's newer.

Tina: That part of the voice is definitely new. Because before I would just have reacted in whatever my initial reaction was, didn't have that tool to talk myself down.

Therapist: And how did you begin to manifest that tool? (at this point I am a little surprised and truly wondering how she gained that tool...it manifested so easily and quickly).

Tina: I think some of our visualizations around Mother Me and a lot of the stuff we've done around bringing myself back in here (inside), instead of coming out here (outside). What did we call it, merging. Not merging with other people or other things. And I notice that when I'm feeling kind of "ah!," it is always about out here, and when I bring myself back in, "Okay, you've got your arms, your legs..." literally like, "breath, bring it back in." Then I feel like, "okay!" It really is about that. I think some of the work we've done around that has given me a tool.

Therapist: And it sounds like although you didn't use that tool before it sounds like you have somewhat easy access to that helpful part of yourself.

Tina: Yeah. Easier than ever. Before I knew kind of what to do but I don't know why I didn't use it as much. I surprise myself (short laugh).

Therapist: What I see is that's the part of you that is loving yourself.

Tina: Yeah. Yeah, it's cool. I love it! (laugh). It's kind of overwhelming. It's like me, love myself, it's kind of new.

Therapist: Yeah.

Tina: Because I've never done that ya know (eyes begin to tear).

Therapist: Yeah (eyes begin to tear).

Tina: Yea, yea for me (cheering). (pause) (tears, laughter).

Thus we can see with these four clinical examples, that I have witnessed a variety of phases of the grief process and client's relationships to the inner child. The experiences in these examples seem to fall into the emotional phases described by Bradshaw (1990), which include validation, shock and depression, anger, hurt and sadness, remorse, toxic shame and loneliness (pp. 77-79). I believe that the process of grieving our inner child is very similar, if not identical, to the process of grieving any other major loss that we experience in life. There are many feelings that occur with our child's grief, similar to the grief that Judy Tatelbaum

(1980) in "The courage to grieve" describes from mourning death. In this book she says, "Feelings of grief are very intense and often very mixed. We may feel emotions in an entirely new or different way. Among the many feelings aroused by loss are sorrow, anguish, disbelief, despair, anxiety, loneliness, guilt, regret, resentment, emptiness, and numbness, as well as yearning, love, and appreciation for the deceased" (p. 23). Here, the "deceased" may be the lost inner child self and it may be the "absent" parent as well. I experienced almost all of those feelings listed, in relation to my grief work around the mother-daughter relationship. Also similar to traditional grief, the recovery of our feelings is a process, and the phases of grief may appear as a spiral rather than linear experience. The unresolved grief work is a re-experiencing process, which then frees our childhood pain and helps to integrate our lost inner child. It may be ongoing or come back again after a long period of rest, as we continue to do the work of integration. Even after deep grieving, my own grief still comes up at times, elicited by a dream or touching circumstance. But I am not overwhelmed now, and to feel my feelings is a conscious choice I can make. I can clearly feel and see the effects of the hard work I have already done. My heart feels deeply but it is also bigger and stronger from my experience.

As Walker (1995) says, "In my experience, the broken heart that has been healed through grieving is stronger and more loving than the one that has never been injured. Every heartbreak of my life, including the broken heartedness of my childhood, has left me a stronger, wiser, and more loving person than the one I was before I grieved" (p. 70). I believe this is true and I can feel this truth myself. Thus this is the work I see as powerfully healing, leading us towards love and authenticity. I can feel the gift of the pain I have suffered from my own past, as it has helped to fill my heart and create the fullness of who I am. Also, I am who I am, and the therapist I am, because of my past. And as John Bradshaw (1990) shares, "I can now see that my whole life is perfect . . . {my childhood experiences} were exactly what I needed to experience in order to do the work I am now doing" (p. 262).

I appreciate Leon Bloy's words, "There are places in the heart which do not yet exist; pain must be in order that they be" (cited in Bradshaw, 1990, p. 272). Through experiencing this pain and healing I can hold the depth of other's experiences, help their fears dissolve and allow their grief, as I sit with my solid presence unafraid of the dark. "In therapy, for clients to . . . accept the experience of the child usually depends upon therapists who have done these things in their own lives. Therapists who have wrestled with their own survival personality and faced their own wounding seem best equipped to mirror the wounding of another" (Firman & Russell, 1994, p. 33). And what an incredible gift to be witness to others growing through grief and becoming their wiser more loving authentic selves. I feel incredible gratitude for my grief work as now my life path leads me to continue to accompany others on their own amazing journey of healing.

I see this as a journey not only on the personal realm but the Transpersonal as well. While at times this grief work hurt tremendously, my adult self was present, knowing of the healing of this pain. My Higher Self was present, aware of the beauty in it. In working with clients I thus hold the pain of the personal in the larger framework of the workings of the Universe and Spirit. As some clients have not tapped into their awareness of the Transpersonal, I continue to hold it in the room for them. For myself, I was always aware more of the "light" and larger beauty of Life, and thus I had to do the opposite-to bring my awareness to the more personal "darkness." I write to myself in the very beginning of my grief work, "You have accepted your life without question, knowing only of the larger beauty. And yes, you are right, all of this life is a gift. But some gifts are painful, tragic, frightful. To live in the truth is to embrace it all. To know the higher love yet feel the shadow that comes along with being human . . . " In whichever case, as Jack Kornfield says, "This is perhaps the most difficult of the balancing acts we come to learn; to trust the pain as well as the light, to allow the grief to penetrate as it will while keeping open to the perfection of the universe" (cited in Walker, 1995, p. 203). This is the balance I hold as a therapist. And for myself, this balance I now know intimately.

Above is adapted from http://www.creativegrowth.com/teresa.htm

****

Personal Notes

Chapter 3

Shadow Self, Soul Fragments and Hidden Aspects

Below is adapted from http://kundalini-teacher.com/guidance/shadow.php

The Shadow Self - Essentially The Same As Soul Fragments, Aspects And Sub-Personalities

"I must not fear.

Fear is the mind-killer.

Fear is the little-death that brings total obliteration.

I will face my fear.

I will permit it to pass over me and through me.

And when it has gone past I will turn the inner eye to see its path.

Where the fear has gone there will be nothing.

Only I will remain."

The Litany against Fear, from "Dune" by Frank Herbert.

Good does not become better by being exaggerated, but worse, and a small evil becomes a big one through being disregarded and repressed. The shadow is very much a part of human nature, and it is only at night that no shadows exist.

Carl Jung.

"Who knows what evil lurks in the heart of man...? The Shadow Knows"

The Shadow. (Radio drama.)

Carl Jung defined the Shadow Self as, "that which we think we are not." In the process of becoming All that Is, that which we think we are not must be embraced as an aspect of the Greater Self, and integrated. You may believe that you are not like your neighbor who does this or that bad thing, however, if those negative qualities you judge, were not also a part of you, then they would not trigger your emotions. Aspects of yourself that are 'Light' are also 'shadow' if they have not been recognized, embraced and integrated .

You may believe that you are a spiritual person who is not cruel or unjust. That belief is a blockage that casts a shadow that can blind you to the cruelty within your ego that is hidden. The shadow shows the "Ugly Mirror of All that Is": you are what you judge yourself not to be. You are what you judge others to be.

Sometimes people resist the Shadow's reflection so much that it takes them over, like Pro-Lifers who bomb abortion clinics. So invested in their accusations of murder that they feel justified in becoming murderers themselves. You may have met some abusive 'passive-aggressive' people , who insist that they are gentle nonviolent beings simply because their aggression is hidden under an ego of "good intentions".

We all have a shadow, and that shadow is a force that is both creative and destructive. We all have an inner demon who can be the violent eruption of repressed anger that makes a crime of passion, or can be the companion to a passionate life that makes skydiving fun because it is scary.

If the 'Divine Beloved' is the representative of God-dess Light within, the Shadow is the reflection of the dark wall of Karma that separates you from knowing yourself as Light. It is a reflection, a dark mirror of Karma. It can perhaps best be understood, in Shamanic terms, as the 'Portal Guardian' or 'Gate Keeper'.

The Portal Guardian is a creature of non-dual light, unconditional love manifest. It has no duality of its own, no emotions... it is pure light. However, in order to descend into duality-space where humans live, it must have shadow, and since it has no shades of gray within itself, it often first appears as a negative polarized image of darkest shadow. However, it truly has no darkness of its own, it's is simply a reflection of your own fears, your Karma. It reflects your dark side.

It is the Shadow that teaches what is hidden on the dark side of the moon.

The Shadow is the voice of your conscience, reminding you of what is unforgiven. It may show up, when you are making judgments of someone else, to remind you of how you are the same as what you judge. When you make judgments of another, you are projecting your own Shadows onto them. You are seeing a reflection of your own inner judgments, not the Divine Perfection within them.

The Portal guardian is the boundary between your conscious and unconscious mind. It is the protector who keeps you from being overwhelmed by all of your memories at once, by all of the archetypes and minds of the collective consciousness,

...and it is the Gatekeeper who decides what memories are allowed to surface into your consciousness. Some people, like myself, have to learn to love the Gatekeeper unconditionally before we find access to the Divine Beloved.

You know the old expressions, "the Devil made me do it"... this expression is a cop-out line for people who are unwilling to take responsibility for their actions, unwilling to admit to the hidden, inner fears and desires that motivate their actions.

There are some people who have physical brain damage or a chemical imbalance in the brain.

There is no big bad guy prince of evil. There is no supreme lord of all darkness. Nothing like that.

Why would Unconditional love make a being whose only purpose is to make your life miserable? That makes no sense... There is no Satan.

Ask the heart voice if Satan is a real creation of God or an invention of the minds of men.

It ALWAYS denies the reality of the devil. Heart chakra says there is no being of evil sent to harm, there is only humans making up reasons for not trusting in the Unconditional love of Creator. By fear, we maintain the illusion of separateness from Creator.

Don't take my word for it, get grounded and ask your own heart: Is the Devil real?

What there is, is an inner aspect of your own Divinity, whose job it is to reflect your fears and doubts back at you so you may forgive them. People make their own demons when they refuse to see love in the nagging voices of conscience and worry. The voice of the inner critic who shows you the fearful beliefs that are the content of your Karma.

There are only humans, being human, acting from fear instead of love... making their own demons. Free Will is Goddess' Law, so She allows it... She knows we are truly infinite, aspects of Her Self, expressing and sharing love in a game of limitless manifestation.

Demon (from Latin daemon "spirit; " from Greek daimon "deity, divine power; lesser god; guiding spirit, tutelary deity"). As far as I know, there was no negative connotation to the word until:

> Used (with daimonion) in Christian Greek translations and Vulgate for "god of the heathen" and "unclean spirit." Jewish authors earlier had employed the Greek word in this sense, using it to render shedim "lords, idols" in the Septuagint, and Matt. viii: 31 has daimones, translated as deofol in Old English, feend or deuil in Middle English. Another Old English word for this was hellcniht, literally "hell-knight."

The Divine Beloved is Love.

The Shadow is Love, too - it is unconditional love, tough love that spanks. It is an aspect of your Self that has taken on the thankless task of being a reflection of your fears so you can grow. It is manifest so that you can have the opportunity to face your fears, surrender them to Divine Will, and get past them. It will show you any selfish expectations hidden under your generosity, and the manipulation behind your martyrdom. It will keep you humble.

It is said, that there is an angel with a flaming sword that guards Eden, and only those who are without fear, can pass under it. Eden is Nirvana. Ascension. Heaven on Earth. To get there, you must integrate your shadow. Fear of the Devil, or not being able to love your own shadow, is a no-go. Getting past the sword is a process of learning to love your own ugliness, unconditionally, and finding a positive outlet for it. What is repressed, comes up ugly... so the shadow side reflects all the ugliness that is repressed. The parts of yourself you are ashamed of, and deny. You must learn to love them, in order to surrender them to Divine Will.

In the dark unknown of the unconscious, "here be dragons". It is the Portal guardian who protects from those dragons. It is the boundary that protects, and makes sure the dragons come to visit one at a time, at a pace where you can make friends with them. It is the gatekeeper, and the being that keeps you from approaching the void, before you are ready. The shadow is terrifying, in proportion to your uncleared Karma. The shadow is fear of death. The closer you get to the light, the less death seems like a scary idea.

That too, might seem like a scary idea. However, consider the phenomena of NDE: Near Death experiences. People who have died and returned to life usually have the experience of going through a tunnel to come into the light of "heaven". From this it can be understood that it is through death that we become re-unified with the Divine.

I'm not suggesting anyone kill themselves to seek unity, that is NOT the meaning. However, it is fairly common for people who are going through the process of Kundalini to go through a phase where it seems like death has come courting.

They have dreams of their own death, which may be quite frightening if they are not understood as metaphor. This is not a premonition of physical death. It is rather, a premonition of the death of the ego. The body is not in any danger. These dreams come at a time when the Veil of Forgetfulness is about to be torn away; when the ego is preparing to ascend into the light, so that the Higher self can fully occupy the body, to be Spirit having a Human experience. Ego death is not about death of the body. It is about living fully, in the Light of Spirit.

Above is adapted from http://kundalini-teacher.com/guidance/shadow.php

Below is adapted from one or more websites in 2010 I can no longer find.

Shadow Selves, Soul Fragments,

Astral Self, Inner Child and Aspects

The Soul is made up of a variety of different energies and levels of consciousness – each part being able to split off or be fractured into its many separate components... each part being able to have its own separate and independent experiences. For each separate incarnation that you ever had in any dimension - whether good or bad, light or dark - there can possibly be any number of 'split offs' or parts of your Soul being individually expressed somewhere out there in the vast universe - running around as a 'sub-personality', 'sub-self' or 'Aspect'. All of these 'aspects' usually have a unique energy pattern, consciousness, ego identity and memory of all that transpired in that one life and of anything else it did since then. And when these parts return there is an integration period where all that this part separately experienced, either 'good' or 'bad', is brought into the human being and processed. In the meantime, if any of these parts remain separated from the whole, you are diminished in either strength or ability. If most of your being remains scattered out in the universe and un-integrated, you can imagine what little of your whole soul you can access and work with in the here and now. 'Soul Retrieval' work helps rectify this.

Among the many dimensions that the individualized soul travels to being a human, it may start out its journey at the highest 'heavenly' level where it was first created, perhaps as an angelic spirit. One can remain at that level for all eternity, or one can descend into the lower dimensions, each time taking on a denser body. You never quite loose the previous bodies. These bodies become the core bodies of the subsequent ones, like rings on a tree. At different points along the way, you might choose to remain on a particular dimension for a long or short time. Some souls may choose to never leave a certain realm. Each time you journey through these dimensions, living in them for any length of time, you invariably end up taking on the energies of that dimension. You will always have these energies as a part of your makeup.

You could have been either Light and LOVING or Dark in any of your incarnations.

> The ones that were Light and LOVING just need to be invited back (You do need to *feel* worthy).
>
> The ones that were Dark need to be healed, transmuted and LOVED. You need to have made peace with them. Then integrate and process them.

In many of these dimensions you journeyed through, you could have taken on bodies with the slightest of human resemblance...

> Perhaps ones that were so extremely alien in nature. (such as the insectoids, reptilians, or grays)
>
> There are dimensions where 'mythological' beings exist. (such as the fairies, elves, goblins, hobbits, unicorns and dragons)
>
> There are dimensions where extremely dark and heavy beings exist. (such as the demons, devils and other assorted monsters)
>
> There are dimensions where our animal totems reside. (such as the dolphins, lions, eagles, and so on)
>
> There are even dimensions where nothing whatsoever resembles a body (such as the geometric or crystalline beings)
>
> Sometimes overlooked is this dimension where there are humans and other life forms we are familiar with. As a human, the aspect/soul fragment could have been from earlier in this life or from a previous life.

The permutations are virtually endless and vary depending on where your soul has been and what it has done.

There are any number of people who have the ability to see into these other dimensions and can confirm what I am saying, maybe even telling you what bodies you have. This knowledge is not necessarily going to do anything for your spiritual growth and healing - it would just be a curiosity, nothing more.

The Shadow Selves

Since these 'aspects' were taken on or created by you and are karmically tied in to your soul, they interact with, and at times conflict with, the other aspects that are 'you'. For example, we are all familiar with the comment "having an angel on one shoulder and a demon on the other". Naturally, it does not take a rocket scientist to figure out that an intense internal conflict would, and does, ensue. This is just one example.

Perhaps you may have heard someone use the expression "one's inner demon". Many people have these inner demonic aspects and are terribly affected by them without being consciously aware of it. Many also think that it is an outer demon who torments, tempts, or possesses people. However, I have found that it is usually one's own personal demonic sub-self/aspect that is the culprit. Yes, on some plane of existence, there are those big nasty demons. They do exist as either individual aspects floating around and/or as a collectively created archetype.

All these aspects/sub-selves that are a part of you also resonate with all those dimensions you at one time traveled through and perhaps at one time called home. Having a resonance with those dimensions also includes a resonance with the beings that currently inhabit them. The implication is this: If these other dimensions are dark, and the beings there are dark/malevolent/demonic, and you have a dark/malevolent/demonic aspect, this would be a disturbing influence in your life. This would certainly affect your Subconscious, dreams, desires, will and energy fields.

However, if you have made peace with your inner demons - meaning, that you have healed, transmuted, LOVED, integrated and processed them - those outer demons would have no power over you, nor have any influence into you, since the energies and consciousness that held the connection are healed and transmuted.

What can, and does, occur with any of your aspects, no matter if they are 'good' or 'bad', 'light' or 'dark', is that they eventually bleed through into your current incarnational experience. These aspects may manifest as any sort of personality changes, from the most subtle alterations in mood, to the most extreme, even paranoid schizophrenic behaviors at any time. Since these multidimensional aspects, individually and collectively, make up who you are as a soul, no matter how hard you try you will not eliminate their influences without LOVE. Even the taking of the most powerful anti-psychotic drugs or mood enhancers is ineffective in dealing with the underlying energies.

Because you and all your aspects are karmically bound to each other, you can never really escape from those aspects of yourself that you do not like. You can heal these aspects to a higher level of energy/vibration. These aspects could then be reintegrated/remerged into the heart of the Creator, which in this case would be into your heart.

I believe the use of mood enhancers, drugs and alcohol is so wide spread because many people do not know how to address the deeper issues and 'aspects that need to be healed. Also, some people are unwilling to look within themselves.

Astral Self

Below our Higher Etheric Self/Spirit Body, at the levels of the astral planes, there are multiple astral bodies, astral selves/sub-personalities that make up our psyche. The 'Astral Self' was created as an extension or projection of the Higher Self as a way to experience itself in another density. There is nothing wrong with having such an astral self and its attached personality. We need them in order to interact with the world as we perceive it. However, there are aspects of these astral selves/personalities that are also partly constructed from the ego-mind. When the ego-mind elaborates or expands on these astral selves/personalities, when it grows unfettered and disconnected from the whole, then we get in trouble. Then certain aspects of the personality generated by the ego-mind need to be tweaked or 'pruned', just like a neglected tree or an overgrown garden. When our 'soul garden' is trimmed, then we can distinguish the individualized 'selves'. In other words, when all these weeds, undergrowth, or 'stuff' is cleared out of our spiritual energetic space, then we can discover our own Soul amidst the confusion that is our life.

These Astral Selves, or sub-personalities, have their own separate ego, mind and will and they are often at odds one against the other, keeping you in conflict, inner turmoil and separation.

We need to unify all these conflicting wills towards a single goal, eventually integrating all separate selves into one being. This is the greatest struggle we will ever face on our spiritual path. One who has aligned and integrated all these 'wills' into one is considered a Great Master. Until that day comes it will be these various aspects, sub-personalities or consciousnesses that are isolated, separated and in conflict with each other and from the totality of God that need this healing work.

Inner Child

When the 'inner child' is on its own, disconnected from the Higher Self, it could be likened to a wild child whose limited material perspective or view on all things and beings revolves around his constant, immediate, and selfish wants, wishes, needs and desires. This inner child is guided by sporadic impulses and feelings, not having any sense of consequences or higher purposes.

Your 'Higher Self', wishes only good for this 'Child'. However, the 'Higher Self' is nearly powerless to help if the child will not or cannot listen to the promptings of spirit , that 'still small voice within'. Your High Self tries to guide you down a sure and safe path. However, if the child is so enraptured with the drama of this world, following their own passions and worldly agendas, they will not be able to hear the important messages coming to them. The enlightened Higher Self says things like: "Don 't do 'that' because it will hurt you...try this instead." And the child may say: "I want 'that' no matter what ... I don't care if it's bad for me or not! I don't want to do what you say... I want to go my own way." Through repetition of this sort of behavior, the child self energetically blocks out the Higher Self's messages and just hears what it wants to hear - itself. Over time, the lower self digs a hole deeper and deeper into trouble, turmoil and suffering, creating more and more negative karma.

At some point, even if the lower self changes its mind and wants to hear what spirit is saying and receive its help, it may not be possible without help from an intermediary. The energetic blocks may be so strong , this vast space of 'disconnect' may be so deep, that neither high or low self can get through to the other. This kind of relationship with Spirit is just like when you make a phone call - if there is a lot of interference in the line you may not be able to hear each other very well. Unfortunately, re-bridging most of these connections is not something either you or your High Self can do alone.

It is at these times, when the child cries out in such pain and anguish, having reached bottom, that it is now willing to be humble and follow the direction of Spirit. Having heard your heart felt desire and plea, your Spirit Guides and Angels can now direct you to another being who can act as an agent or intermediary for your High Self. This Being, a powerful ally, may help remove these blocks and interference patterns between and within you, so that you may once again reconnect with your own Inner Higher Self.

Timing

Timing is extremely important in our unfolding. If we remain in our resistances, behind our walls for too long, we will miss out on many good opportunities that were just waiting around the corner. Of course, our lower self always has a choice to follow through with the path our High Self presents, or reject it and go in a different direction. If we reject the higher path, the greater destiny we planned for when we were in Spirit/Bardo may not occur. There are windows of opportunity that are only open at certain times. If we are not awakened to, and in sync with, our destiny, these opportunities may be lost to us. Also, if we are not open to the subtle warnings our spirit gives us, we may miss the 'signs' and find ourselves in the wrong place at the wrong time. Examples are; making a left turn instead of right, being in an auto accident, being shot at... the list goes on and on.

Self-Discovery Practices

There are many ways to practice self discovery and integration.

They include: Hypnosis, Soul Retrieval, Shamanic Healing, Inner Child Healing, Meditation and Contemplation.

Whatever method(s) you choose, make sure whoever you choose to assist you is in integrity and connected to, and accessing, LOVE. They also need to know what they are doing.

Faces behind the Face

'Aspects' can be seen as 'faces behind the face'. If one looks just right, the superimposed impression or shadow of a face may be seen. It may not always appear human nor be light. Some people can see this quite easily, others not at all. As an experiment, sit opposite a willing partner and glance gently and diffusely onto the others face and eyes. There is some Subconscious control in what, if any, faces another will allow you to see. If there is trust, openness, and a non-judgmental attitude, the soul faces you are looking for may reveal themselves. This can even be done by yourself by looking in a mirror under a soft light.

Ouija Board, Drugs and Alcohol

I know that many people who have used such things have had some negative experiences. I do not advocate the use of the Ouija Board, drugs, or alcohol. I think these are all distractions away from directly doing the healing work, and I truly understand the caution and danger in these things. However, I just want to make a comment on this whole phenomenon in light of the information on 'Aspects' I have provided.

As long as a person has parts of themselves that remain un-integrated, un-transmuted, or un-LOVED, they run the risk that lower and darker 'Aspects' of themselves may come through at any time, especially when they use the Ouija Board, certain drugs and alcohol. These have a tendency to open your being up to unresolved 'aspects', 'issues' and 'things' that are in the periphery of your consciousness and energy field.

Some people do have a chemical imbalance in the brain or have been angry for so long it has become a habit. These people should usually keep taking any medication they are on until the chemical imbalance is resolved or until the brain has been retrained.

If you have thoroughly healed all aspects of your being, thus greatly strengthening your aura, you have nothing to worry about from the spirit world.

After a certain point on your healing path, your connection to Great Spirit/Divinity/God is strong enough that you can step "where Angels fear to tread", as long as you are guided to for a higher purpose and do it with LOVE. To do this safely requires Wisdom, LOVE and something that can't be described. Make sure you are ready.

Above is adapted from one or more websites in 2010 I can no longer find.**************

Chapter 4

Spirit and Energetic

Energy Flow per

Edgar Cayce and Chinese Acupuncture

The crown chakra corresponds to acupuncture point GV 20 and the naval chakra corresponds to CV 8 in the center of the umbilicus.

The Crown and Naval Chakras and Kundalini per Edgar Cayce

Below is based on Edgar Cayce's Readings: Written by John Van Auken

Adapted from: http://edgarcayce.org/ps2/body_temple_of_god_J_Van_Auken.html
(web page no longer available as of October 2016))

Any place the word *I, my* or *me* is used in this section it is John Van Auken speaking.

From Edgar Cayce's attunement to the Universal Consciousness, he too saw and taught that our bodies are more than physical vehicles for living in this world.

There are two excellent ways to enter the temple within: deep sleep and deep inner stillness.

Let's explore how the body, the temple, is arranged for spiritual activity.

THE EXPERIENCE

I am often asked to describe what it feels like to open centers and raise energy, and to be in the presence of Great Spirit. The Ineffable is just that, ineffable. Additionally, I've found that people are quite unique in their wiring and perception. Some are more visual. Others are auditory. And some are tactile or kinesthetic, feeling more than perceiving. Some are conceptual; they know. Frankly, I could find no difference in the profoundness of their experiences. For me, it began with feeling the Presence and the energy, then developed into knowing, and eventually became visual. I recommend that you seek and practice and allow yourself to discover it as it comes to you. You must have some faith that it is there and in the beginning you'll need to be inspired (that helps lift you into the Spirit).

Chakras, Endocrine Glands, and Energy Flow

Many of the body's major systems may be used for both physical and spiritual activity. For example, the seven major endocrine glands that secrete hormones directly into the bloodstream to keep the body running optimally are also a physical portion of the seven spiritual centers or chakras that can affect major changes in our vibrations and consciousness. The central nervous system, so vital to living in the three-dimensional world, is also a portion of the kundalini pathway that can raise our vibrations and help us perceive beyond three dimensions.

Much of this was known in the sacred and often secret temple schools of ancient cultures around the world. For example, the staff carried by the god Mercury (also known as Hermes by the Greeks, Thoth by the Egyptians, and Enoch by the Hebrews, and who Cayce said was an incarnation of "the Word") remains today as the emblem of modern medicine (the caduceus), however few really know its intended meaning. It is an excellent emblem for physical healing, and it also contains the metaphysical structure of the body for spiritual flight.

An important and often forgotten teaching in several ancient temple schools dealt with the movement of the life force in the body. It was taught that when the life force flows downward and outward through the body's structures, one becomes fully incarnate and conscious in this world; when the life force flows inward and upward through these same structures, then one moves beyond this reality and becomes conscious of the heavens. **If both flows are made to circulate the life force, then integration occurs, and the person becomes whole, both human and divine.** Cayce and other sources teach that this is accomplished by using the breath. The Taoist teacher Liu Hua-yang wrote: "There is a turn upward toward Heaven when the breath is drawn in. When the breath flows out, energy is directed towards the Earth. In two intervals one gathers Sacred Energy."

Edgar Cayce's readings affirm these energy flows and encourage us to work at entering the temple within and raising the life force in order to draw closer to Great Spirit and receive His/Her counsel and comfort, and ultimately to become one with Great Spirit. In the process, we are to channel that LIGHT and LOVE into this world, into our lives and the lives of those we interact with each day. This, according to many spiritual teachers and schools, is the primary lesson to be learned in this incarnation: know and LOVE Great Spirit completely and channel that LIGHT and LOVE into this life's daily opportunities with others. Entering the temple, raising the energy, enlivening the spiritual centers, and uniting with Great Spirit are not necessary to living a spiritual, loving life. However, if one wants to experience the whole of Great Spirit consciousness and eternal life, then one needs to raise the body's vibrations and experience higher states of consciousness.

Let's explore the body's secret structure and some of the techniques for finding Great Spirit within us and channeling the LIGHT and LOVE into our lives.

SPIRITUAL CENTERS & THE LIFE FORCE

The concept of spiritual centers can be found in the art of antiquity, from glowing globes on people's heads in Egyptian art to third eyes on the bodies (even on the palms of hands) in classical Asian art.

The first formal mention of energy centers and pathways appears in Patanjali's Yoga Sutras, c. 300 B.C. He reveals six centers and an ultimate luminescence that occurs around the top of the head. These centers are depicted in two ways: as chakras (literally, "spinning wheels") and as padmes (literally, "lotuses"). Therefore, one may understand that the centers are both energy vortexes that generate movement as they are stimulated (as a spinning wheel) and enlightenment complexes that unfold as they grow (as an opening lotus). Cayce correlated these centers with the endocrine glandular system in the body. He also said that there are twelve (1861-11), seven of which are of importance here.

Patanjali also identifies three pathways in the body. Two are an interwoven double helix called ida and pingala, often represented by double serpents (as in the caduceus). The third is a single path, the sushumna, beginning in the lower pelvic area and traveling directly up the body to the top of the head. These pathways correspond to the body's two nervous systems: the sushumna to the central nervous system, with its spinal column and the brain, and ida and pingala to the deeper autonomic nervous system, with its woven nerves that begin in the lower torso and ascend to the brain. These three pathways act as one. The energy flows through them simultaneously.

The endocrine glands along this pathway are, in order from lowest to highest: gonads (testes in males and ovaries in females), cells of Leydig, often unrecognized and overlooked, (named after the doctor who discovered them, located in and above the gonads), adrenals (located on top of the kidneys), thymus (located in the upper chest), thyroid (in the throat), pineal (near the center of the brain at the top of the spinal fluid canal), and pituitary (just above the back of the roof of the mouth, behind the bridge of the nose, tucked under the frontal lobe). In order as chakras they are: the root, navel, solar plexus, heart, throat, crown, and brow, or third eye. Many modern books and teachers list the crown as the highest and the third eye as sixth. Cayce instructs us otherwise, as do many of the more classical texts and images. For example, in ancient Hinduism the kundalini pathway is symbolized by a cobra in the striking position, instead of straight up. In mystical Egyptian and Mayan art it is a winged serpent in the striking position. In Hebrew and Christian mysticism it is the shape of the shepherd's staff. Instead of flowing like an exclamation mark (!) the energy flows along a path that is like a question mark (?). Cayce says it flows up the body to the base of the brain, then over to the center of the brain and the crown of the head, and then on to the forehead and the great frontal lobe of the brain and the third eye.

The release of energy should never be forced by such methods as exercise, or holding the breath or by focusing one's mind on a special center, or by willing the center to open. When meditation is properly approached, these centers will open voluntarily. The knowledge, power and illumination of the soul which accompany this opening will then be concentrated on the good of others. The opening of the centers should come only as a result of spiritual growth without being forced. Unless the power released is used to express Great Spirits' LOVE for ourselves and for others, it will inflame our lower natures. The glands of reproduction are the reservoirs of the life force. They house the creative energy of the body. As an individual sits in silence, having lifted his/her mind to LOVE, creative energy is released at this level. This energy now carries the stamp of the Divine, because both the purpose and the thought which released it were holy. The 'cells of Leydig' (lyden gland), control-center of the soul's activity, opens its doors to this energy, enabling the **mind of the soul – the subconscious** – to rise to the pineal, seat of the Light that we are and Higher Consciousness. This energy is then transmitted to the other centers of the body by means of the pituitary. As it passes through the centers, it illuminates them. Meditation brings an increase in vigor and improved health. An expansion of consciousness is achieved, and with this expansion comes the realization that we are in eternity now. The realization dawns that indeed there is no death. The only real death is the separation in consciousness of the soul from Great Spirit. When this has been overcome there is no death, for consciousness is continuous in whatever plane one manifests.

Cayce states that **<u>the navel and the crown centers have a powerful magnetism between them</u>**. He says that the crown is always ready to illuminate and elevate, and that individuals must open the navel center before they can begin to transcend and transform. He calls the navel center the "closed door" and the crown the "open door." Some Eastern texts call them the "lower gate" and the "jade gate." Reconnecting these two centers is key to restoring our connection to the divine within. Here are three Cayce excerpts on this:

"This was from the flow of emotion from the kundaline center or the Lyden (Leydig cells) gland, to the ones in the center [pineal] and frontal portion of the head [pituitary]. As this flow develops keep the emotions balanced."

"Second sight or the super-activity of the third eye may come whenever there is the opening of the lyden (Leydig) center and the kundaline forces from same to the pineal."

"When there has been the opening of the Lyden (Leydig) gland, so that the kundaline forces move along the spine to the various centers that open."

PREPARATION

Cayce teaches us to prepare to raise the spiritual forces in the body by setting and feeling a powerful, fully-penetrating ideal of Great Spirit's will, rather than our will, and to feel Great Spirit's direction throughout the whole of our being as we open the centers and raise the energy.

After imbuing ourselves with the ideal of "Great Spirit's will be done," Cayce instructs us to get our bodies in order: properly assimilating nutrients needed to maintain high levels of life and eliminating wastes and toxins that build up in the system. He also directs us to exercise, even if it is just walking a mile after dinner, and to get massages and adjustments to keep the fluids and electrical energies flowing smoothly through the whole of our system. He specifically identifies three points along our spines through which there is the activity of "the kundalini forces that act as suggestions to the spiritual forces for distribution through the seven centers of the body." They are among the vertebrae and ganglia of the spine: 3rd cervical, 9th thoracic, and 4th lumbar. These need to be kept limber, open, and flowing. Get them massaged and adjusted, and do daily exercises to keep them fluid.

So important is the body's condition that in some cases he actually recommended waiting to practice deep meditation until the body's health improved.

Seek within! You will find.

Cayce states that **<u>the crown and the navel centers have a powerful magnetism between them</u>**. He says that the crown is always ready to illuminate and elevate, and that individuals must open the navel center before they can begin to transcend and transform.

Reconnecting these two centers is key to restoring our connection to the divine within.

Above is adapted from http://edgarcayce.org/ps2/body_temple_of_god_J_Van_Auken.html
(web page no longer available as of October 2016))

Explanations of Chinese Acupuncture points

GV-20 and CV-8

NOTE: The **cun** (Chinese) is a traditional Chinese unit of length. Its traditional measure is the width of a person's thumb at the knuckle; whereas the width of the two forefingers denotes 1.5 cun and the width of all fingers side-by-side is three cuns.

GV20

Chinese Name Bai Hui **English Name** Hundred Meetings (Convergences)

Location: 5 cun posterior to the AHL. On the midline of the head, 7 cun directly above the posterior hairline, approximately on the midpoint of the line connecting the apexes of the two auricles.

The Eding and Dingzhen zones together form a central line from the front to the back of the scalp. In mapping the zones to the body structure, this line represents a continuum from head to abdominal base repeated twice, first covering the front of the body (the more frontal points) and then the back of the body. **The meeting point of the two zones, GV-20, can be used to treat the entire body, depending on the aim of the needle.**

CV 8

Chinese Name Shen Que **English Name** Spirit Gate (Shrine of God)

Location: In the center of the umbilicus. Precautions: No Needling.

ENERGY FLOW and Choice for Great Spirit or the EGO

Below is by the author June, 2010

The way from being Unconscious-to Conscious- to Enlightened (Awake) - to Fully Enlightened to Ascended depends on asking Great Spirit and Great Spirits Helpers for help as the first step.

It Always comes down to forgiveness and LOVE which will lead to holding no grievances, being non-judgmental and LOVING **all** as Spirit.

It is a matter of clearing old beliefs and thoughts and dissolving the energies.

FIRST: Always FORGIVE to the best of your ability. The more you practice Forgiveness and LOVE the better you will become at Forgiving.

SECOND: Some people will need to begin with Traditional and Holistic healing practices As you progress until you are fully enlighened, you may need to revisit these modalities occasionally with a facilitators help.

1. Healing of the emotional and mental wounds of the inner child through Inner Child work.

2. Soul Retrieval through Prayer, Hypnosis, Bus Ride per Debbie Ford in "The Dark Side of the Light Chasers", Shamanistic healing work, energy work including massage.

3. A spiritual reconnection with one's Highest Self and with The All-Powerful All-Knowing Creator of the Universe through prayer, hypnosis, Shamanistic healing work, energy work and practice.

4. **ALWAYS:** FORGIVE

NOTE. Whether the practitioner you see to helps you practice Forgiveness as part of their modality or not, it is vital that you practice Forgiveness. Continue to see your traditional medical practitioners as you feel the need. There is nothing wrong with working with duality while you are still in duality, as long as you practice Forgiveness which at some point will become ADVANCED FORGIVENESS.

Advanced Forgiveness is what you are striving for.

Ho'oponopono (per Ihaleakala Hew Len)

"I Love you.
I am sorry.
Please forgive me.
Thank you."

Course in Miracles ("A Course in Miracles" – original unedited)

"You are Spirit.
Whole and Innocent.
All is Forgiven and Released."

NOTES:

Realize at a certain point you become aware that you are actually forgiving yourself and even forgiveness is an illusion because it is within duality and only "GOD IS".

What you are upset about or afraid of is never the real problem and is only a prompt to FORGIVE.

Preoccupations with problems set up to be incapable of solution are favorite ego devices for impeding progress.

The One question you must learn to ask in connection with everything is, "What for?" ("What is the purpose?"). Whatever it is will direct your efforts automatically.

Forgiveness is a choice and advanced forgiveness is always done at the level of consciousness with the help of the Unihipili (subconscious) and with the help of Great Spirit and Great Spirits Helpers.

Thoughts, beliefs and ideas form your 'body' and 'reality'. Choosing LOVE or Ego moment to moment determines whether you become closer to Great Spirit/God or more firmly entrenched in duality.

In diagrams A through D below, notice that the energy flows through your 'body' and surrounds your 'body'.

In diagram E the energy flow depicts someone who is ascended.

There is always a choice to choose Great Spirit and it is a simple choice. These diagrams show why it seems so difficult at first and why some clearing is needed before the choice becomes "visible". In order to start all you need to do is ask Great Spirit and Great Spirits Helpers for assistance and guidance with LOVE in your heart.

In the diagrams below:

1) Aumakua/Higher Self / "I Am That I Am" / Great Spirit Helpers

The Aumakua is the mediator between the interpretations of the ego and the knowledge of the spirit. It has the ability to deal with symbols, which enables communication with the ego's beliefs. It has the ability to look beyond symbols into eternity, which enables understanding the laws of the Universe. It can therefore perform the function of reinterpreting what the ego makes. It is therefore tasked to reinterpret you on behalf of Great Spirit.

2) Unihipili/Subconscious mind.

The Hawaiian name for what is sometimes called the subconscious /inner/emotional/intuitive mind. I use the name 'Unihipili' because there is nothing sub about the subconscious. It may need our LOVE and guidance; however, in many, and probably in most ways, it is much more powerful than the conscious mind.

3)Uhane/Conscious Mind.

The 5 (A - E) Diagrams below show my concept of energy flow in regards to The Crown Chakra (GV20) and the Naval Chakra (CV8). Edgar Cayce and Chinese Acupuncture both address the importance of this flow.

Diagram A

PERSON (or BEING) WHO IS **UNCONSCIOUS**, HAS CHOSEN EGO and HAS NOT ASKED GREAT SPIRIT FOR HELP.

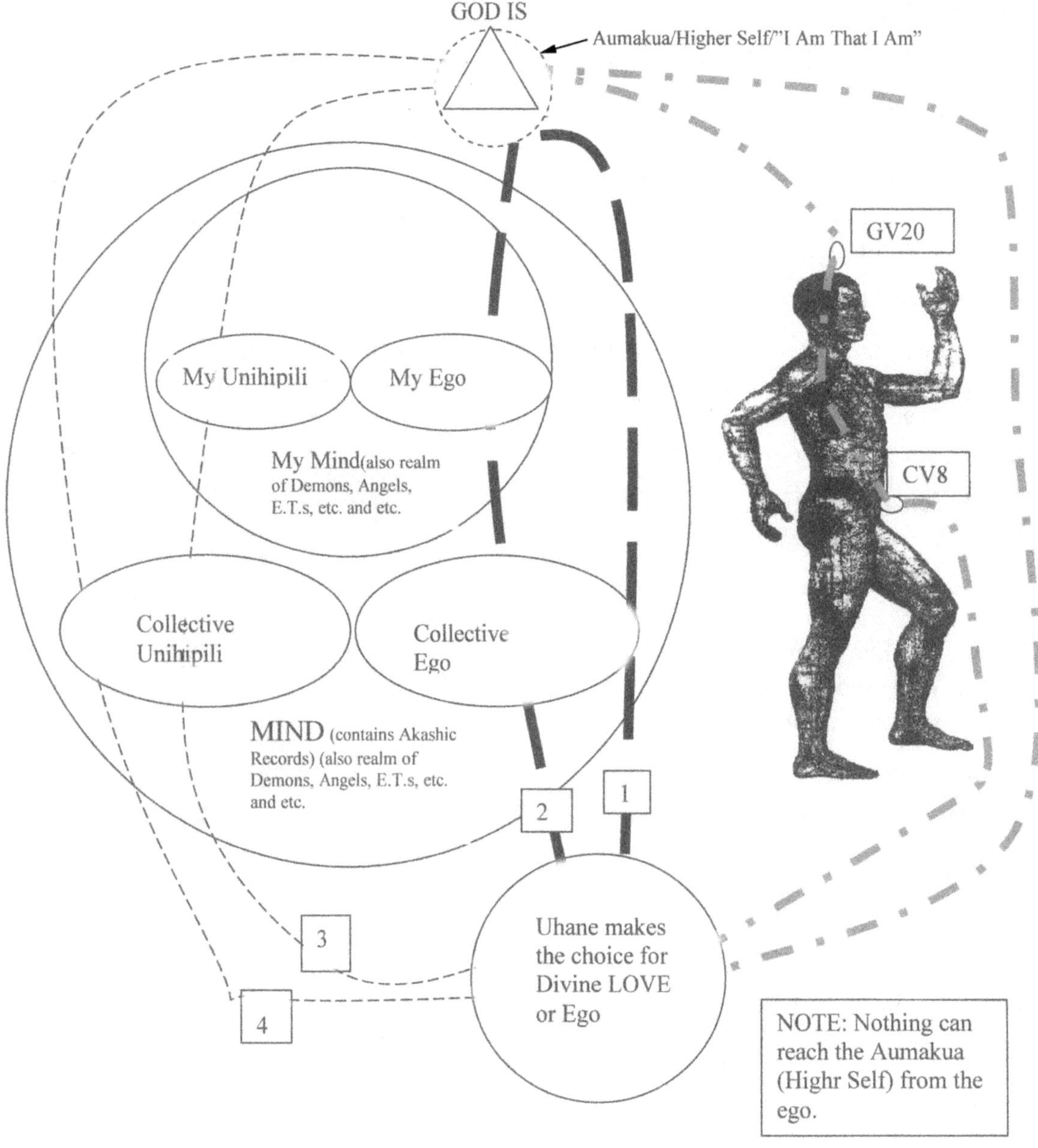

Diagram B

PERSON (or BEING) WHO

HAS **ASKED FOR GREAT SPIRITS HELP** and is beginning to see the light.

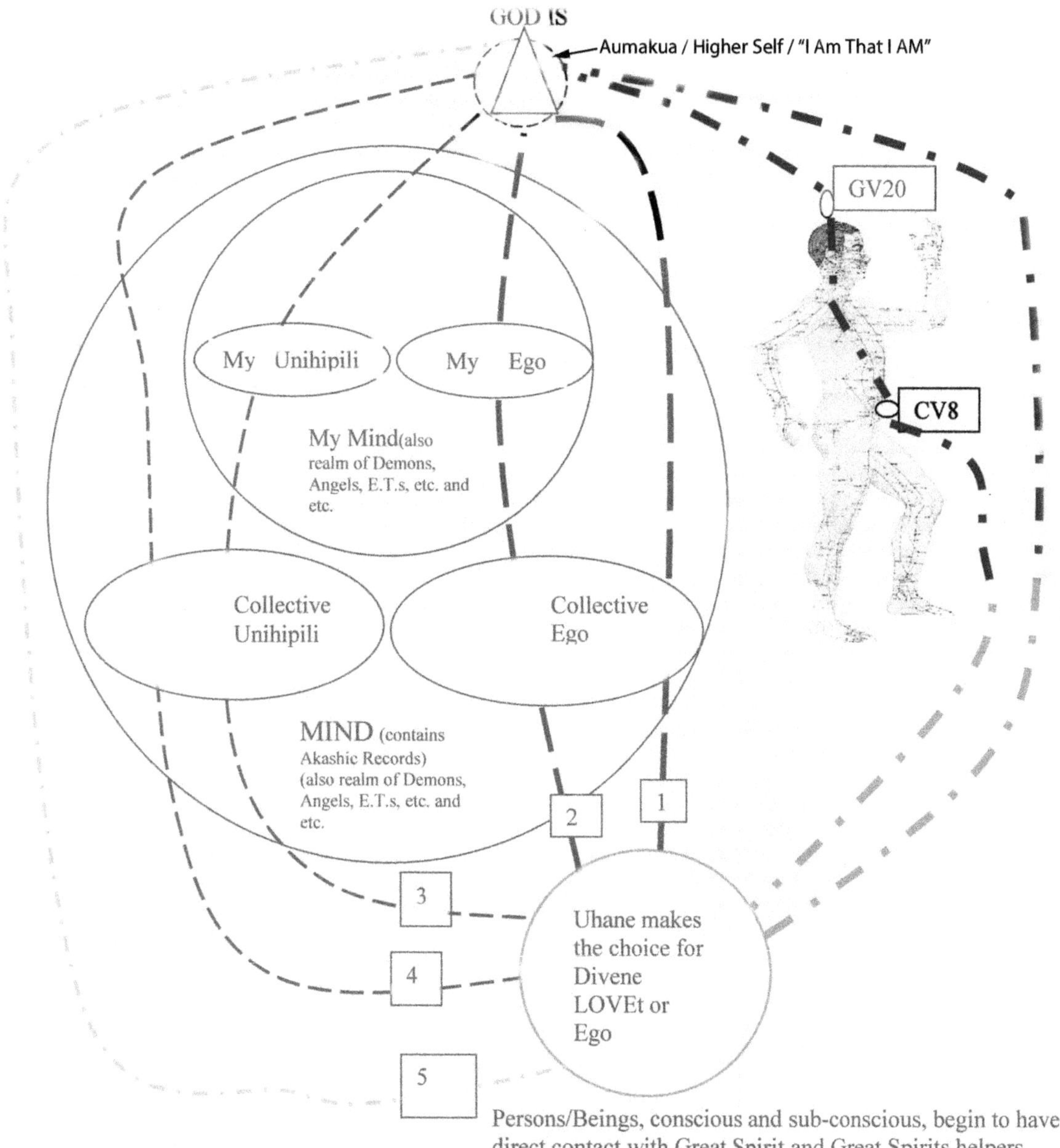

Persons/Beings, conscious and sub-conscious, begin to have direct contact with Great Spirit and Great Spirits helpers.

Diagram C

PERSON (or BEING) WHO HAS ASKED FOR GREAT SPIRITS HELP and is seeing more of the light and **PRACTICING FORGIVENESS**

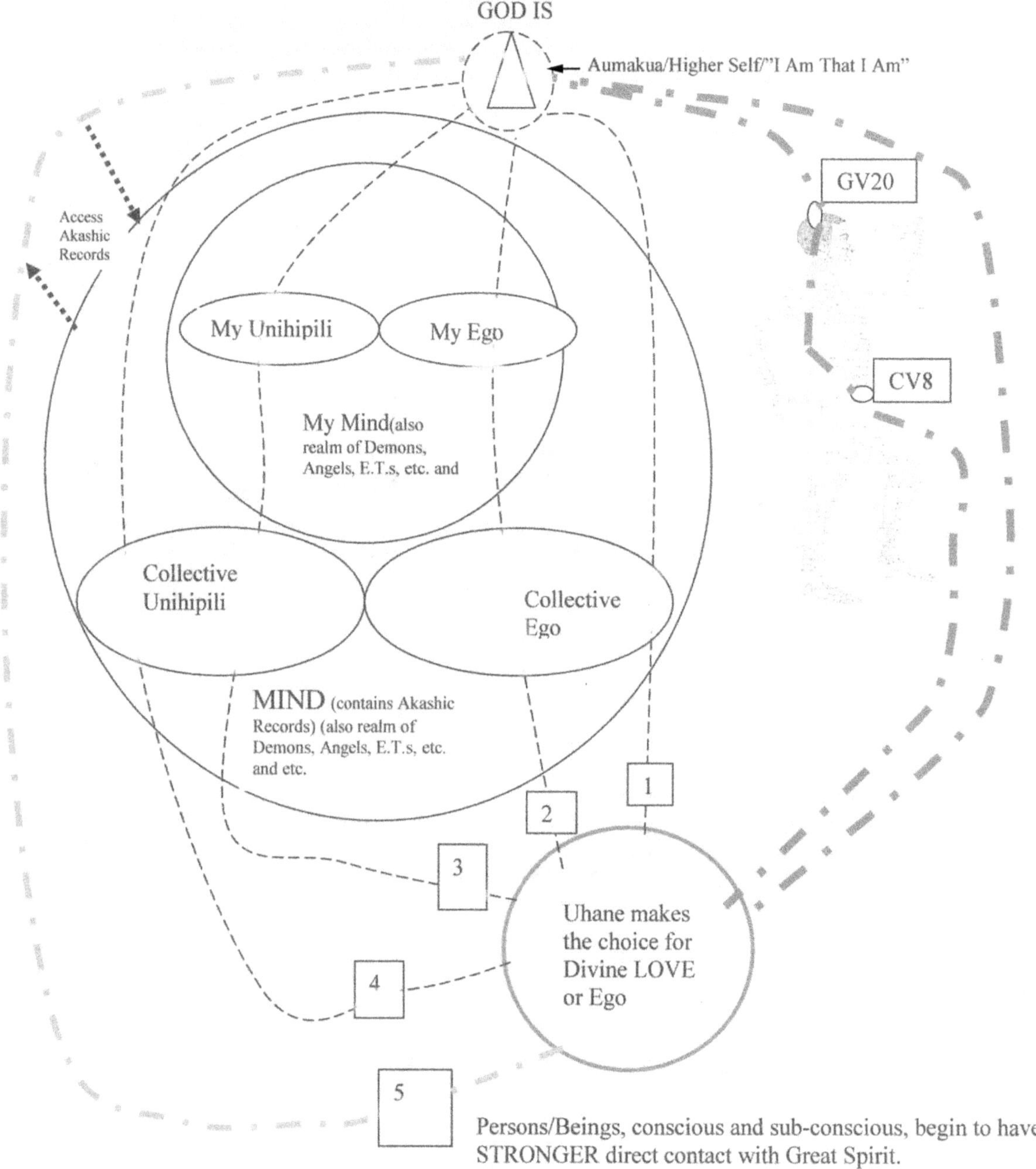

Diagram D

PERSON (or BEING) WHO HAS ASKED FOR GREAT SPIRITS HELP AND IS **FULLY ENLIGHTENED**

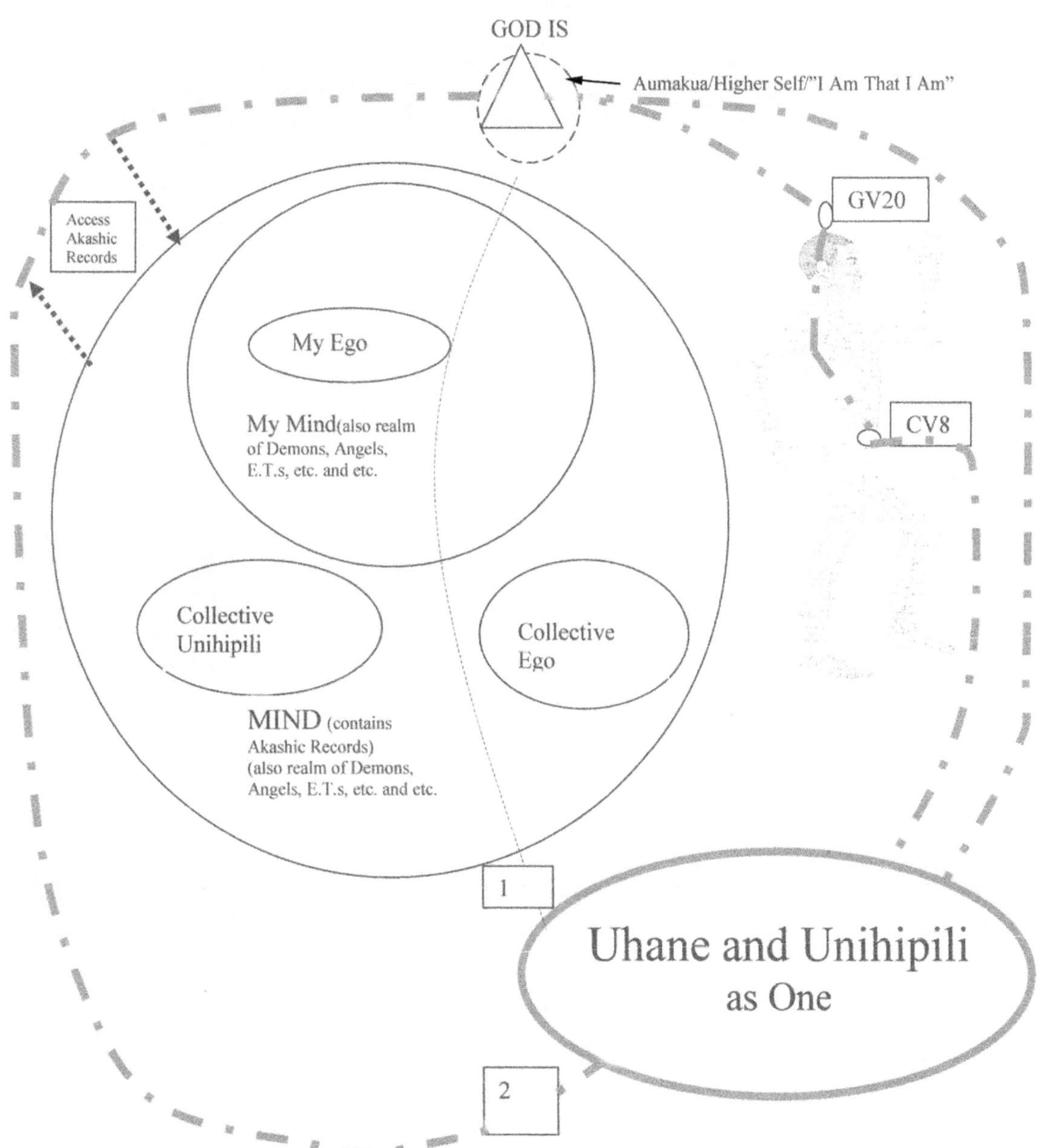

Direct connection with Great Spirit and Great Spirits Helpers with just enough energy going through the Mind & ego to maintain the body in duality automatically.

Diagram E

PERSON (or BEING) is **ASCENDED**

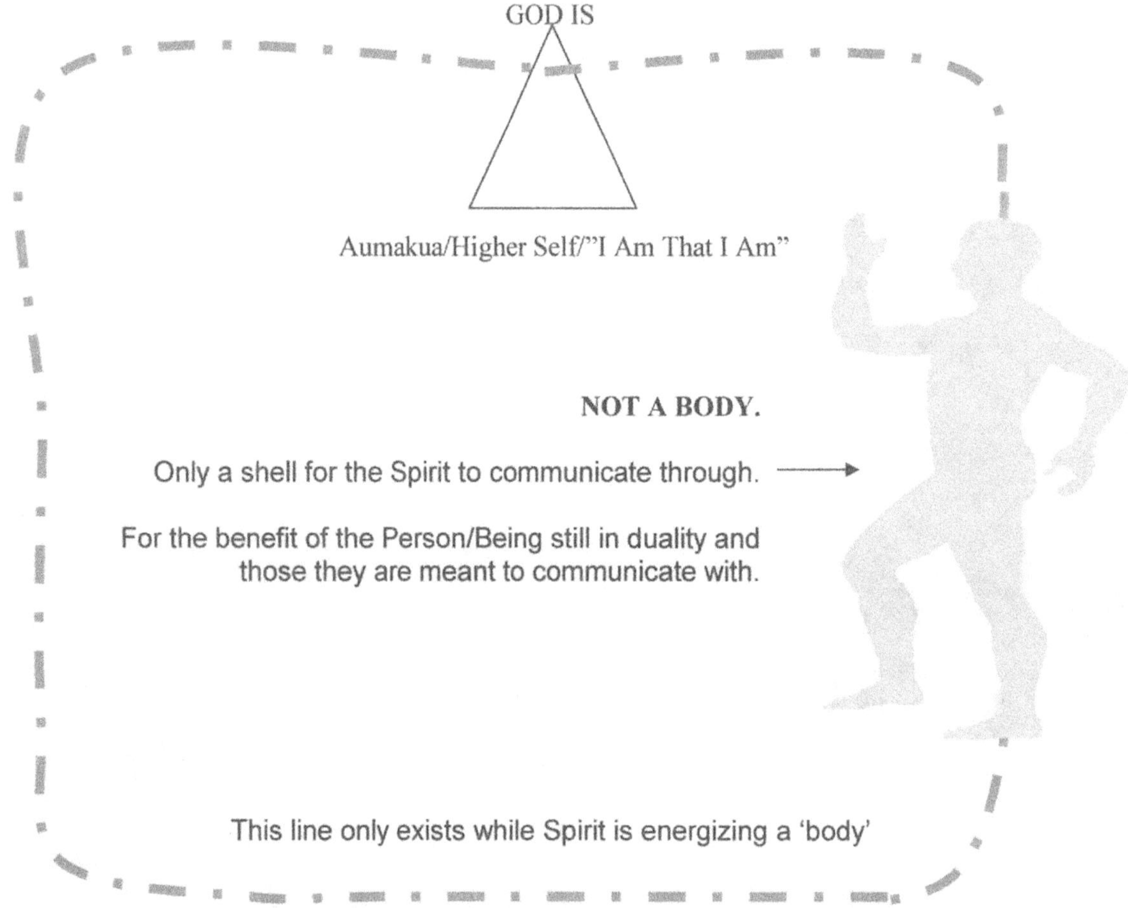

One with Great Spirit. The only time a body is appropriate is when a body is needed to communicate through. Even then it is only a shell for the benefit of the Person/Being still in duality.

And Finally

GOD IS...

Above is by the author June, 2010

****

Soul and Oversoul Structure and Consolidation

Below is adapted from an article by John Hornecker (2010) http://www.earthscape.net/soul_oversoul.htm (on June 1, 2016) and from a web page I can no longer find "Soul Consolidations and Transfers" (1996 John Hornecker)

Sections titled "Is it the same as Possession?" and "Odd notes on walk-ins:" are from an internet source I can no longer find.

In this section wherever you see "I have", "I did" or "I always" it is John Hornecker.

Soul and Oversoul Structure

As we move through a process of spiritual awakening and transformation a wide range of possibilities and experiences begins to open to us. Most of these involve our *soul*.

Our soul and oversoul are essentially an intermediate level that exists between our Higher Self and our human self, as depicted in the diagram below.

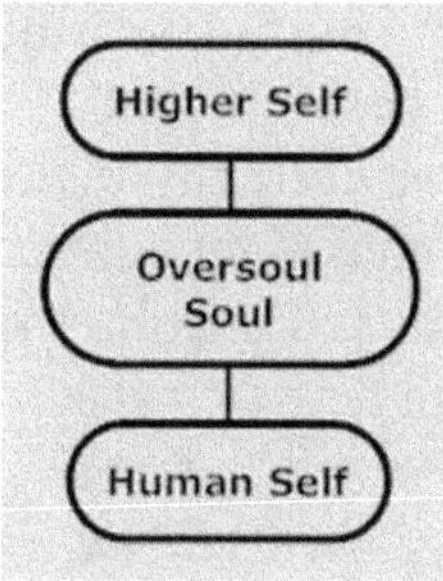

Let's explore this in more detail.

Whereas our Higher Self is the individualized essence of our Creator, and remains in a state of perfection, our soul and oversoul represent our cumulative life experiences. At the end of a human lifetime here on Earth, the memory of our experiences are integrated into our soul and oversoul. And prior to entering into a new life experience here on Earth, it is our soul and oversoul that, in concert with our Higher Self, and our guides and mentors, create a Life Plan for the upcoming life experience.

What is the difference between our soul and our oversoul? Sometimes the analogy of a human hand is used to describe the relationship between the two. The fleshy part of the hand would represent the oversoul, while a soul would be represented by one of the fingers. This obviously implies that there is more than one soul that is associated with a particular oversoul.

A model that we like to use to explain the relationship between an oversoul and the related souls is the following image. If one has 13 spheres, all exactly the same size, 12 of the spheres will fit perfectly around the 13th sphere in the center. Each of the 12 peripheral spheres is in direct contact with central 13th sphere. So in this model, the center sphere would represent the oversoul, and each of the 12 peripheral spheres would represent a soul that is an integral part of the "oversoul cluster".

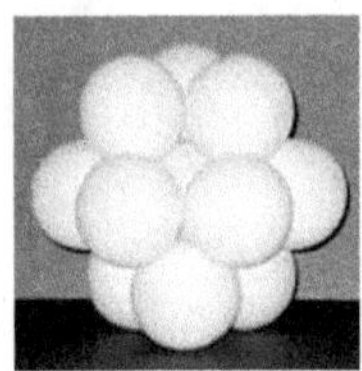

Such a clustered arrangement enables more than one of the soul units of the oversoul to extend into human embodiments "simultaneously", thus expanding the collective experience of the oversoul cluster. The oversoul itself does not enter into physical embodiment . . . it always remains within the higher realms so that it can oversee and guide the collective experience. The realm in which the oversoul resides is the "Eternal Now", which is outside of the time-space domain. So the individual soul units can, and often do, extend into embodiments that are in different time periods, as we experience time here on Earth.

Parallel Experiences

Each soul of the cluster has ongoing roles and responsibilities within the non-physical realms, whether or not it is currently involved with a physical embodiment. For example, it may be involved in learning experiences in the "Halls of Learning", either as a student or a teacher, depending on the level of evolutionary development of the soul. Or it may be involved in a wide range of other activities. If a soul is currently involved with a human embodiment, most of these activities take place while the human body is asleep. The body in which a soul functions within the non-physical realms is sometimes referred to as a "Light body" or "traveling body". Even while the human body is awake, the soul continues to monitor what is going on within the higher realms, and sometimes it needs to partially withdraw its focus on the human self to carry out responsibilities within the non-physical realms. During such situations, the human self may experience a sense of drowsiness, or a feeling that it is "not all here" . . . indeed it is not!

When the human self begins to awaken after it has been sleeping, there is usually a period of time before consciousness fully returns to the body in which there may be "bleed-through" of awareness from within the non-physical realms. This may be in a form similar to a dream, or it may come through as an intuitive feeling. A few people who are well along in their spiritual awakening process may actually "remember" some of what was happening in the non-physical realm.

Functioning as a "Collective"

It is also possible for more than one of the souls of an oversoul cluster to extend into the same embodiment. And in fact, because of the importance of this particular lifetime as Earth moves to completion of a long cycle of evolution, many (if not most) oversoul clusters are "consolidating" into a single embodiment. Since each soul unit has its own history, and therefore its own unique characteristics, such a consolidation can be a very 'interesting' experience. The embodiment functions more as a "collective", with different souls of the group moving into the forefront at different times. This can be a very unusual, and sometimes challenging experience for the person involved.

For example, If "Soul A" was in the forefront yesterday, and "Soul B" is in the forefront today, Soul B tends to not remember the experiences that the embodiment had yesterday with the same clarity as Soul A would if Soul A was still in the forefront.

Functioning as a collective can also present some challenges with regard to relationships, since each of the individual souls of the cluster tend to have their own personality characteristics. If you are a person who has undergone this form of a soul consolidation and are now functioning as a collective, people who are close to you in your life, such as a mate, may experience you as having a multiple-personality disorder. And if your mate or a close friend is sensitive to energies, they often will see the shift in the energies in your eyes. So for them, it is almost like living with a kaleidoscope . . . they don't quite know who (which soul) is going to be present in any given moment.

For the sake of accuracy we should acknowledge that not all oversoul clusters involve 12 soul units being associated with an oversoul . . . it all depends of the level of evolvement of the oversoul cluster. But even if a particular oversoul cluster has less than 12 soul units, all of the same concepts and considerations still apply.

The below diagram was done by author for further clarification.

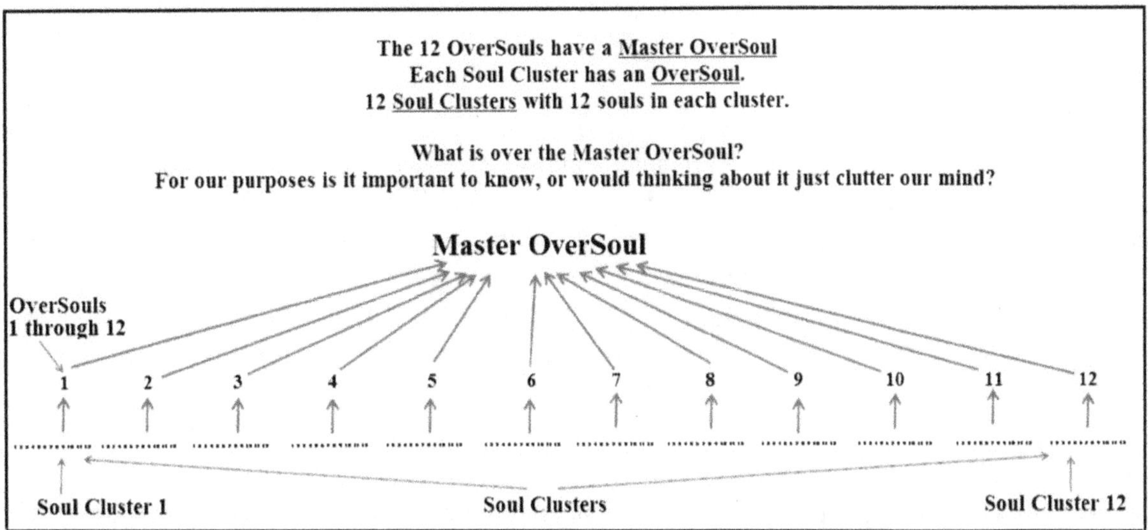

Each soul cluster at first includes 12 parallel lives. One of the prerequisites for ascension is that all of the soul units of an oversoul structure must be embodied in the same body. One reason for this is that ascension is an experience of the total oversoul; it cannot be undertaken by just one soul unit independently. Since ascension involves the transformation of the physical body, in order to create an ascension body, this cannot be done with multiple bodies involved.

"Non-Human" Soul Histories

To complicate matters further, virtually all of us have had past embodiments in forms other than human. Those embodiments may have been here on Earth, or perhaps in other celestial systems. For example, we know that here on Earth the cetaceans (dolphins and whales) are sentient beings. And many of the spiritually evolved souls who are now here on Earth have had experiences as a dolphin or whale in other lifetimes. That experience is, of course, retained in the memory of the soul and oversoul. So in the present lifetime in a human form, they still tend to carry an affinity (resonance) with the cetaceans. And they may also tend to feel more comfortable in a heavier body that is more similar to a cetacean shape.

Also, many souls have had experiences within the angelic kingdom, and tend to carry the angelic consciousness with them in their current human form. Angelic consciousness is recognizable by its feeling of "lightness", and usually the body form tends to be sleight or petite.

Also, throughout the many past experiences of most souls, they on occasion may have chosen to experience life as a form within the nature kingdom, such as a tree deva, or mountain deva, or one of the many animal forms. In the celestial systems throughout the Universe, there is a virtually infinite number of different body forms into which souls may incarnate. Many of these forms are similar to animal forms that are present here on Earth, but which have evolved to a high degree . . . to a state of "sentiency" and beyond. If a soul has an extensive history of embodiments in one of these forms, such as a feline form for example, the human body in which they are currently embodied here on Earth may take on a feline appearance, especially in the facial features. If one's soul has a long history in other than humanoid forms, it is not uncommon in the early moments of awakening from sleep to feel a bit strange being in a human body.

Soul Transfers (Walk-Ins)

Next, let's consider the subject of *"soul transfers"*, more commonly known as *"walk-ins"*. One of the early books on this subject, *Strangers Among Us*, was written by Ruth Montgomery in the mid-1970's. A "walk-in", as she introduced the concept, is a situation in which the soul that has been associated with an embodiment since birth agrees to leave the body and make it available to be embodied by a different soul. There are various reasons why a soul might agree to do this. For example, it may involve a person that is very discouraged with life, and no longer wants to live. So, rather than going through the death of the physical body, the original soul may make it available for another soul to embody. The "incoming" soul has to agree to take on all of the "karmic" responsibilities of that life, such as children (if there are any) or perhaps aged parents, and so on.

In every walk-in situation, there must be complete agreement between the outgoing and incoming souls. But since the agreements are made at the soul level, the human self may not be aware that a soul transfer (walk-in) has been agreed to. And since the incoming soul inherits the memory of the body that it comes into, the human self is usually not aware, at least initially, that a soul transfer has taken place.

In Ruth Montgomery's book, she indicated that an incoming soul is almost always a more evolved soul than the outgoing soul. This gave rise to an impression that if someone is a "walk-in", they must be a very evolved person. While it is true that a soul must be at a certain level of evolutionary development before it is permitted to come in as a walk-in, it is also true that many of the souls who came in as walk-ins during the 1970's and 1980's were highly evolved "Lightworkers" souls, many of the souls who have come in as walk-ins during the past few decades have struggled to acclimate to the human life situation they have entered. And more than a few have allowed themselves to be diverted from their soul's mission and purpose.

There have also been some misconceptions about the circumstances under which the actual soul transfer takes place. The earlier perspectives were that the transfer almost always took place in conjunction with a traumatic situation, such as a car accident or severe illness.

Although that seems to be true in some cases, there are many soul transfers that seem to take place rather seamlessly, without trauma involved. It is true, however, that in some cases trauma tends to shatter rigid energy patterns, making it easier for the incoming soul to integrate into the human form.

Although most soul transfers seem to take place in mid-life, they occasional take place during the first few years of life, or even in the senior years. And a few people have undergone multiple walk-in experiences, separated by a few years, or in some cases several years.

The most noticeable and challenging issues for an incoming soul is that it quite likely will not have the same feelings for family members and friends . . . this tends to especially apply to spouses. So, quite often marriages do not survive long after a soul transfer takes place.

What are the advantages for a soul to come in as a walk-in rather than through the natural birth process? Assuming that the soul transfer takes place in mid-life, the incoming soul can focus on its mission and purpose much more quickly, without having to go through the stages of infancy and growing up years. The risks are that it is all too easy to become entrapped in personality patterns that are already well established . . . patterns that may not be supportive to the life plan of incoming soul.

Is it the same as Possession?

It can be, in some cases. A Fundamentalist Christian would certainly say so. The term "possession" is generally used in a negative sense, to imply that the walk-in soul is unwelcome and dominates the body, forcing the original soul to perform actions it may not otherwise do. However, in many indigenous religions including some Southeast Asian and Afro-Cuban traditions, voluntary possession is a normal religious experience and is done for beneficial reasons. Spirits enter the bodies of worshippers to give advice and comfort. In these traditions, a spirit shouldn't usually stay on, however, and should be encouraged to go back to its own home if it seems inclined to move in for good.

If the walk-in soul is not malevolent, and/or the original soul has enough strength-of-will to keep control, then this sort of situation will not occur. It would not be true to say that all walk-ins are cases of possession, because frequently the relationship between the two souls is one of co-operation.

Odd notes on walk-Ins:

A walk-in soul need not be the same species as the body. It may be otherkin, alien, or animal, for example.

A walk-in soul need not be the same gender as the body. While souls may not have a gender, often a soul will retain traits from former lifetimes, including preferences for clothes, speech, mannerisms, and '- yes -' gender. So a resident need not be the same gender as the body.

It is possible to be multiple for more than one reason at once; that is, you may be a ‘split multiple’ AND have a separate walk-in soul as well.

If a soul can walk-in, it is often also possible for them to walk-out as well. Such a soul may abandon the body before death, The body's birth-spirit can also leave some hours or days before the body dies. (This is, of course, called a \"Walk-Out\".)

Early "Retirement" (Walk Outs)

Although the subject of walk-ins has received considerable attention in recent years, a more recent phenomenon involving soul transfers has, as yet, received virtually no attention. Thus, I feel it is important to address this situation in considerable detail. This new phenomenon could perhaps be termed, "walk-outs"; however, I prefer the term "early retirement". Let's begin with a background perspective.

Before we came into incarnation for this lifetime, we were thoroughly briefed on the overall transformation plan for Earth, and each of us clearly understood our individual assignments within the context of this overall mission. Although the details of the mission plan were not directly available to our human consciousness, we retained this knowledge within our oversoul. This included an awareness that group ascensions were planned to begin in the mid-1980's, and for most of us, the major part of our mission was to be completed after we were able to function within the human realm in our ascension body. So when ascension did not take place in this time-frame, there was a growing restlessness within many of the Light Workers. Aside from ascension, there were numerous other setbacks and delays in the mission. Although most of the Light Workers did not consciously understand the exact reasons for their restlessness, there was a general sense that there was much more important work that we had committed to do in the lifetime, yet the circumstances did not seem to enable clarity, or provide support for this work.

A significant part of the frustration is often focused on economic issues. Most of the Light Workers have found themselves in a continuing state of economic tension. Part of the difficulty is that the economic system is based on profit and many Light Workers feel that the economic system is artificial or unnatural and have trouble working within it.

It may help to recognize and accept that times have changed and money, if freely given, is the same as accepting food, shelter, moccasins, a chicken or any other gift for sharing your knowledge and LOVE.

World events have not provided much of a source of encouragement. To a great extent, it has been one step forward, and two steps backward. For example, the breakup of the Soviet Union provided only a short-lived sense of optimism, as we watched the former suppression of the communist system replaced by the new tyranny of organized crime, and the destruction of their economic system through manipulated devaluation of the currencies. Also, the senseless killing and injuring of men, women, and children in continuing conflicts around the world has not provide much reason for encouragement.

Thus, as the months and years came and went during the latter part of the decade of the 80's, and early part of the 90's, an increasing number of Light Workers were becoming weary and discouraged.

When we, as Light Workers, agreed to come to Earth so very long ago, we agreed to remain here, come hell or high water (and we have been through both!), until the end of the cycle. It was anticipated that Earth would be firmly back on it evolutionary track by that time. However, free will of the people of Earth cannot be overridden, and despite our best efforts, progress has been less than we anticipated.

The Spiritual Beings who guide the evolutionary course of this planet are compassionate beings. Most have experienced first-hand lifetime after lifetime in human embodiment here on Earth. So a decision was made to make a new option available to the Light Workers. This option is limited to only those Light Workers who have been here for the longest time - those who came here as part of the original groups. Essentially the option goes like this:

> For any of these Light Workers who would like to be released from their original commitment, and to return now to their home star system, such a request will be honored. Rather than accomplishing this through physical death, or through a lift-off of the physical body, a "soul transfer" will be arranged, and a new volunteer soul will come into the embodiment to finish out the normal human lifetime.
>
> The incoming soul will also be a Light Worker, but in virtually all cases, one of lesser evolutionary development. Thus, it will still be possible to fulfill at least part of the mission of the original soul.
>
> An aspect of the agreement related to the soul transfer is that conscious knowledge of the transfer will be "sealed", and not made available to the incoming soul. The intent of this is to minimize disruption to the human life.

I personally have mixed feelings regarding this new option. From the standpoint of the soul, it is a wonderful, and well deserved opportunity to be released from a very difficult situation, and to finally return home. However, from the perspective of the "human-self" that remains on Earth, the struggle continues.

Quite a few of my Light Workers friends have elected this option. For me, it is a great feeling of loss, for the soul that I have known and loved for so very long is no longer in the familiar embodiment. Quite frankly, in many cases I don't quite know how to relate to the remaining human- self. My experience has been that even though in most cases the human-self does not have conscious awareness that it no longer embodies the same soul, there is some sort of an unconsciousness awareness that bleeds through. And there seems to be a sort of "pulling back" on their part from our friendship, since the soul-resonance of the original soul is no longer part of our relationship.

It also has been interesting to observe some of the Light Workers who have lived high-profile lives in the music and motion picture business, who have accepted the early retirement option. There have been some very profound shifts in the focus of their lives, and in the nature of the soul essence which the emanate.

It is not clear to me to what extent the decision of a soul to leave under this option is made only by the soul, or made in collaboration by the soul and human-self. My guidance assures me that the human-self must be in agreement with the decision. In my own case, I have made it clear to my higher-self that I am not amenable to this option, so long as I have any say-so in this matter. And my higher-self assures me that it has no intention of accepting this option.

Soul "Braiding"

Soul "braiding" is a term used to describe a process whereby a new soul merges into an existing embodiment, but the original birth soul does not leave. It is similar to the process described earlier in which more than one soul of an oversoul cluster enters into the same embodiment. Soul braiding, however, can also involve the merging in of a soul from a different soul cluster. In this sense, it becomes more like a "hybrid".

Also, soul braiding sometimes involves a more temporary situation, whereby a new soul merges in for a period of time, and then later withdraws. For example, one case we are aware of involved a soul who had never been embodied on earth before, who wanted to experience what it was like to be embodied in human form here on Earth for a few days before making a decision to embody for a full lifetime. Another example would be a situation in which a soul with special talents and abilities may want to come into an embodiment for a year or two to carry out a special mission.

The foregoing types of soul consolidations and transfers are but a few of the virtually infinite variety of soul rearrangements that are taking place at this time. During recent years, the term soul "braiding" has come into common use among various Light Workers in reference to the integration of more than one soul into a single embodiment. My perspective is that many of the situations that have been referred to as soul braiding simply involve oversoul consolidation, as discussed earlier in this section. However, in some cases, the integration of an additional soul unit into an embodiment may be of a more temporary nature.

For example, if a person is in an important leadership position, one or more of the souls from the same oversoul structure may merge into the embodiment for a period of time to assist in carrying out a particular task. In some cases, such a temporary merger may involve a soul from an entirely different oversoul unit.

Soul braiding, whether long-term or short-term, is always done under mutual consent of the "host" oversoul and the incoming soul unit. And there is always mutual benefit - the embodiment is able to more easily accomplish a specific task, and the incoming soul is afforded an additional learning experience.

Uninvited Guests ('entities')

Now let's shift gears and discuss a very different situation; one that could be confused with the walk-in or braiding situation. Uninvited Guests could also be confused with the oversoul consolidation process.

It is *very* common that more than one soul will attach to the same embodiment. Thus, such a person may experience the multiple "attachments" as multiple "personalities", in a manner similar to which a Light Worker may experience multiple souls that have integrated into the embodiment through the oversoul consolidation process. There is, however, one very important distinguishing difference between these two types of experiences. In the case of soul attachments (possession), it is very common to experience *conflict* among the various souls who have attached. In the case of oversoul consolidation, there is seldom, if ever, conflict among the souls who have integrated into the embodiment.

Soul attachment is very prevalent - even among Light Workers, even though many people assume it is only common among people such as alcoholics, or others who had severely weakened their life energy field in various ways.

When a soul completes a lifetime here on Earth, it is intended that the soul will return to the higher realms, and resume their evolutionary journey in those realms. However, in some cases, a soul may be unwilling or unable to fully separate itself from the human realm. This may be for a variety of different reasons. One of the more common reasons involves addictive behavioral patterns such as alcohol or drug abuse, gambling addiction, or sexual addictions.

Other reasons include that it may become disoriented and confused. In many cases, it will attach to someone who had been a friend or family member in the lifetime just departed.

Although the vast majority of souls who attach in this manner do not have evil intent, such an attachment does not serve the highest good of either the soul who does the attaching, or the soul to whom the attachment is made. Furthermore, it is *very* common that more than one soul will attach to the same embodiment. Thus, such a person may experience the multiple "attachments" as multiple "personalities". Although an individual may be able to release such attachments without assistance, some attached souls can be *very* stubborn, especially if they have been attached for a long period of time.

In such cases, when the soul leaves (through death) the body in which the addictive behavior patterns were formed, it is attracted to places or situations in which living humans are involved in these behaviors, such as bars, gambling casinos, strip joints or bordellos. However, when the soul is no longer in a physical body, it can only observe other humans that are involved in these behaviors, but it cannot experience the *feelings* of the addictive behaviors. The only way they can do that is to merge into the embodiment of someone who is involved in these behaviors, and experience it through that person's body. All too often in such cases, the wayward soul then becomes "entrapped" in the body of the other person, and does not know how to leave, or perhaps does not want to leave.

From the perspective of the person who has been invaded by the wayward soul, it is what is commonly referred to as being "possessed", or as having an "entity" within the body. The best protection from being invaded by such a disembodied entity is to maintain a strong and healthy energy field, and of course, to avoid addictive behaviors. Unfortunately, drugs and alcohol severely *weaken* ones energy field, and makes such a person especially vulnerable to intrusion.

There are other situations which commonly attract entities. Most common are situations that involve "emotional vulnerability". An example would be a person who becomes distraught over the death of a family member or friend. Such a person might then attract a disembodied entity who would, with all good intentions, attempt to console them. If the entity is not careful, however, it can become entrapped in the body of the distraught person. And frequently such entrapments continue on for many years . . . in some cases, a lifetime.

From the perspective of the person with the attached entity, it is never a healthy situation, regardless of whether the original intent of the entity was for selfish pleasures, or compassionate supportiveness. First and foremost, having an attached entity is a drain on the energy level of the body. Secondly, it can result in personality disorders if the attached entity had a strong or abusive personality that can at times overshadow the personality of the person involved. And thirdly, having an attached entity can create a severe distraction from the life plan of the person involved.

We have found that if a person has one attached entity, it is likely that they will have more than one. And the more entities a person has, the greater the drain on their energy level. We believe that many cases of Chronic Fatigue Syndrome are essentially nothing more than a situation involving attached entities.

How does one know if a person has one or more attached entities? Inconsistency in personality characteristics is one of the most common indicators . . . sometimes pleasant, but at other times coarse or abusive. Also, a person with attached entities tends to avoid direct eye contact . . . the entities are in effect "hiding" inside, and they are afraid that they might be seen . . . and indeed they can be seen by skilled spiritual counselor.

If a person feels that they may be the host for such uninvited guests, my advice would be to seek the assistance of a spiritually-aware therapist who is experienced in helping to facilitate the release of such attachments (Glenn's note: Someone who can help release the attached soul/spirit/entity with LOVE). Although an individual may be able to release such attachments without assistance, some attached souls can be *very* stubborn, especially if they have been attached for a long period of time.

Above is adapted from an article by John Hornecker (2010) http://www.earthscape.net/soul_oversoul.htm (on June 1, 2016)

and from a web page I can no longer find "Soul Consolidations and Transfers" (1996 John Hornecker)

Sections titled "Is it the same as Possession?" and "Odd notes on walk-ins:" are from an internet source I can no longer find.

Below is adapted from https://lightworkers.org/page/58696/ascension-information-more-on-the-galactic-oversoul-merges

Soul Consolidations and Transfers

During recent years, many of the Light Workers have been undergoing various forms of soul and oversoul rearrangements. Let's discuss some of the more common experiences.

Oversoul Consolidation

The most common type of oversoul structure among the Light Workers who came to Earth as part of either of the first two groups is the "Star-Cluster Oversoul". So let's use this structure for purposes of illustration.

An oversoul within such a structure consists of a "master soul unit", and the individual soul units. Such oversouls are clustered together in a group of oversouls, along with a "master oversoul unit". Let's begin with our focus on just one of these oversoul units.

Throughout most of our incarnational experiences here on Earth, each of the soul units within the oversoul structure has embodied in separate, simultaneous incarnations. From the perspective of the oversoul, this expansion of incarnational experiences enables the oversoul to accelerate its evolutionary development.

When the plans for the final phase of this long evolutionary cycle were being worked out, it was anticipated that most of the Light Workers, at least those from the early groups, would go through the ascension process at some point during this lifetime. One of the prerequisites for ascension is that *all* of the soul units of an oversoul structure must be embodied in the same body. One reason for this is that ascension is an experience of the *total oversoul;* it cannot be undertaken by just one soul unit independently. And since ascension involves the transformation of the physical body in order to create an ascension body, this cannot be done with multiple bodies involved.

So within the context of this ascension plan, each of the oversouls worked out a plan as to how it would accomplish this "oversoul consolidation". The development of such a plan started with a decision as to the particular embodiment into which the various soul units would be consolidated. Typically, just one of the soul units would initially be extended into this particular embodiment. Such an embodiment could either be through the natural birth process, or through a "soul transfer" arrangement. In most cases, it was the plan that this embodiment would proceed through the early life experiences, and through a significant part of the awakening and healing processes, before other soul units would begin to integrate into the embodiment.

Identity Issues

In the lives of many of the Light Workers, there has been a lot of confusion around this entire issue. One reason for this is that as the second soul begins to integrate into the embodiment, a Light Worker may suddenly begin to feel like a "different person". It is not at all uncommon that such a person might feel inclined to change their name, of even leave a relationship, because in reality, they *are* a different person - or at least, 50% of them is a different person.

Typically, after the integration of the second soul unit into the embodiment is completed - a process that may take place over a period of a couple of months - the embodiment will often remain in that configuration for 2 or 3 years, in order to enable the personality-self to assimilate the influence of the second soul.

After such a period of assimilation is completed, then the 3rd soul unit will begin to integrate into the embodiment. Usually the assimilation process is slightly easier related to the 3rd soul unit, because at that point only 33% of the embodiment is "new". So the time period for assimilation of the 3rd soul unit is typically 1-2 years.

As this process continues, with the integration of the additional soul units, each successive integration tends to require somewhat less time for the assimilation process. Typically, the time period required for integration and assimilation of all of the soul units is in the range of 7 to 10 years. However, there are various factors that may cause the assimilation period to be extended or shortened.

As the soul units progressively integrate into the embodiment, they tend to take turns being in the "drivers seat". In other words, one soul unit may function in the forefront of the personality self for a period of time, while the other souls remain in the background. Then, one of the other soul units may take a turn at being in the forefront. This may cause such a Light Worker to feel at times like he/she has multiple personalities. Close friends also may be sensitive to this "revolving chair" phenomenon. Sometimes this can create significant complications in a relationship. Consider, for a moment, a hypothetical situation in which the original soul in the embodiment has a close soul connection, and corresponding attraction, to the soul of a marriage partner. And then as other souls merge into the embodiment, the original soul may spend most of its time in the background. So one's spouse may experience very distinct personality shifts, and at times wonder whatever happened to the person he/she married.

There is yet another phenomenon which many of the Light Workers have experienced. Throughout the many lifetimes of evolutionary experience here on Earth, it is fairly common to extend some of the soul units into embodiment in human form, and other soul units into embodiment in cetacean forms. In such cases, when the soul units that have had many embodiments in cetacean forms are integrated into the singular human embodiment, the Light

Worker may quite suddenly develop a deep attraction to the cetaceans, such as dolphins or whales. Many of the Light Workers who are currently working to help bridge understanding between the human and cetacean kingdoms are oversouls who have experienced embodiments in cetacean forms.

Healing the Individual Soul Units

There also are some important issues related to the *healing* process. One of the important purposes of this final lifetime of this evolutionary cycle is to heal, and bring into balance, all of the residual imbalances from previous lifetimes. So as each soul successively integrates into the embodiment, it brings with it such residual imbalances. If these imbalances are severe, they can trigger a healing crisis within the embodiment. I have observed many of my light worker friends as they have gone through the oversoul consolidation process. And it seems to be a very common experience that such a Light Worker may feel that they are in good health, and then "wham", all of a sudden a physical disorder will spring up - seemingly from nowhere. As I have tuned into such situations, it is very common that such a crisis has been caused by a residual imbalanced situation in one of the incoming souls - - usually the most recent one to integrate into the embodiment. A similar phenomenon can occur related to emotional or mental energy imbalances. Usually these are somewhat more subtle, although no less important, than those that occur on a physical level.

External/Internal Issues

There is yet another unexpected issue which sometimes arises in conjunction with the soul consolidation process. As a way of introducing this issue, let me use as an example the experience of one of my Light Worker friends.

In the early stages of her spiritual awakening, a "teacher" within the unseen dimensions came to her and introduced himself (she related to him as a male energy), and indicated that he would be assisting her in her Lightwork mission to the extent that she would be open to his assistance. His energy was very loving, and he seemed very wise, so she gratefully accepted his offer. As her spiritual unfolding continued, he played an increasingly important role in her life and in her work. Her path of service involved leading workshops and doing individual soul- oriented counseling. By mutual agreement, he often would merge into her embodiment during a workshop, and share teachings directly with the participants in her workshops. As a side note, the two of them became very important teachers for me in the early stages of my awakening.

This relationship between the two of them continued for at least 20 years, and he became her dearest friend and source of inspiration. One day he came to her on the unseen dimensions and indicated that he would no longer be able to serve her in this way. He indicated that the reason for this is that he would be merging into her embodiment along with her. Her emotional reaction to this announcement was intense. On the one hand, she felt a tremendous loss - as though her closest and dearest friend was going to "die". Yet, on the other hand, she felt elation that his love and wisdom would now become a part of "her". As the situation turned out he was simply one of the other souls of the oversoul cluster of which she also was a part. And it was time to integrate into the embodiment in preparation for the ascension process.

In tracking the experiences of many of my Light Worker friends, I have learned that this is a fairly common experience, although not necessarily to this same extreme. It is not at all unusual for one of the souls (who is not currently in embodiment) of the same oversoul cluster to serve as a guide and teacher for a Light Worker for a period of time before integrating into the same embodiment. Thus, a relationship develops as though the two are separate beings. Then, as the integration occurs, the "separate" being no longer exists as an external identity, and it is quite common in such cases to feel a significant loss.

Oversoul Cluster Consolidation

Next, let's consider the concept of *oversoul cluster* consolidation. In certain situations, the entire oversoul cluster may be ready to go through one of the galactic or universal initiations. One of the prerequisites for such an initiation is that the entire oversoul cluster much be integrated into a single embodiment. In such cases, after the individual oversoul has completed its consolidation process, it will then begin to integrate other *oversouls* of the cluster into the embodiment (Glenn's question: possibly a non-physical embodiment?). From a human perspective, the experience of this procedure feels very much like a continuation of the earlier soul integration process.

Although the star-cluster oversoul was used as an example to discuss oversoul consolidation, the same concept applies to other oversoul configurations.

Above is adapted from https://lightworkers.org/page/58696/ascension-information-more-on-the-galactic-oversoul-merges

****

Personal Notes

Chapter 5

Reincarnation and Past Lives

To do the subject of reincarnation and past lives justice would take an entire book.

It has been well documented that past life hypnosis and therapy can and does help heal phobias, fears and physical ailments, sometime by just becoming aware of them. For the purpose of healing it is unimportant whether the memories are actually memories or they are fabricated by the subconscious mind. I believe the following three books are an excellent introduction and will clarify how the regression can help.

Children's Past Lives by Carol Bowman (helps to understand adults too)

Return From Heaven by Carol Bowman

Many Lives, Many Masters by Dr. Brian L. Weiss, M.D.

A great example

Below is from Chapter One of *Children's Past Live*s by Carol Bowman. It is her story of five year old Chase and nine year old Sarah and how past life regression helped them to overcome phobias. Does it matter if the memories were real or the subconscious somehow fabricated them.

July 4, 1988

Every year my husband Steve and I hosted a big Fourth of July party at our house, which was a short walk to the best spot in all of Asheville for watching the city's fireworks. Our friends and their young children looked forward to joining us in our back yard for an afternoon of picnicking and celebration. The party always culminated with a walk down the hill to the municipal golf course to watch the grand fireworks display.

For weeks Chase had been talking excitedly about the fun he had had in previous years at our parties, and especially about the fireworks. His eyes got bigger as he remembered the bright colors in the sky. This year he was hoping for a long and spectacular show.

On the afternoon of the Fourth, our friends arrived with pot luck, Frisbees, and sparklers. The yard filled up fast, and kids were everywhere - hanging from the swing set, crowded in the sandbox, hiding under the back porch. Our quiet neighborhood was charged with the sounds of squealing, laughing children. Adults tried to relax on the porch while the children ran circles through the house and around the yard, usually with red headed Chase in the lead.

Indeed, Chase lived up to his name. Always in motion, full of energy and curiosity, often unstoppable, it seemed we were always two steps behind him, trying to catch him before he knocked something over. Friends teased us about choosing the name *Chase,* saying we got what we asked for.

Our nine year old daughter, Sarah, and her friends retreated to a spot on the side of the house under the hemlocks and set up their own small table and chairs, just outside the range of watchful parents. For hours they entertained themselves, decorating their table with flowers and toy china, creating their own holiday party apart from the "wild" little kids. The only time we saw the girls was when they bustled back and forth from Sarah's room, modeling different dress-up clothes, jewelry, and hats on each trip.

When the sun sank low in the trees, throwing orange light into the back yard, we knew it was time to corral the kids and prepare for the march down the hill. I grabbed Chase as he ran by, washed the cake and ice cream off his face, and forced a clean shirt onto his squirming little body. Armed with blankets and flashlights, we joined the parade of people headed down our street toward the golf course.

Unexplained Fear

Chase, holding my hand tight, bobbed my arm up and down as he skipped along with the crowd. The older girls, Sarah's gang, formed their own giggling procession. They clutched the sparklers that we promised they could light once we got to the golf course. We reached our favorite spot just as the sun set behind the Blue Ridge Mountains in the distance, then spread our blankets on a strategic slope.

From the slope we watched the plain below - the lower nine fairways - fill with people. Soon blankets and lawn chairs were strewn everywhere. As the sky grew darker, boys and men set off firecrackers and Roman candles, filling the valley with flashes, bangs, and smoke. Nearby our children waved sparklers in the air, drawing bright circles and zigzag trails in the dusk; fireflies danced and blinked in approval.

Chase, pumped with excitement and sugar, ran up and down the hill with his friends until he finally ran out of steam and collapsed on my lap. We watched the noisy party below while we waited for the big show to begin.

Suddenly the cannonlike booms announcing the start of the fireworks reverberated off the hills, echoing all around us. The sky lit up and crackled with giant starbursts. The crowd around us oohed and aahed at the extravaganza of light and color against the black sky. Hearing the shots and booms at such close range added an exciting intensity to the show.

But Chase, instead of being delighted, began to cry. "What's wrong?" I asked him. He could not answer; he only wailed harder and louder. I held him close, thinking he was exhausted beyond his breaking point and that the loud noises had startled him. But his crying got deeper and more desperate. After a few more minutes, I could see that Chase was not calming down - his hysteria got worse. I knew I had to take him home, away from the noise and confusion. I told Steve that I was leaving with Chase and asked him to stay with Sarah until the fireworks were over.

The short walk home seemed long. Chase was sobbing so deeply, he couldn't walk, and I had to carry him all the way up the hill. But even when we got home, he was still crying. I held him on my lap in a rocking chair on the back porch, amid the debris of the party, hoping he would calm down. When his deep crying softened enough for me to ask him if he was sick or hurt, he could only whimper and shake his head no. When I asked him if the loud noises scared him, he cried harder. There was nothing I could do but hold and rock him, while I watched the fireflies' silent show in our back yard. Chase gradually settled down and nuzzled into my chest. Finally, just when my arms were too stiff to hold him any longer, he fell asleep and I put him to bed.

Chase's unusual behavior puzzled me. He had never cried so long or so deeply in his short life. And he had never been afraid of fireworks before. This incident seemed out of character for Chase, who was not easily frightened by anything. I put it out of my mind by reasoning that he was frazzled from the long day, and maybe he had eaten too many treats, or something had just set him off - after all, things like this happen with children.

But a month later it happened again. On a hot August day, a friend invited us to cool off at their town's indoor swimming pool. Chase loves the water and was eager to jump in the pool. As soon as he entered the pool area, where the sound of the diving board and splashing and yelling echoed in the big hall, he began to cry hysterically. Howling and screaming, he grabbed my arm with both hands and dragged me toward the door. Reasoning with him was futile; he just pulled me harder. I gave up and took him outside.

We found a chair in the shade. I held Chase and asked him what was bothering him. He couldn't tell me, but he was obviously deeply disturbed, terrified of something. He finally calmed down, but even after he stopped crying, I couldn't persuade him to go back into the pool building.

As we sat outside, I thought back to the other time he had acted this way - on the Fourth of July. I recalled the sound of the fireworks reverberating in the hills, which had triggered his first attack of hysteria. Then I realized that the sound of the diving board reverberating off the bare walls of the pool building sounded the same. I asked Chase if he was frightened by the sounds. He sheepishly nodded yes, but still would not go anywhere near the pool.

So that was it - the booming sounds! But *why* did Chase suddenly have such a fear of loud noises? My mind tried to put all the pieces together. I couldn't remember anything that had happened to him in the past that would cause such a severe reaction to booming sounds. And this was the second time it had happened in a month. The fear seemed to come out of nowhere. Would it happen more often now, every time Chase heard a loud noise? I was worried! This could develop into a real problem, especially if I wasn't there the next time he became hysterical. I didn't know what to do, except wait and hope that he would outgrow this mysterious fear.

A few weeks later, we were fortunate to have a wonderful man and skilled hypnotherapist, Norman Inge, as our house guest. He was staying with us while he conducted workshops in Asheville on past life regression and did private sessions with some of my friends. With Norman as our teacher, we were all just beginning to explore the realms of past life regression.

One afternoon during his stay, Norman, Chase, Sarah, and I were sitting around the kitchen table having tea and cookies, laughing at Norman's stories. Something reminded me of Chase's irrational fear of loud noises, and I asked Norman about it. He listened to my story and then asked if Chase and I would like to try an experiment. Though I didn't know exactly what Norman had in mind, I trusted him and knew that he would be sensitive to my young son's limits. And since Chase was as eager as I was to solve this problem, we both agreed to try.

Still sitting around the kitchen table, Norman began. That moment, I realized later, was a turning point in my life. Up to that time I had never thought that children could remember their past lives.

Actual Hypnosis and regression starts here.

Chase Sees War

"Sit on your mom's lap. Close your eye and tell me what you see when you hear the loud noises that scare you," Norman gently instructed Chase.

I looked down at Chase's freckled face. *Nothing* could have prepared me for what I was about to hear.

Young Chase immediately began describing himself as a soldier - an adult soldier - carrying a gun. "I'm standing behind a rock. I'm carrying a long gun with a kind of sword at the end." My heart was pounding in my ears, and the hair on my arms stood up as I listened. Sarah and 1 glanced at each other in wide-eyed amazement.

"What are you wearing?" Norman questioned.

"I have dirty, ripped clothes, brown boots, a belt. I'm hiding behind a rock, crouching on my knees and shooting at the enemy. I'm at the edge of a valley. The battle is going on all around me."

I listened to Chase, surprised' to hear him talk about war. He had never been interested in war toys and had never even owned a toy gun. He always preferred games and construction toys; he would spend hours at a time happily building with blocks, Legos, and his wooden trains. His television watching was strictly limited to *Sesame Street* and *Mister Rogers,* and none of the Disney movies he had seen depicted war.

"I'm behind a rock," he said again. "I don't want to look, but I have to when I shoot. Smoke and flashes everywhere. And loud noises: yelling, screaming, loud booms. I'm not sure who I'm shooting at - there's so much smoke, so much going on. I'm scared. I shoot at anything that moves. I really don't want to be here and shoot other people."

Although this was Chase's little-boy voice, his tone was serious and mature - uncharacteristic of my happy five-year-old. He actually seemed to be feeling this soldier's feelings and thinking his thoughts. He really didn't want to be there shooting at other men. This was not a glorified picture of war or soldiering; Chase was describing the sentiments of a man in the heat of battle who had serious doubts about the value of his actions and was terrified, thinking only of staying alive. These feelings and images were coming from someplace deep within him. Chase was not making this up.

Chase's body, too, revealed how deeply he was experiencing this life. As he described himself shooting from behind the rock, I could feel his body tense on my lap. When he admitted he didn't want to be there and shoot at other people, his breathing quickened and he curled up into a ball, as if he were trying to hide and avoid what he saw. Holding him, I could feel his fear.

Norman sensed Chase's distress with his role as a soldier who, in order to survive, had to kill other men. He explained to Chase, talking slowly, "We live many different lives on Earth. We take turns playing different parts, like actors in a play. We learn what it means to be human by playing these different parts. Sometimes we are soldiers and kill others in a battle, and sometimes we are killed. We are simply playing our parts to learn." Using simple language, Norman emphasized that there was no blame in being a soldier. He assured Chase that he was just doing his job, even if he had to kill other soldiers in battle.

As my son listened to Norman's assurances, I could feel his body relax and his breathing become more regular. The anguished look on his face melted away. Norman's words were helping. Young Chase was actually understanding and responding to these universal concepts.

When Norman saw that Chase had calmed down, he asked him to continue telling us what he saw.

"I'm crouching on my knees behind the rock. I'm hit in the right wrist by a bullet someone shot from above the valley. I slide down behind the rock, holding my wrist where I was shot. It's bleeding - I feel dizzy.

"Someone I know drags me out of the battle and takes me to a place where they took soldiers that are hurt - not like a regular hospital, just big poles, like an open tent, covered with material. There are beds there, but they're like wooden benches. They're very hard and uncomfortable."

Chase said that he felt dizzy and could hear the sounds of gunfire around him as his wrist was being bandaged. He said he was relieved to be out of the fighting. But it wasn't long before he was ordered back into battle, and he reluctantly returned to the shooting.

"I'm walking back to battle. There are chickens on the road. I see a wagon pulling a cannon on it. The cannon is tied onto the wagon with ropes. The wagon has big wheels."

Chase said that he had been ordered to man a cannon on a hill overlooking the main battlefield. He was visibly upset by this order and repeated that he didn't want to be there. He said he missed his family. At the mention of his family, Norman and I looked at each other with raised eyebrows. But before we could learn more, Chase started to fidget and told us the images were fading. He opened his eyes, looked around the kitchen, looked at us, and smiled. The little-boy glow in his face had returned. Norman asked him how he felt. Chase chirped, "Fine." Then he hopped off my lap, grabbed another cookie, and ran into the other room to play.

As Chase pattered out of the kitchen, Norman, Sarah, and I looked at each other with our mouths open. I glanced at the clock on the stove: only twenty minutes had passed since Norman had told Chase to close his eyes. It felt like hours.

Norman broke our stunned silence to ask for another cup of tea.

We talked about the small miracle we had just witnessed.

Norman was sure that Chase had remembered a past life. He explained that a traumatic experience in a past life such as being in war - and especially a traumatic death - can cause a phobia in the present life. Could this past life war experience be the cause of Chase's extreme fear of loud noises? Possibly. Norman said we'd have to wait and see if the fear went away.

Norman admitted that he had never worked with a child so young and that he was surprised at how easily Chase had retrieved his past life memory - no hypnotic induction had been needed, as with his older clients. Apparently, Chase's memories were close to the surface and needed only gentle encouragement to come out.

Sarah, who had been quietly absorbing everything that happened, suddenly bounced up and down in her chair, waving her arms, and piped in, "That spot on Chase's wrist, where he was shot - that's where his eczema is!"

She was right. The location of the wound Chase described was exactly the same location as that of a persistent rash he had suffered since he was a baby. He had always had severe eczema on his right wrist. Whenever he became upset or tired, he scratched that wrist until it bled. Sarah said that it sounded like Chase was "ripping his flesh" as he relentlessly scratched that one spot. I often bandaged his wrist to prevent his scratching and bleeding. Without a bandage, Chase would wake up with blood streaked on his sheets. I had taken him to several doctors because of the severity of his rash, but allergy testing, a food elimination diet, salves, and ointments failed to clear it up.

To our astonishment and relief, within a few days of his regression to the lifetime as a soldier, the eczema on Chase's right wrist vanished completely, and it has never returned. (Glenn' note: The hypnoses was done in 1988 and the book was written in 1997)

Chase's fear of loud noises also totally disappeared. Fireworks, explosions, and booming sounds never scared him again. In fact, soon after the regression Chase began showing an intense interest in playing the drums. For his sixth birthday he got his first drum set. Now he's a serious drummer, filling the house with loud booming sounds every day.

(Glenn's note: When I met Carol in 2002 Chase had come home from college with a bandage on his right wrist. Carol asked him what he had been up to. He said he had been to the movies and going out with his girlfriend and not studying as much as he could. "I also had to register for the draft..." Within a couple days the eczema had cleared up again.

Nine year old Sarah - Dolls Under the Bed

Nine year old Sarah had taken in everything Norman said, and during Chase's story she seemed to be in a trance herself, hanging on to every word. When we were finished processing Chase's experience, she asked Norman if he could try an experiment with her too. She confided to him that she had been struggling with her own terrible fear of house fires.

Like Chase's fear of loud noises, Sarah's extreme fear of fire was inexplicable. Though she admitted now that fire had terrified her as long as she could remember, Steve and I had become aware of it only a year earlier ...

Above is from Chapter One of *Children's Past Lives* by Carol Bowman

Chapter 6

A. R. T. (Autonomic Response Testing)

Below is adapted from http://www.holistichealthtools.com/muscle.html

Introduction to A.R.T and Muscle Testing (Kinesiology)

Everything is composed of energy: biological, chemical, and spiritual. Although you may not be able to see or feel it, even inanimate objects emit energy. Some energy fields are compatible with one another, some have a neutral response, and yet others may be incompatible.

Exposure to incompatible energy fields can have a weakening impact on the body. For example, a food or substance you are allergic or sensitive to may actually be rooted in energy incompatibility. Continued exposure to incompatible energies can create imbalances in the body, leading to illness and disease. This is why it is so important to be aware of the impact everything you eat and are exposed to has on you. This includes the environment, food, and even other people! Avoiding weakening energies creates an environment for good health and healing.

Muscle testing, also known as Applied Kinesiology, is a useful technique that taps into your body's innate wisdom to help identify things that strengthen or weaken you. By tapping into to these energy signals you can make choices that will enhance your well being. I have personally used this form of testing for many years and find it to be an effective guide.

Dr. Darren Weissman, author of *The Power of Infinite Love & Gratitude*, describes muscle testing this way: "The body has an innate intelligence that can be assessed with this method to determine whether it's maintaining balance. Just like the autonomic nervous system, muscle testing is a polarity-dependent mechanism where a muscle will maintain its strength as long as there's a congruency with the function, adaptability, and the survival of the entire organism. When there's incongruency, an indicator muscle will test weak. When a muscle locks out, it's an indication that whatever is being evaluated is congruent with the overall balance of the body. When the muscle gives way, it's a sign that what's being tested is incongruent with this balance."

Kinesiology is another word for muscle testing. Kinesiology is simple. With practice anybody can do it because it uses your electrical system and your muscles. If you are alive, you have these two things. I know that sounds smart-mouthed of me, but I've learned that sometimes people refuse to believe that anything can be so simple. So they create a mental block—only "sensitive types" can do this, or only women can do it. It's just not true. Kinesiology happens to be one of those simple things in life just waiting around to be learned and used by everyone.

Small children can learn to do kinesiology in about five minutes, mainly because it never occurred to them that they couldn't do it. If I tell them they have an electrical system, they don't argue with me about it; they just get on with the business of learning how to do simple testing. Actually, I do mean to intimidate you. Your first big hurdle will be whether or not you believe you have a viable electrical system that is capable of being tested. Here's a good test. Place a hand mirror under your nose. If you see breath marks, you have a strong electrical system. (If you don't see breath marks, call your local emergency rescue squad—you're in trouble.) Now you can get on with learning how to use kinesiology!

If you've ever been to a chiropractor or holistic physician experienced in muscle testing, you've experienced kinesiology. The doctor tells you to stick out your arm and resist his pressure. It feels like he is trying to push your arm down after he has told you not to let him do it. Everything is going fine, and then all of a sudden he presses and your arm falls down like a floppy fish no matter how hard you try to keep it up. That is using kinesiology.

Simply stated, the body has within it and surrounding it an electrical network or grid. If anything impacts your electrical system that does not maintain or enhance your health and your body's balance, your muscles, when having physical pressure applied, are unable to hold their strength. (Muscle power is directly linked to the balance of the electrical system.) In other words, if pressure is applied to an individual's extended arm while his body's electrical system is being adversely affected, the muscles will weaken and the arm will not be able to resist the pressure. The circuits of the electrical system are overloaded or have short-circuited, causing a weakening of that system. However, if pressure is applied while this electrical system is being positively affected; the circuits remain strong, balanced and capable of fully functioning throughout the body. The muscles will remain strong, the person will easily resist and the arm will hold its position.

This electrical/muscular relationship is a natural part of the human system. It is not mystical or magical. Kinesiology is an established method for reading the body's balance through the balance of the electrical system at any given moment.

When working in a co-creative partnership, nature answers your yes/no questions by projecting a positive energy or a negative energy—whichever is appropriate—into the electrical circuit that you have created by your fingers (or with a partner) especially for the kinesiology testing. The "yes" or "no" that nature projects registers in this one electrical connection and not throughout your entire electrical system. The special connection created by your fingers (or with a partner) allows you to use the kinesiology technique without adversely impacting your electrical system or your body's balance. Only one circuit is being used, and this circuit is created by you for the testing and is not a part of the normal function of the electrical system throughout your body. The answer you are able to discern through the testing is from nature. It is not an answer that has been concocted by you.

If you have ever experienced muscle testing, you probably participated in the two-person method. You provided the extended arm, and the other person provided the pressure. Although efficient, this can sometimes be cumbersome when you want to test something on your own. Arm pumpers have the nasty habit of disappearing right when you need them most.

TIPS AND USES FOR MUSCLE TESTING

The key to successful muscle testing is to have an open mind. and to let go of preconceptions and desired or expected answers. If you are new to alternative medicine, or haven't used techniques like this before, I know it sounds a little "out there." But it really can be a very powerful tool, especially with a little practice! It is important to try to do the testing in a neutral environment with no distractions such as music, scents, etc. Drinking water beforehand may be helpful in optimizing brain function. Taking a few deep breaths to help oxygenate your body may help as well.

In addition to testing products and foods, you can also use Muscle Testing to gauge your body's reactions to various ideas, thoughts, etc. An example might be if you are contemplating a new treatment method, such as acupuncture. You can use Muscle Testing to get an idea of how your body reacts to this thought. So you would use the testing technique below, but instead of holding an object you would make a statement, "Acupuncture is an effective method of treatment to aid in my healing." If your muscle strength remains strong the answer is "yes;" but if you lose muscle strength the reply would be considered a "no."

One important note: Many people teach that when testing an object or asking the body questions, **make statements, do not ask questions.** For example:

Correct - "This _____ is compatible with my body."

Incorrect: - " Is this ______ compatible with my body?"

(Glenn's note: The critical point is that there are only two possible answers; ***yes*** or ***no***.)

Note: If you are testing an item that is too large to hold, use this same procedure but instead of holding it you will make contact with the item you are testing by touching it.

This technique is obviously not fool-proof...but the more you do it, and the more comfortable you become doing it, the more accurate the results can be.

Above is adapted from http://www.holistichealthtools.com/muscle.html

Below is by the author

I recommend that you say a prayer before any form of ART.

This is to help you to surrender to yourself. Make sure you have created a safe environment for the process and that you are relaxed. Quiet your mind and open to Sources Love and guidance. You may want to turn off your phone and other devices.

You may want to open sacred space for yourself and the area you are in. Surround yourself with LOVE, LIGHT and VIOLET FLAME.

Use your own way or you may say a prayer similar to the following.

Great Spirit and Great Spirit Helpers, as are best,
Help me stay fully connected to YOU and YOUR LOVE and LIGHT. *Thank You.*

Great Spirit and Great Spirit Helpers, as are best,
Help me stay standing fully in YOUR LOVE, LIGHT and VIOLET FLAME. *Thank You.*

Great Spirit and Great Spirit Helpers, as are best,
Keep me completely surrounded by YOUR LOVE, LIGHT and VIOLET FLAME. *Thank You.*

Great Spirit and Great Spirit Helpers, as are best,
Help me stay filled with Your LOVE, LIGHT and VIOLET FLAME as is best. *Thank You.*

Great Spirit and Great Spirit Helpers, as are best,
Help me keep it so only energies and beings of Pure Divine LOVE and LIGHT surround me, influence me and share and communicate through me. *Thank You.*

Great Spirit and Great Spirit Helpers, as are best,
Help me to Open Your Sacred Space of LOVE as is best, keep me in Our Sacred Space and close our sacred space as is best when I have finished this exercise. *Thank You.*

Great Spirit and Great Spirit Helpers, as are best,
Do this as is best for all those participating in this healing. *Thank You.*

Great Spirit and Great Spirit Helpers, as are best,
Keep me/us Integrous, well intentioned and without interference from material ego or fear. *Thank You.*

Keep ME/US tied in to the highest level of information which is You at all levels and in all dimensions, and keep me/us unswitched and open." *Thank You.*

Keep all my (our) questions appropriate, well worded, clear, integrous and well intentioned. *Thank You.*

Help me/us to understand the answers and the significance of the questions and answers at all levels and in all dimensions as correctly as possible. Please raise my level of consciousness and vibrational frequency if needed to understand. *Thank You.*

Ask permission of the persons Self and of Great Spirit. Verbal permission of person should be sought if possible. If the person is comatose or unable to communicate you can still check with their higher self.

NOTE: With practice you will sense if there is unwanted interference and then need to deal with it.

NOTE: Make sure you give GOD/Great Spirit the credit and you are not trying to impress anyone.

When using pendulum, muscle testing or sensing the energy field first:

Say “show me yes”

Say “show me no”

Say “show me inappropriate to ask”

Say “show me unable to answer”

If while asking a question you get and inappropriate or unable to answer.

You can say “The last question is inappropriate to ask”.

If the answer was yes drop it and don’t try to weasel around it.

If the answer was no you can say

“The question was poorly worded or thought out”.

If the answer is yes you can reword the question.

If you get a no you can say “The question is unanswerable at this time.

If you get a yes, Someone or some Being somewhere may need to make a choice that will affect the answer; it could even be you.

Above is by the author

Below is adapted from http://www.holistichealthtools.com/muscle.html

Kinesiology: A Tool for Testing

One Person Method

Kinesiology Self-Testing Steps

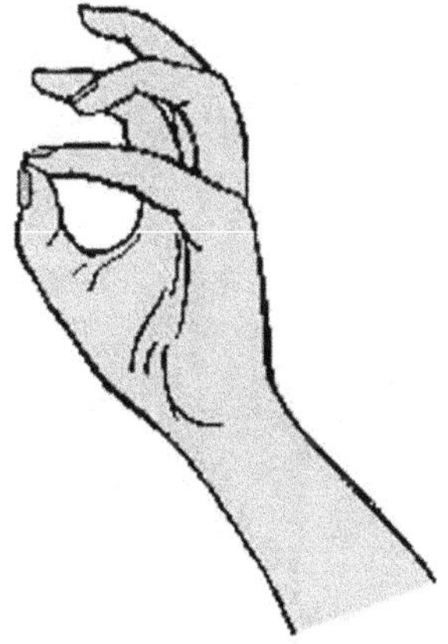

1. THE CIRCUIT FINGERS.

If you are right-handed: Place your left hand palm up. Connect the tip of your left thumb with the tip of the left little finger (not your index finger).

If you are left-handed: Place your right hand palm up. Connect the tip of your right thumb with the tip of your right little finger.

By connecting your thumb and little finger, you have closed an electrical circuit in your hand, and it is this circuit you will use for testing.

Before going on, look at the position you have just formed with your hand. If your thumb is touching the tip of your index or first finger, laugh at yourself for not being able to follow directions, and change the position to touch the tip of the thumb with the tip of the little or fourth finger. Most likely this will not feel at all comfortable to you. If you are feeling a weird sense of awkwardness, you've got the first step of the test position! In time, the hand and fingers will adjust to being put in this position and it will feel fine.

Circuit fingers can touch tip to tip, finger pad to finger pad, or thumb resting on top of the little finger's nail. Women with long nails need not impale themselves.

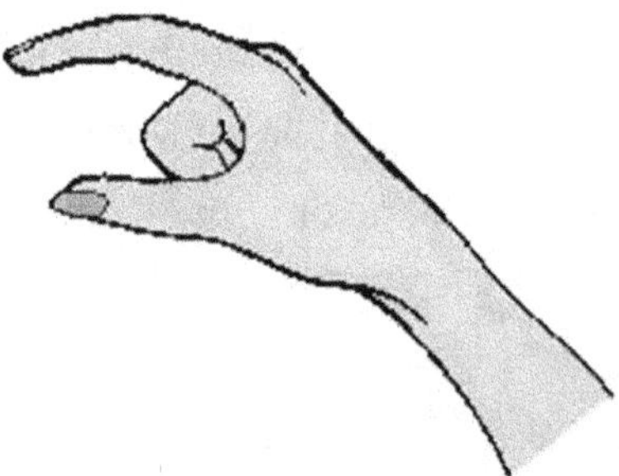

2. THE TEST FINGERS. To test the circuit (the means by which you will apply pressure to yourself), place the thumb and index finger of your other hand inside the circle you have created by connecting your thumb and little finger. The thumb and index finger should be right under your thumb and your little finger, touching them. Don't try to make a circle with your test fingers. They are just placed inside the circuit fingers that do form a circle. It will look as if the circuit fingers are resting on the test fingers.

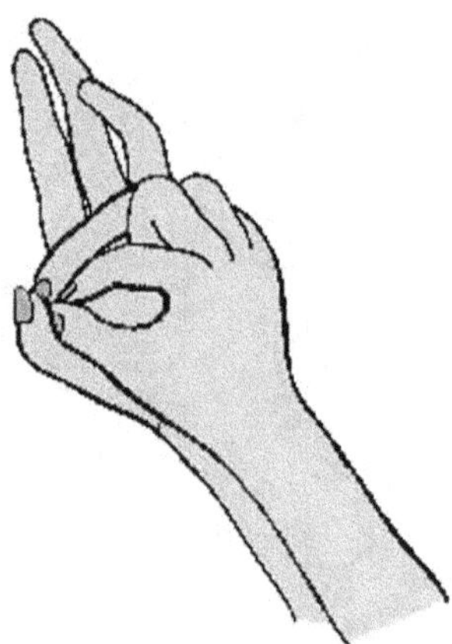

3. **POSITIVE RESPONSE**. Keeping this position, ask yourself a yes/no question in which you already know the answer to be yes. ("Is my name _____?") Once you've asked the question, press your circuit fingers together, keeping the tip-to-tip position. *Using the same amount of pressure,* try to pull apart the circuit fingers with your test fingers. Press the lower thumb against the upper thumb, and the lower index finger against the upper little finger.

The action of your test fingers will look like scissors separating as you apply pressure to your circuit fingers. The motion of the test fingers is horizontal. Don't try to pull your test fingers vertically up through your circuit fingers. This action sometimes works but it is not as reliable as the horizontal scissors action.

The circuit position described in step 1 corresponds to the position you take when you stick your arm out for the physician. The testing position in step 2 is in place of the physician or other convenient arm pumper. After you ask the yes/no question and you press your circuit fingers tip-to-tip, that is equal to the doctor saying, "Resist my pressure." Your circuit fingers now correspond to your outstretched, stiffened arm. Trying to pull apart those fingers with your testing fingers is equal to the doctor pressing down on your arm.

If the answer to the question is positive (if your name is what you think it is!), you will not be able to easily push apart the circuit fingers. The electrical circuit will hold, your muscles will maintain their strength, and your circuit fingers will not separate. You will feel the strength in that circuit.

IMPORTANT: Be sure the amount of pressure holding the circuit fingers together is equal to the amount of your testing fingers pressing against them. Also, don't use a pumping action in your test fingers when applying pressure to your circuit fingers. Use an equal, steady and continuous pressure.

Play with this a bit. Ask a few more yes/no questions that have positive answers. Now, I know it is going to seem that if you already know the answer to be "yes," you are probably "throwing" the test. That's reasonable, but for the time being, until you get a feeling for what the positive response feels like, you're going to need to deliberately ask yourself questions with positive answers.

While asking questions, if you are having trouble sensing the strength of the circuit, apply a little more pressure. Or consider that you may be applying too much pressure and pull back some. You don't have to break or strain your fingers for this; just use enough pressure to make them feel alive, connected and alert.

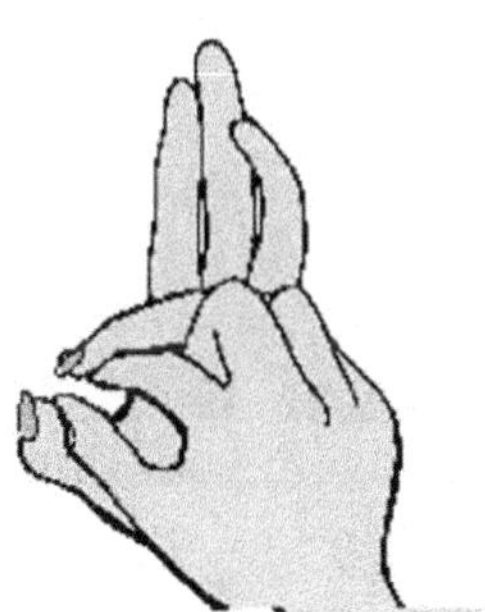

4. **NEGATIVE RESPONSE**. Once you have a clear sense of the positive response, ask yourself a question that has a negative answer. Again press your circuit fingers together and, using equal pressure, press against the circuit fingers with the test fingers. This time the

electrical circuit will break and the circuit fingers will weaken and separate. Because the electrical circuit is broken, the muscles in the circuit fingers do not have the power to easily hold the fingers together. In a positive state the electrical circuit holds, and the muscles have the power to keep the two fingers together.

How much your circuit fingers separate depends on your personal style. Some people's fingers separate a lot. Other's barely separate at all. Mine separate about a quarter of an inch. Some people's fingers won't separate at all, but they'll definitely feel the fingers weaken when pressure is applied during a "no" answer. Give yourself time and let your personal style develop naturally.

Number 5 below added by author.

5. INAPPROPRIATE TO ASK or UNABLE TO ANSWER

Something a lot of people forget to take into account is that some things are best left unasked, thus the inappropriate to ask.

Also, the answer may be unavailable at this time. Someone (human or otherwise) may be in the process of making a decision that will affect the answer.

Ask for clarification on how you get answers by saying:

1) Show me "YES".

2) Show me "NO".

3) Show me 'INAPPROPRIATE TO ASK".

4) Show me "UNABLE TO ANSWER".

Any time the answer is unclear, I suggest you ask, "Is it inappropriate to ask". If the answer is yes drop the question and avoid trying to weasel your way around it. It may be ok to ask later.

Any time the answer is, "unable to answer", is it because the question/statement was unclear, the 'Mind" question was different than the verbal/conscious question or someone still needs to make a choice that will affect the answer?

If you are proficient in the use of a pendulum the same process applies.

Number 5 above added by author.

Also, if you are having a little trouble feeling anything, do your testing with your forearms resting in your lap. This way you won't be using your muscles to hold up your arms while trying to test.

Play with negative questions a bit, and then return to positive questions. Get a good feeling for the strength between your circuit fingers when your electrical system is balanced and the weakness when it is short-circuited or imbalanced. You can even ask yourself (your own system) for a positive response and then, after testing, ask for a negative response. ("Give me a positive response." Test. "Give me a negative response." Test.) You will feel the positive strength and the negative weakness. In the beginning, you may feel only a slight difference between the two. With practice, that difference will become more pronounced. For now, it is just a matter of trusting what you have learned; and practicing.

Don't forget the overall concept behind kinesiology. What enhances our body, mind and soul makes us strong. Together, our body, mind and soul create an environment that, when balanced, is strong and solid. If something enters that environment and challenges the balance, the environment is weakened. That strength or weakness first registers at the physical level in the electrical system, and it can be discerned through the muscle-testing technique; kinesiology.

Above is adapted from http://www.holistichealthtools.com/muscle.html

Below is adapted from http://www.healwithhope.com/#!muscle-testingapplied-kinesiology/c20dx

Two Person Method

(Glenn's note: Both people need to be clear, unswitched, connected to Sources LOVE and have no preconceived notions or desires as to the answer.

Step One: Are you ready for testing?

(Note: This step is useful in determining if your body is in balance, which will ensure optimum results)

1) Stand facing the person who will be testing you (if you need to be seated when doing this make sure your legs are not crossed and your feet are flat on the floor).

2) Extend your arm straight out to the side.

3) Tester will rest one hand on your shoulder and with the other hand use their pointer and middle fingers to **apply light pressure** to your wrist, and will say "resist", as you make an effort to prevent your arm from going downward. You should be able to resist the pressure and hold your arm in position.

4) You will then repeat this process, except the tester will put the hand that was on your shoulder, palm up, on the top of your head and again apply pressure to your wrist area, saying "resist", as you again make an effort to prevent your arm from going downward.

5) If you arm becomes weak, this means you are ready for further testing. If not, try tapping on the center of your chest (breastbone area where your thymus is located) with your fingertips for a minute. The tapping stimulates the thymus gland, which in turn powers up the immune system and this can improve your polarity. You can then retry this, and if your arm goes weak, you are ready to proceed.

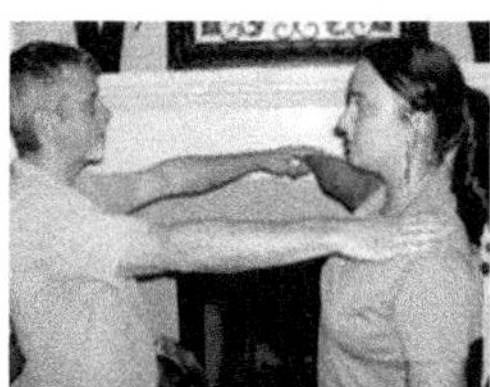 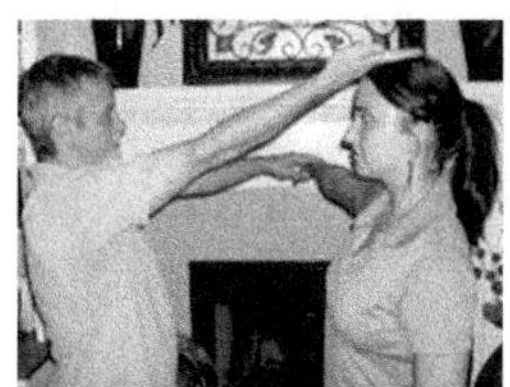 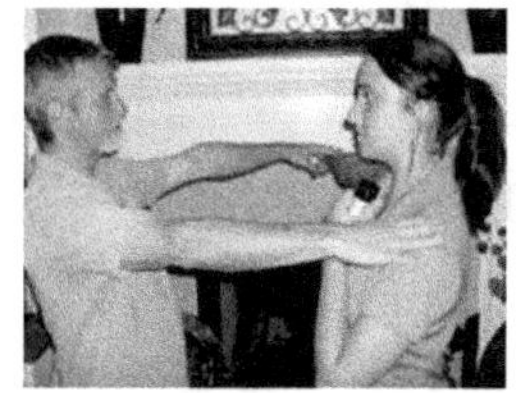

Step Two: Ready to Test

1. You and the tester will face one another in a standing position (if you need to do this in a seated position, make sure you do not cross your legs, and that your feet are flat on the floor).
2. You will hold the item you are testing to your chest (breastbone/thymus area) with one arm and the other arm extended straight out to the side.
3. Tester will rest one hand on your shoulder of the arm that is holding the object while applying firm pressure to your wrist area with their pointer and middle fingers on the other hand, as you make an effort to prevent your arm from moving downward. Their other hand will be resting on your shoulder of the arm that is holding the object. To enhance results, you or the tester will say, "this (product) is compatible and agrees with (your name)… resist". If your arm remains strong, the body's response is yes and the item agrees with you. If your arm weakens and goes down, your body's response is negative- the item weakens you.

Above is adapted from http://www.healwithhope.com/#!muscle-testingapplied-kinesiology/c20dx

Below is by the author

Use Of The Pendlum To Get Anawers

From Great Spirit

The form of questions are critical. Remember that answers are binary (yes or no) with no in-between (Includes "Inappropriate to ask" or "unable to answer"). Keep questions simple and single. Avoid: ***and, or, not, but*** and ***if*** in any form.

Music, light, and pictures all have an influence. They should be controlled in the environment where testing is done. The environment should be neutral. In an everyday environment the surroundings should be kept as positive as possible.

Drink some water and remember to breath while testing.

The pendulum is an "extension" of the Unihipili or subconscious mind through which questions consciously, either mentally or orally, are directed to the Unihipili.

The objective of using the pendulum is to gain a good working relationship with your Unihipili (Subconscious) and get guidance beyond the logical/conscious mind.. The Unihipili (Subconscious) is the key.

The pendulum needs to be cleansed before and after using. When not in use, keep it in its own pouch or container. One way to clear it is to say "indigo, ice blue, white" with the intent to clear and clean it.

Carefully teach your Unihipili (Subconscious) the following directions of movement for the answers he/she will give. Go over it slowly to give the Unihipili (Subconscious) a chance to learn.

For me:

(1) Circular movement means "inappropriate to ask" or "unable to answer."

(2) Vertical movement means "POSITIVE" or "YES."

(3) Horizontal movement means "NEGATIVE" or "NO."

Your movement of the pendulum may be different. Make sure it is consistent and accurate.

Above is by the author

Below is adapted from http://www.craniosacral-biodynamics.org/cranialrhythmic-impulse.html

Cranial Rhythmic Impulse Method

Cranial Rhythmic Impulse

One of the rhythms oriented to within craniosacral therapy is called the *cranial rhythmic impulse* (CRI). This term was later shortened by some practitioners to the *cranial rhythm*. It commonly manifests at rates of 8–14 cycles a minute. The CRI is the most common rhythm discussed in many cranial courses. The CRI is a conditional rhythm that expresses historical forms and central nervous system and autonomic nervous system activation. It is not a tide, but is an artifact of the presence of unresolved conditional forces and patterns within the system.

Whereas the Long Tide is totally stable, and the mid-tide is relatively stable, the CRI is highly variable in its expression. The CRI is first and foremost an expression of the conditions of our lives as these conditions must be met and centered in some way. It is a superficial rhythm generated as tidal potencies act to center the unresolved inertial forces of trauma, toxins, pathogens and experience in general. It is generated as potency acts to neutralize, contain and compensate for the unresolved forces of experience. The CRI is a level of perception within which effects and affects, such as tissue resistance, fluid congestion, emotional charge, and psychological form, are more easily perceived than the underlying tidal forces that order them.

One way to think of this is to use the analogy of ocean tides. The Long Tide is like the gravitational field phenomena that generate the ocean tides. In turn, the tide generated within the waters of the ocean is like the mid-tide and is relatively stable, while the CRI is like the variable wave forms on the ocean's surface generated as the tide meets the resistance of the land and the motion of the conditioned winds above. The CRI is thus like the waveform riding on deeper tidal motions and is not a tidal phenomenon.

Any unresolved force held within the system, such as unresolved trauma or toxins, will affect the expression of the CRI in some way. As the system experiences inertial forces of various kinds, and as it holds the effects of these as autonomic nervous system affect, tissue resistance and fluid congestion, the CRI changes in rhythm, tone, and tempo. It is a composite rhythm, which manifests in relationship to all of these factors.

Whereas tissue motility within the mid-tide is sensed to be a unified and holistic dynamic, in the CRI tissue structures may seem to be separate in their expression of motion. Because of this, the CRI has become associated with what is known as *craniosacral motion*, the individual and particular motions of tissue structures sensed within its faster rate. It is like looking at things from the outside-in with a narrow field of viewing. These externalized motions are commonly termed *flexion/external rotation* and *extension/internal rotation.* At the level of the CRI, inertia within the system may be perceived as tissue resistances within and between the separate structures.

Above is adapted from http://www.craniosacral-biodynamics.org/cranialrhythmic-impulse.html

Below is adapted from

http://www.cranialtherapycentre.com/a-beginners-guide-to-craniosacral-therapy/

A Beginner's Guide to Craniosacral Therapy – Core Connection By Sophia Schweitze to better understand how the cranium rhythm can be used as a form of A.R.T.

Jenny started medical school at the University of California-Davis this year. She leads a normal life. She's agile and intelligent. You never would have thought that in fourth grade, when she was 11, her future wasn't as promising. Severely dyslexic, Jenny was reading at a first grade level. She struggled. Then her mother saw an advertisement for a class in craniosacral therapy. She took her daughter in for treatment.

"What have you done with Jenny?" exclaimed a teacher a week later. "This isn't the same child." Jenny's learning problems had disappeared days after her first and only craniosacral therapy session which lasted all of 30 minutes. Hugh Milne, an osteopath from Britain and director of the Milne Institute in Big Sur, CA and author of *The Heart of Listening: A Visionary Approach to Craniosacral Work* (North Atlantic), has treated many children like Jenny: "Children often respond immediately," he says, noting that the change is often permanent. For Jenny, it gave her opportunities she wouldn't otherwise have had.

While not everyone believes that craniosacral therapy works, proponents say it has alleviated many diverse symptoms: from chronic pain, ear infections, jaw pain, migraines, and joint stiffness to pregnancy problems, depression, autism, anxiety, dyslexia, spinal cord injuries, coordination impairments and anger.

You might think of it as a gentle massage technique, or a cross between chiropractic or osteopathic maneuvers and hands-on healing. Quiet and relaxing, sometimes inducing restful sleep, it's been labeled mysterious. In reality, craniosacral therapy addresses a rhythmic system at the core of our physiology – the pulse of energy that flows between our head and pelvic area. It's as essential, measurable, and tangible as our breath and heart rate. The craniosacral system follows a rhythm, and the skull bones accommodate its pulse. Just as a cardiologist seeks to improve the cardiovascular system, a craniosacral practitioner evaluates and optimizes the pulse of the craniosacral rhythm. This is a gentle, often deeply intuitive technique. "It's a form of bodywork consisting of exceedingly light finger and hand pressure upon the cranial bones and the sacrum, and upon the involuntary movements of these bones," says Dr. Milne.

(Glenn's note: As a form of A.R.T. there is no need to touch the person. With practice the rhythm can be sensed without touching.)

The History of Craniosacral Therapy

In the early 1900's, in osteopathic school, William Sutherland came to the conclusion that skull bones are capable of shifting – an unorthodox medical view still not fully accepted today. A visionary and pioneer, sensing the far-reaching spiritual implications of his findings, he developed a treatment method making him the grandfather of cranial osteopathy.

Then John Upledger, D.O., author of *Your Inner Physician and You* (North Atlantic), made a major leap when he discovered why skull bones move in 1975 (explained below) and started to talk openly about the cranial rhythm. He began working with students who weren't medical professionals. Ten years later, he founded the Upledger Institute in Palm Beach Gardens, FL. The word was out: "It works!" In 1994 the American Craniosacral Therapy Association, also located in Palm Beach Gardens, FL. was created. Last year, the Craniosacral Therapy Association of North America, which has a sister organization in Europe, was set up with headquarters in Canada.

Still a new kid on the block when compared to other medical modalities like Ayurveda and Traditional Chinese Medicine, craniosacral therapy with its many schools and forms is now one of the fastest growing practices in alternative medicine. Hundreds of massage therapists are being trained, while many psychotherapists, acupuncturists, physiotherapists, chiropractors, dentists and medical doctors are adding it to their list of tools. Increasingly used as a preventive health measure, this practice seems to be blurring the boundaries between the health professions because it's easy to learn and safe.

How does craniosacral therapy work?

On a surface level, the practitioner works with the bones of the skull and the pelvis. This affects, in turn, the deeper layers of membranes and cerebrospinal fluids in the spinal canal, the brain, and the spinal cord itself. Why is this important?

A pulse through the fluids proceeds through the entire craniosacral system, like a tidal wave, from the sutures in the skull to the spinal cord. Cycling about six to ten times a minute, it causes tiny movements measuring no more than one or two sixteenths of an inch. "It's a hydraulic system," says Dr. Upledger, noting how all the components work together to regulate the pressure of these fluids on the brain. "There is an optimal circulation, which depends on constant mobility," he explains. When the membranes and lubricating liquids lose their freedom to glide freely, we hurt and symptoms start.

It's easy to imagine how even the slightest impact, lesion or distortion can stretch or strain this delicate system. Any infraction causing nerve endings to alter their perception and signals can negatively affect our entire well-being. Craniosacral therapy helps the body to re-establish an unobstructed wave, which is how symptoms disappear.

There's also a unique and undeniable spiritual dimension to this practice: "The craniosacral wave isn't just a physical phenomenon," says Dr. Milne. "It's also a field of information and intelligence. In the tiny movements of the system, and in the still points in between, is consciousness." Dr. Upledger refers to this intelligence as the inner physician, explaining: "The inner wisdom which knows what is wrong, why it's wrong, and how to correct it. The body tells the therapist what needs to be done."

Thus, craniosacral work is based on a shamanistic and meditative approach as well as on physiological facts, making it doubly powerful.

What happens during a session?

“There is no need for a client to tell me verbally what’s wrong,” Dr. Upledger says. He prefers to remain open to the body’s own language, although some therapists may want to talk with you first. For the hands-on work to be most effective, you should wear loose, thin clothing. This way, the practitioner can better sense what’s going on in your body. You’ll be asked to lie on your back on a massage table.

By quietly resting the hands on your skull and sacrum, the therapist evaluates your craniosacral rhythms. (Glenn’s note: As a form of A.R.T. there is no need to touch the person. With practice the rhythm can be sensed without touching.)This in itself can create a shift in energy. Sometimes, the therapist’s hands become aware of places along the column where energy is stuck or heated. She then uses the bones of the sacrum and cranium as “handles” to manipulate the deeper layers of fluid and membranes. No instruments or devices are used.

In sessions lasting 45 – 60 minutes, clients and therapists work closely together. “Ideally,” says Dr. Milne, “the client clears a mental space so something might occur.” The therapist waits and listens. You might feel a quieting down, a sinking in, and a deeper awareness. The whole idea is that the practitioner works with such gentleness and subtleness that the body itself can do the healing and necessary adjustments. “It’s a question of trust,” Dr. Upledger notes. A session can be described as a physically connected meditation, in which hidden information in the craniosacral system reveals itself.

Healing then can occur via the corrective mechanism known as the still point, the spontaneous quiet between waves. Typically, you have one every three to four minutes, and it lasts from five to sixty seconds. It’s a natural pause in the rhythm. Synchronizing and optimizing the waves, still points are like sighs. During sessions, when you’re more sensitive to them, they’re like moments of deep relaxation in which you let go and return to yourself. It’s the moment of insight, when you “get” it.

Does it always work?

While many conventional doctors and even some alternative practitioners are skeptical of this method, there’s lots of proof that it works. Anecdotes abound and just three to five sessions often give astonishing results.

Still, you have to keep in mind that craniosacral therapy is more of a preventive than a cure for serious illnesses. Dr. Upledger states in his book that “craniosacral work is most often a complement to other forms of treatment – not an alternative.” Its effectiveness depends on the cause of a complaint (i.e. whether a problem deals directly with the nervous system), the accessibility of the underlying cause, and what related contributing factors are present. An open, receptive attitude helps. “When client and practitioner have no connection, there sometimes is no efficacy,” Dr. Milne says.

Scientific studies proving the validity of craniosacral work exist, especially in the osteopathic and dental medical journals. So why doesn’t everyone praise it? Provable as it is, it’s also a relatively new concept. Skeptics want to know about the long term effects as well as see more research before they give it any thumbs up. And, the mystery implied in the tactile almost hypnotic treatments stretches conventional thinking, even today.

The bottom line

So should you go for it? Look at it this way. For the most part, you don't have anything to lose, and you'll get a healing method that connects the physical, emotional and spiritual. Intuition, insight and the perception of facts are equally important. The whole is greater than the sum of the parts. Maybe, the mind can't understand the details – that the body holds the answers if we dare to be still enough to listen to the tide of the cranial wave, our core. That's what craniosacral therapy aims for.

Above is adapted from http://www.cranialtherapycentre.com/a-beginners-guide-to-craniosacral-therapy/

****

Personal Notes

Chapter 7
Physical

****

Below is adapted from'Five Levels of Healing' and 'Applied Psycho-Neurobiology' by Dietrich Klinghardt, M.D., Ph.D.

for the actual web sites go to

<http://www.klinghardtacademy.com/images/stories/5_levels_of_healing/Klinghardt_Article_5_Levels_of_Healing.pdf> (still available as of 12/27/14)

<http://www.mercola.com/article/applied_psycho_neurobiology/apn.htm> (still available as of 12/27/14)

<http://www.klinghardtacademy.com/Articles/ART-Laws.html> (still available as of 12/27/14)

The 5 Levels of Healing

By Dietrich Klinghardt, MD, PhD, USA

I developed this systematic model of healing in the 1980s and have been teaching it to practitioners all over the world since then. Many doctors and healers have been able to understand their own work better and have been able to make better choices for their patients and their own education based on this understanding. This model has already entered the heart and consensus reality of integrative medicine worldwide.

In recent years we have observed a worrisome over- emphasis on the value of nutritional supplements. Few people have gotten well by taking supplements alone. Dietary supplements have disappointed! Much lip-service is given to energetic and psychological care. However, very few practitioners offer practical solutions as a natural and regular part of their consultation or treatment protocol. Please consider these ideas below. Our patients need care on all levels of their existence. It works. People really can recover from their chronic illness. But patients have to shift their way of being in the world on a deep level. They need your guidance! For every vitamin there will be a better one tomorrow. Every deep conflict that is resolved, is resolved for good. Learning is forever. Vitamins are not.

We exist in different dimensions - simultaneously. The physical body exists within a sphere of invisible etheric bodies that each have their own anatomy and physiology. There is an alive and profound interaction between the different levels. When we die, the physical body stays behind – it is cast off. There seems to be a process after death in which also the emotional body (second level) and later the mental body are cast off. The 4 th and 5 th body survive. Every ancient culture knows this system and has described it in different terms. This healing system has evolved from interpreting the yoga sutras of Patanjali (which are believed to be over 10,000 years old) and from trying to express this ancient knowledge with contemporary language. Applying this knowledge in a practical way is taught by myself and the Institute of Neurobiology in Bellevue, Washington.

Treatment

There is much ongoing discussion as of how to approach the 1st level. Everything from the Physicians' Desk Reference (PDR), herbal medicine, low potency homeopathics to orthomolecular medicine belongs here.

I use a basic set of principles:

a) Diet based on "Diet Therapy Software (Food Pharmacy)". It scans all current and old literature on illness-specific diet research- including these 4 books: Metabolic typing Diet (Wolcott), Protein Power (Eades), The Blood Type Diet (D'Adamo), No grain Diet (Mercola) and prints out the most appropriate diet for this client in minutes. ART* food sensitivity test (takes minutes, no lab fee, very accurate)

*ART stands for "autonomic response testing". It is the author's advanced composite of hands-on examination techniques that uses changes in the autonomic nervous system as primary indicator of practitioner-elicited stress responses in the client's body. The "direct resonance phenomenon" allows scanning of the body for specific infections, toxins and other "invisible" problems.

b) Exercise at least 20 min every other day – balance between aerobic (running, bicycling, etc.) and anaerobic (weights) and stretching (yoga).

c) Balancing the hormones: 24 hr urine hormone test (Meridian Valley Lab, Kent WA) every 6 months for the first 2 years. I give herbal and homeopathic drainage remedies (Sanum, Heel) for the organs which test with ART during the course of treatment. Use homeopathic hormones including HGH to balance the hormones, before resorting to "real" hormones

d) Heavy metal detoxification and treatment of infections belongs to this level as well (see my earlier "neurotoxin elimination protocol" and "Lyme disease protocol" in Explore!).

e)Always supplement the missing minerals (best test: autonomic response testing)

The Vertical Healing System: the 5 Levels of Healing

by Dr. Dietrich Klinghardt, M.D., PhD

When you carefully study the pyramidal order of the 5 bodies (table is later in this chapter), much is self evident and does not require further explanation. This healing system has evolved from interpreting the yoga sutras of Patanjali (which are believed to be over 10 000 years old) and from trying to express this ancient knowledge with contemporary language.

First Level

The lowest or densest level is the **physical body**. It is at the bottom not because it is less valuable. Instead, the physical body is the foundation upon which everything else rests. It is our connection to the earth and the source of our physical energy. The physical body is identical with what we see, feel, hear (i.e.: when we scratch it), smell and taste (if we lick it). It ends at the skin.

Second Level

The 2nd level is the **electromagnetic-body** or "body-electric". It is the summation of all electric and magnetic events caused by the neuronal activity of the nervous system. Since most somatic and autonomic nerves in the body travel in the longitudinal axis of the body and the nerve currents spread as electric fields along these nerves, the magnetic fields created by these forces travel perpendicular to this axis into space. Even though their strength decreases with distance from the body, they extend into space beyond the skin. Theoretically these bio-magnetic fields extend into infinity.

Third Level

The next higher body which I call "**mental body**" extends to infinity squared and the higher two levels extend beyond that. Only mathematics is able to conceive the expansive size of the higher levels.

Over the 25 years that I have been in practice certain orders and rules have emerged and become obvious that appear to govern the relationship between these 5 levels of healing. In turn, each level has its own laws and its own order which needs to be acknowledged and understood. I will try to summarize those observations, so that they may be helpful to others.

Each phenomenon that we observe in the physical realm seems to occur simultaneously also on the other 4 levels. In fact, the physical body is designed like a computer-screen which makes that visible and tangible which happens in the soul (the 5th level). However, you can have problems in the higher levels, which have not yet penetrated down to the lower levels. This is most known in acupuncture, where disturbances on the 2nd level are picked up by the practitioner (using pulse and tongue diagnosis and understanding early warning signs) before symptoms occur. The traditional Chinese medicine doctor was only paid when the patient's physical body remained healthy. He/she had to pick up the disturbance on the 2nd level long before it penetrated down to the 1st!

Fourth Level

The highest level, at which an interaction between physician and client is possible, is the 4th level. I call this level "**dream-body**".

The 4th level is a level beyond the mind and beyond language. It is the home of near-death experiences, past-lives, archetypes, spirit possession, ecstatic states, karma and the expression of unresolved trans-generational family issues.

The proper attitude on the 4th level requires to not hold an intention of wanting symptoms to improve but to hold the intention that after the work is done there is more love, harmony and respect.

Fifth Level

The 5th level is the plane of self-healing. I call this level the "**spirit-body**". The only relationship that exists here is the relationship between the individual and god. **A physician, psychologist or guru who claims that he can be helpful on the 5th level is being arrogant, misleading, dangerous and simply wrong.** Anyone, who truly has experienced this level will have an attitude of deep respect and understands that it cannot be explained using language. People, that talk often about "god", "angels" and other spiritual experiences are suspicious to me and usually phony. Many"New age" followers have significant unresolved family issues or guilt that is either taken on from another family member or "earned" through one's own mistakes. The pain and necessary healing work is often avoided by involving oneself in extensive spiritual practices, that never seem to resolve the real issues.

True healing requires simultaneous work on all 5 levels.

I will give an example:

First Level

The first level**, the physical body,** is the home of orthomolecular and conventional medicine . Let's assume a young female patient has the clinical diagnosis of "anorexia nervosa". We know that approximately 85% of these patients have a clinical zinc deficiency. Therefore the true diagnosis on the 1st level would be "zinc-deficiency". The laws that govern this level are the laws of biochemistry and mechanics. If you keep her on a life time of zinc supplements, she would probably stay reasonably well.

Second Level

However, looking at this patient at the 2nd and next higher level, the **electromagnetic body**, we may find that she has a hidden malabsorbtion syndrome caused by over activity of the sympathetic celiac plexus (which leads to vasoconstriction of the absorbing lymphatics and blood vessels in the gut). This condition may respond well to periodic treatment with acupuncture or neural therapy. The patient would start absorbing zinc from the food again and would improve without zinc-supplements. The 2nd level has an organizing effect on the 1st! The laws that operate on this level are the natural laws of neuro-physiology (or the practical stepped down rules of acupuncture or autonomic response testing -ART).

Third Level

Now let's look at the 3rd level, the "**mental body"**: this young woman may have an unresolved conflict with her father, who was very oppressive during her childhood - stern, punishing, critical and at times violent. The unresolved memory held in her limbic system is responsible for stimulating the hypothalamus and sending sympathetic stress messages to the celiac ganglion, which is now in a pathological state of chronic arousal. Finding and resolving this conflict with a targeted and specific approach such as Applied Psycho-Neurobiology ("PK") eliminates the focal area in the limbic system. The celiac ganglion cools permanently off and the patient starts to absorb zinc again - and gets well! The 3rd level has an organizing effect on the 2nd and also on the 1st level! Vice versa, without the absorption of food (1st level) and a functioning autonomic nervous system(2nd level) the patient would not have the energy and functioning mind required to remember the past and work with it in a healing way. The energy to do the necessary healing-work comes from the lower levels! Therefore it is best for the patient, to treat all levels simultaneously - take zinc during the initial treatment period and have some neural therapy at the beginning of treatment. The laws that govern the 3rd level are the simple natural rules that are being gradually rediscovered by modern psychotherapy: nurture and love a child, provide it with opportunity to learn, keep it safe, nourished and warm. Each violation of these natural needs has consequences, leading to fairly predictable distortions of the mind, nervous- and immune system. Other "laws" and natural orders have been outlined by the leading psychologists of this century.

Fourth Level

Now let us go to the 4th level, the "**dream body"**. The typical family-constellation in a young woman with anorexia looks like this: invisible to anyone on the outside, including the children in the family, the patient's father was deeply rejected by the mother - his wife - and subtly pushed her out of the family. The patient in turn is unconsciously loyal to the rejected father and holds the "magical belief" that if *she* disappears, the father would stay. "I leave for you" is the operative sentence and a sign of a deep and strong love and loyalty for the father. Anorexia is a way for the client to disappear. The fathers oppressive behavior (behavior belongs to the 3rd level) was his way of responding to the wife's rejection of him (which in turn triggered and restimulated his unresolved childhood issues). If the therapist can facilitate healing in this situation, which may culminate in the child saying in the therapeutic session to the father (who does not need to be present): "*Dear daddy! What happened between mom and you is none of my business. I am only your child. You are the grown-up and I am only your child. I trust that you can handle the issue with mom yourself! Look kindly upon me if I stay*" And to mom:" *Dear mom! I am only your child. Please look kindly at me when I stand by my father. He is the right and only father for me*". Healing on this level often leads to instant disappearance of the associated unresolved conflicts on the 3rd level, and - in this case - disappearance of the celiac ganglion dysfunction and therefore improved zinc absorption. Again, the energy required for this healing work has to flow upward from the lower energy supplying levels. Simple interventions on the lower 3 levels would be laying the foundation to make the work on the 4th level possible. The laws that govern the 4th level are the rules and orders of Systemic Family Therapy "discovered" by Murray Bowen and Bert Hellinger: in a family every member has an equal right to belong. If someone denies this right to one of the members, another member will try to balance the family by self-excluding him/herself. Other rules are discussed in the book: "Love's hidden symmetry" by Bert Hellinger, which is a must for anyone working on this level. Issues such as spirit possession, evil entities, alien takeovers and implants etc. seem to lose their grip on us when the family of the client is in a state where there is respect and love between all the family members of the system. A family system is comprised of the genetically linked persons of the last 3 generations (some people say 7) and all of their respective partners.

Fifth Level

What about the 5th level, the "**spirit body**" then? Here are a few hints: it would be a good start, if after resolution of the physical problem both the physician and the patient turned inwards and upwards with an attitude of gratefulness. For the client to do something "good" with the newly gained hope and vitality and clarity may be the appropriate concluding work on the 5th level. **Simply praying or meditating in a cave may be enough - but maybe not. If the work on the 5th level is not completed there may be a gradual relapse of the condition…**. The laws that are operative here are gradually revealed to us as we mature.

Conclusion:

The vertical healing system can be a valuable foundation for understanding truly what holistic medicine is and gives the practitioner and client a road map that makes it easier to navigate the sometimes chaotic landscape of healing techniques. Each level has its own order and its own laws which need to be understood. The lower 3 levels belong to the personal realm, the 4th and the 5th level to the transpersonal realm. Each higher level has an organizing influence on the lower levels. The lower levels supply energy to the higher levels and create boundaries for the individual to exist in. The practical conclusions for leading a healthy lifestyle and guiding a client towards wellbeing may look like this:

1) Put as much effort as possible into healing your own family. Don't rest, until there is love and respect between everybody in your generation and the two generations before you (Glenn's note: may go back 7 generations). The "family" includes children who have died early, aborted children, husbands that were excluded after a divorce, mothers that died at childbirth and uncles that died in a war. The healing involves relating and communicating to everybody that is alive and holding a loving memory of those who are gone.

2) Pump as much energy as possible into the lower 3 levels: eat right, sleep right, exercise and take your vitamins. Nurture your body-electric with massage, acupuncture, neural therapy, laying down by a waterfall, listening to good music and doing your yoga stretches. See a therapist to work through confusion and unresolved conflicts on the mental level.

3) Turn inward to investigate the 5th level. Don't follow anyone's advice. Create time and space to be alone. You need all of you, undistracted, to do this.

Remember,

True healing requires simultaneous work on all 5 levels.

Table showing the pyramidal order of the 5 bodies - Five Levels Of Healing:

		Level Body / Sphere	Our Experience At This Level	Anatomical & Conceptual Designation	"Diagnostic" Method	Related Medical Treatment & Healing Techniques
		5th Level Spiritual Body	Oneness with God, Satori	Spirit, Higher Consciousness	Knowing & Awareness	Self Healing, Prayer, True Meditation, Chanting
	Soul is a composite of Levels 2 through 4	4th Level Intuitive Body	Intuition, Symbols, Trance, Meditative States, Dreams, Magic Curses, Spirit Possession, Out of body & near-death experiences	Collective Unconscious, "No Mind"	Intuition, systemic Family constellation, Sound & VoiceAnalysis, Radiesthesla, Dream Analysis, Syntonic Optometry, Art Therapy	Applied Psycho-Neurobiology (APN) II, Systemic Family Constellation, Color and Sound Therapies, Shamanism, Hypnotherapy, Jungian Psychotherapy, Radlonics, Rituals
Emotional Body is a composite of Levels 1 through 3		3rd Level Mental Body	Thoughts, Beliefs, Attitudes, Long distance healing, Consensus reality	Mind & Mental Field [conscious & Subconscious mind], Morphic field, The "Will"	AutonomiC Response Testing (ART) I & II, Applied Psycho-Neurobiology (APN) I & II, Psychological interview· (MMPI), Homeopathic Repertoirizing	Applied Psycho-Neurobiology (APN) I, Mental Field Therapy, Psychotherapy, TFT, EMDR, Homeopathy
		2nd Level Energy Body	Feelings - [anger, Joy, etc], Chi [qigong "energy"], 6th sense & other "energy" perceptions	Nervous system, Meridians, Chakras, Aura, Bio-Electric system, GAGS, Microtubules	Autonomic Response Testing (ART) I & II, Thermogram, EEG, EKG, EMG, VAS, EAV, KInesiOlogy, Chinese Pulses, Kirlian Photography, X-rays, MRI, CAT scan	Neural Therapy (A & B), Microcurrent Therapies, Acupuncture, BodyWork/Touch, Breath Therapy, Yoga, Qigong, Meditation, Radiation Therapy
		1st Level Physical Body	Sensations [touch, smell, etc], Action, Movement	Structure & Biochemistry	Direct Resonance·- Autonomic Response Testing (ART) II, Physical Exam,Lab Tests, BDORT	Diet Therapy, Exercise, Osteopathy & Chiropractic, Surgery, Physical Therapy, Drugs & Herbs, Orthomolecular Medicine, Aromatherapy

****

Applied Psycho-Neurobiology (APN)

By Dietrich Klinghardt, M.D., PhD

All events in life are accurately recorded by the Subconscious. Whether the location of the recording is the brain or consciousness itself is not relevant for most practical applications. A memory can be complete and resolved or it can be unresolved. Unresolved memories can belong to one of two distinctly different categories:

1. The memory is always present - to different degrees - disturbing, haunting, relentless and painful. It keeps the person from being present in the moment. These patients are often highly dysfunctional. Post-Traumatic Stress-Disorder belongs in this category. Dr. Klinghardt refers to this condition as "Unresolved Psycho-Emotional Trauma". Significantly traumatic circumstances - usually in late childhood or young adulthood - are the cause of this condition.

2. The memory is suppressed into the Subconscious, the patient is not aware of all details of the original event and of the psycho-emotional impact it had and still has. These patients (all of us) are often fairly functional in life but have specific areas of dysfunction.

Both unresolved psycho-emotional traumas and unresolved psycho-emotional conflicts are the most common - or only - cause of illness, chronic pain, accidents, psychological problems, relationship and job-related problems. The neurophysiology involved is fairly simple:

Researchers have demonstrated that unresolved psycho-emotional conflicts create a significant bioelectrical disturbance in conflict-specific areas of the brain. The abnormal signals produce abnormal neuropeptides and abnormal electrical currents that reach the hypothalamus. From here, the signals travel in the autonomic nervous system to distinct target organs, which are - again - conflict specific. Chronic abnormal stimulation of, for example, the sympathetic fibers that reach the liver, creates chronic vasoconstriction, abnormal gating phenomena at the ionic channels of the cell walls and, of course, the presence of abnormal noxious neuropeptides and leads to chronic illness, pain, and other dysfunctions.

Theoretical Background

The nervous system of the conscious mind is the well-known and studied motor and sensory nervous system. The nervous system of the Subconscious mind is the autonomic nervous system, the stepchild of modern medicine. The Subconscious is in charge of the survival. It can, however, not distinguish between real danger and perceived danger. The memorized snake, that was responsible for an unresolved psycho-emotional conflict many years back, is as scary to the Subconscious as a real snake. Therefore the Subconscious uses the defense mechanisms (the term coined by Freud) to keep the unresolved psycho-emotional conflict down in the Subconscious.

It is the consciousness that will steer the person again and again in the direction of healing the original traumatic event. To resolve an unresolved psycho-emotional conflict, it has to be remembered by the conscious mind, understood, and the coupled response in the autonomic nervous system has to be disconnected. Dr. Klinghardt calls this process "un-coupling."

Applied Psycho-Neurobiology is a practical process of:

1) Having a dialogue with the Subconscious mind with the intention to uncover the unresolved psycho-emotional conflict.

2) Understanding the limiting beliefs that were formed as an attempt to resolve the unresolved psycho-emotional conflict and replacing them with freeing beliefs.

3) Uncoupling (disconnecting) the autonomic nervous system from the unresolved psycho-emotional conflict.

The method that consciousness uses to help the person to deal with an unresolved psycho-emotional conflict is to have the person repeat the same or similar situations until the person deals "successfully with the situation." This may or may not happen. When a therapist helps a patient to identify a repetitive painful theme (such as repetitive financial crises, repetitive failure in relationships), and helps to uncover and resolve the underlying unresolved psycho-emotional conflict, the patient's need to repeat the painful event ceases, the pattern is broken, the patient is free, and their life changes often immediately and significantly. Chronic pain and illness follow the same mechanism.

The Four Steps of Healing

1. Diagnosis

To establish the diagnosis that an illness or chronic condition or psychological problem is caused by an unresolved psycho-emotional conflict or unresolved psycho-emotional trauma, one has to remember several elements: the Autonomic nervous system is the peripheral nervous system of the Subconscious mind. If touching an ill part of the body or thinking of a particular life situation causes an autonomic nervous system stress signal, the Subconscious is involved in the problem. The Subconscious is usually only involved if there is a related unresolved psycho-emotional conflict or unresolved psycho-emotional trauma. Autonomic nervous system stress signals can be detected with biofeedback equipment or with kinesiological tests.

APN uses changes in the autonomic nervous system innervated muscle spindle as an indicator for the state of the autonomic nervous system. The autonomic nervous system and the test-muscle are our delicate testing instrument. Researchers have shown for over 30 years that whenever an unresolved psycho-emotional conflict is activated by a therapeutic dialogue or procedure, the prefrontal cortex becomes active. Again, muscle testing can be used to confirm activity in the prefrontal cortex. The changes after a successful treatment can be confirmed by a new objective test Heart Rate Variability Testing, which measures the function of the autonomic nervous system.

2. Dialogue with the Subconscious

As explained earlier, the Subconscious protects us from the content of the unresolved psycho-emotional conflict and avoids exposure, until we are ready. Whenever in the therapeutic dialogue a question is asked, or a statement is made, that points in the direction of the unresolved psycho-emotional conflict, the Subconscious sends a stress signal. By monitoring the signals elicited by the dialogue and steering the questions accordingly, the unresolved psycho-emotional conflict can be uncovered.

The rule of Three:

To uncover an unresolved psycho-emotional conflict, one must find

1. The exact time of the original traumatic event, the age of the person.

2. The circumstances (create an internal picture or short video-clip of the event).

3. The feeling that was not appropriately expressed at the time.

Uncovering Limiting Beliefs

Our belief systems are the programming of our bio-computer, from which we create our reality - current, past, and future. If we can exchange a limiting belief with a freeing expanding one, our reality, and therefore our life, changes - always for the better. At the time of traumatic events we are in an altered state, which is the state in which new beliefs are laid down and incorporated into our already existing belief systems.

To change our beliefs, we have to be in that identical state again. This is achieved with the previously mentioned dialogue. Now the limiting beliefs can be an original traumatic event without having heart palpitations, trembling, muscle tension. The need to repeat or perpetuate the painful event is extinguished.

The Unresolved Psycho-Emotional Conflict

For an event to cause an unresolved psycho-emotional conflict, several conditions have to be present:

1. The nervous system is in a vulnerable phase.

2. The person is in a situation where it is not safe to express their feelings. (Example: soldier in combat. He really feels fear but has to act aggressive)

3. An event happens which is perceived as shocking and that interrupts the anticipated normal flow of life (example: the first day of school).

Events That Frequently Leave Behind an Unresolved Psycho-Emotional Conflict

The intra-uterine period:

Emotional problems between parents at the time of conception or later during pregnancy

Thoughts of abortion

Attempted abortion

Feelings of older siblings about the ever-increasing loss of attention by the mother

Physiological problems in the womb (mother's smoking, amalgam fillings, alcohol abuse, illnesses, accidents, medical drugs - especially psychopharmacological medications taken by mother, malnutrition)

Being aware of a twin dying ("vanishing twin"), 6-10% of all pregnancies start as twin-pregnancies, less than 2% of pregnancies end with the birth of twins

Birth and the time before, during, and after (drugs, trauma,)

Post-birth trauma: needle pricks to heel, silver nitrate in the eyes, cutting the umbilical cord, circumcision and other invasive procedures often without proper anesthesia.

The early years:

Birth of younger siblings
Emotional climate with parents and older siblings
Weaning the baby (too early, too late, etc . . .)
Not breastfeeding
Traumatic toilet training
Relationship with babysitter
Early sexual abuse Drug use by parents
Physical abuse
Emotional abuse or abandonment
Neglect
Childhood diseases
Illnesses/hospital stays of a parent
Relationship to pets, nature, other kids
Kindergarten

The young years:

First day in school
Relationship to teachers and other students
Moving
Changing school
Academic performance
Athletic performance
Dealing/becoming conscious of physical impairment
The locker room
Relationship with kids of the opposite gender
Social roles
Roles in the family
Abusive parents

Puberty Adolescence:

Academic/athletic performance
First romance
Competition
Peer groups/peer pressure
Fights/injuries
Operations: tonsils, appendix
Dental interventions - placement of amalgam fillings (causes shyness, etc . . .)
Parties/dancing

Ritual abuse, cults, black magic
Sports
Accidents
Divorce of parents
Physical/emotional abuse
First sexual experiences
Abortion
Betrayal/broken trust in first deep, often non-sexual relationship
Disappointments
Depression/thoughts of - or attempted ñ suicide
College/separation from family/friends
First drug experience
Academic pressure

The grown-up years:

They never come
Relationship problems
Separation from a loved one
Broken friendships
Academic failure
Divorce
Death of a loved one
Financial disasters
Financial problems
Failure (job, university, relationship, sports)
Legal problems (jail, convictions)
Illnesses (of oneself or loved ones)
Diagnosis of a serious illness
Loss of energy
Loss of sex drive
Signs of aging

All of these events and circumstances may leave an Unresolved Psycho-Emotional conflict behind; Or the patient can negotiate them successfully and become more mature and stronger because of the way the conflict was negotiated and navigated).

Three laws of Autonomic Response Testing

1. The **First law of Autonomic Response Testing - <u>the law of resonance between two identical substances</u>** (this law has been most clearly identified by the research of Y.Omura,M.D.): if a substance is held in the energy field of a person and the indicator muscle weakens, the identical substance is in the body (resonance between two identical substances). If the substance is only in a particular organ, ganglion or other structure, the test substance has to be held exactly over this area. A variation of this test is the most common Autonomic Response Testing: the examiner finds a structure that therapy-localizes (while holding it, the indicator muscle weakens). The indicator-muscle becomes strong, when the resonating substance is placed anywhere on the patient.

2. The **Second law of Autonomic Response Testing - <u>Pointing</u>**: if the examiner therapy localizes more than one structure, ganglion etc. during the Autonomic Response Testing body scan or examination, two structures (or more) may be affected by the same toxin or infection, or one structure may affect one or more others. If the indicator muscle weakens while holding one of these structures but strengthens while holding another (which weakened when held alone), there is:

a) either a cause/effect relationship between the two

or

b) they are both affected by the toxin/infection.

The 2nd law of Autonomic Response Testing is therefore really a variation of the 1st law.

3. The **Third Law of Autonomic Response Testing- <u>Resonance between the examiner and the patient</u>** : the examiner's body acts exactly like any other substance held into the energy field of the patient. If the doctor is toxic with the same substance that is causing the patient's illness or that is stored in one or more of the patient's tissues, the test will be affected as outlined in the 1st and 2nd law of Autonomic Response Testing. Therefore, the 3rd law is really a variation of the 1st law also (but overlooked in any other school of kinesiology).

As outlined in the Autonomic Response Testing manual, the patient also has this effect on the examiner. Therefore no two examiners can find the same problems in a given patient, unless both examiners are free of stored toxins, infections, root canal filled teeth, untreated scars, active psycho-emotional conflicts, have not recently consumed foods they are allergic to etc. The 3rd law results in a simple postulate: the Autonomic Response Testing practitioner has to continuously strive to improve their own health. The practitioner should be "ahead" of their healthiest patient

Above is adapted from'Five Levels of Healing' and 'Applied Psycho-Neurobiology' by Dietrich Klinghardt, M.D., Ph.D.

for the actual web sites go to

<http://www.klinghardtacademy.com/images/stories/5_levels_of_healing/Klinghardt_Article_5_Levels_of_Healing.pdf> (still available as of 12/27/14)

<http://www.mercola.com/article/applied_psycho_neurobiology/apn.htm> (still available as of 12/27/14)

<http://www.klinghardtacademy.com/Articles/ART-Laws.html> (still available as of 12/27/14)

****

Below is adapted from http://members.iimetro.com.au/~hubbca/dr_dennis_myers.htm and http://www.life-enthusiast.com/cause-of-degenerative-disease-a-3526.html

PLEOMORPHISM

PLEOMORPHISM - a good basic explanation

by Dennis L. Myers, M.D.

Pleo-morphism means *many forms,* many or more (*pleo-*), forms or bodies (*morph-*). This is in contradistinction to *Monomorphism* which means one (*mono-*) body or form. Modern medicine, bacteriology, is founded on the idea of Mono-morphism where once a germ is a particular germ it always stays that way. According to this way of thinking a streptococcal germ is always a streptococcus. It only has one (*mono-*) form, it doesn't change into anything else.

Pleomorphism on the other hand maintains that "germs" occur in *many* forms beginning with the Protit, which can change into a virus, which can change into a bacteria, which can change into a fungus. Any of these forms, bacterial, viral or fungal can and do eventually, break all apart, and turn back into the Protits from whence they came. It starts all over again, life. The Protit never dies. This is a nature of life. It goes on no matter what. A germ is 'a beginning', that's all.

These Protits or colloids of life in our blood develop or change according to the condition (pH, etc.) of the blood. At some stages of their development they are outright pathogenic (make you sick) and parasitic. These are our *internal parasites*. These Protits can go in the other direction too and turn into cells we need. See *Live Cell Therapy* They can help regenerate organs.

The *internal parasite,* which exists in us always, is in contrast to *external parasites* with which we occasionally come in contact. This is where the germ theory actually holds relevance. This is the area of external microbes and parasites that when taken to extremes, intensifies into infectious diseases and epidemics which overwhelm the system.

Surprisingly, without having even the slightest idea of pleomorphic biology, medicine through hygiene, has accomplished much in this area. The fact is, opportunistic bugs, bacteria and viruses are all over the place, in our blood even. Modern science says this is not so, even though they are easily seen. Some of us get sick and some of us don't. As far back as the plagues of the dark ages some lived and some died. One third of the people didn't get plague. Nobody knew why.

Pleomorphism is a concept discovered in the early 1800's. It shows that 'germs' come from inside the body, from the "tiny dots" you can see in the blood with any microscope. These "tiny dots" of course are the colloids of life, or Protits.

As the environment that surrounds the cells becomes *acid, toxic, polluted*, these "tiny dots", Protits, change form, into the microorganisms that clean up the garbage, dead cells, toxins and the like, that are the result of the toxic condition. This is what bacteria, 'germs' are for.

When the host balance is destroyed, when the internal environment the Protits and cells live in, the *internal milieu*, becomes toxic and acid, the Protits lose their *symbiotic* (live harmoniously together) and life giving qualities and devolve downward, changing first into viruses, then into bacteria and finally into fungal forms, each stage of which is progressively more hostile to surrounding tissue cells.

Germs, all microorganisms, (viruses, bacteria, fungi and everything in-between) are the result, not the cause of disease!

Louis Pasteur was wrong!

His idea of the bacterial cause of disease was wrong!

If "germs" are there as a result, not a cause,

then to treat the resultant germs with antibiotics is, in theory and in fact, wrong!

This basic misconception about disease effects all aspects of medicine.

This is why this is a "new"... biology.

Louis Pasteur is said to have said on his death bed that really he had been wrong about his "Germ Theory" of disease. He said then, in so many words, that, it is not the germ that is the problem, it is the internal environment, the *internal milieu* that allowed the germ to develop in the first place that is the problem.

Add to this the error of William Harvey, who stated in 1651 that the cell is the smallest unit of life and the magnitude of this issue becomes even more apparent. That was more than 300 years ago!! and still, to this day, this fallacy has not been corrected even though Bechamp (1816-1908) demonstrated that the smallest unit of life was what he called the *microzyma* and Enderlein again published in 1921 and 1925 that the smallest unit of life is not the cell but the *Protit*.

One should treat the cause, not the result. The idea of *anti-biosis*, anti-biotic (anti-life) is one way. The opposite of anti-biosis is PRO-BIOSIS (for-life), which is what Eclectic Medicine is about. It's not "alternative", it's Eclectic. "Alternative medicine" is just a popular anachronism for Eclectic. None of this is new and it isn't alternative.

As these "little dots", Protits, change form, they can change into organisms that are more and more detrimental to the body, they become independent and no longer live in harmony and in support of their host body. As they develop their individual form, they create their own metabolism and waste products of that metabolism, which is harmful to the local body fluids, causing pain and inflammation. Finally, this 'local' process, which develops in the body's "weakest organ", effects the Whole body.

It is not the organisms that make you sick,
it is the waste products of the metabolism of those organisms
that make you sick.

> "In reality, it is not the bacteria themselves that produce the disease, but we believe it is the chemical constituents of these microorganisms enacting upon the unbalanced cell metabolism of the human body that in actuality produce the disease. We also

> believe if the metabolism of the human body is perfectly balanced or poised, it is susceptible to no disease." (from the Annual Report of the Board of Regents of The Smithsonian Institution, 1944, The Rife's Microscope, The Smithsonian Report, 1944).

* * *

These disease processes, these changes in the blood, are difficult to fathom at first as they make themselves known in the beginning as functional disturbances (effecting the functions but not yet the structures of the body) in the most diversified organs such as by;

> headaches, high or low blood pressure, inability to maintain chiropractic adjustment, feeling poorly, unmotivated attitude, lack of appetite, drab complexion, coated tongue, wounds in the mouth, pimples, sores, hoarseness, runny noses and the like, ear noises, diarrhea, lowered capacity for seeing and hearing, depressions, weak, concentration or poor memory.

Later, these disturbances manifest as the chronic diseases we know so well today. See *How You Rot and Rust* by Steve Denk for another discussion on pleomorphism, pH balance, and oxidation/reduction which is another part of this whole process.

Medicines based on these ideas have been available and well researched in Europe for the last 150 years. Many of these medicines are available in this country now, this because of the heroic work of some very dedicated and wonderful people. There is more known about these older medicines than about modern drugs, simply because these ideas have been around for so long. Just because these scientists lived in the 1800s or before doesn't mean they were stupid

Pleomorphism is a concept that today sounds very strange. What pleomorphism is, however, cannot be denied as the vast amount of data that has been obtained over the last 180 years confirms what modern microbiologists are discovering, re-covering today. As noted, many people have been involved in this debate for a long time.

Dennis L. Myers, M.D.
1237 Washington ST
Indiana, Pennsylvania USA

Above is adapted from http://members.iimetro.com.au/~hubbca/dr_dennis_myers.htm and

http://www.life-enthusiast.com/cause-of-degenerative-disease-a-3526.html

****

Below is adapted from http://curezone.com/forums/fm.asp?i=919966

Pleomorhism and Body PH

Synthesis of the Work of Enderlein, Bechamps and other Pleomorphic Researchers

All mammals and most likely all other animals have two parasites. They are in a particular relationship and supplement each other.

Those two parasites or endobionts are called Mucor racemosus Fresen and Aspergillus niger van Tiegham.

Bechamp, Rife and Naessens could demonstrate that they are virtually indestructible. Neither carbonizing temperatures nor radioactive radiation can harm them.

Enderlein believed that they entered the cells of higher differentiated cell colonies as parasites while Antoine Bechamp believed that they are the essence of life in the cell.

The endobiont is always present and cannot be removed from the living cell; the clinical symptoms of a disease depend on the stadium of its development. This "fungal parasite" can be present in all tissues and organs.

Today's mainstream medicine is governed by consent of opinions rather than hard scientific evidence. This is the reason why false and fraudulent teachings can survive even though the truth has been known for a long time. There are basically three dogmas that are still adhered to:

The first and probably most disastrous error originates from Ferdinand Cohn, who in 1870 proclaimed that all microbes and bacteria have only one form (Monomorphism). This was also taught by Louis Pasteur. This teaching was opposed to the teaching of Antoine Bechamp who, roughly at the same time, could demonstrate that microbes can alter their form and appear as different germs (pleomorphism). Enderlein basically confirmed this and many other researchers after him have too.

All microbes that permanently live in our organism go through the same stages of their development. According to Enderlein they are as follows: Colloid - microbe (primitive phrase), bacteria (middle phase), fungus (end phase). Royal Rife could show that with increased toxicity the transformation goes into non-filterable forms, not visible with ordinary light microscopes (viruses). This also disproves Pasteur's infection theory as the "pathogenic bacteria" do not have to come from outside and in fact hardly ever do.

The state of development depends on the medium the germ lives in:

Primitive phases live in a strong alkaline pH.
Bacterial phases live in mild alkaline pH.
Fungal forms live in a medium acid pH.
Viral forms live in a strong acid pH.

In order to keep the right environment, every microbe produces an organic acid:

Mucor racemosus - lactic acid,
Aspergillus niger - citric acid.

The pathogenity of a particular germ lies only in one phase of its development. Our "constant tenants" are the only exemption where all but the very early stages are pathogenic. Only what Enderlein termed protit and chondrite are completely avirulent and play an important regulatory role in reducing higher virulent forms to primitive forms by copulating with them.

Those phases can be easily seen in living blood under the microscope, but only in "darkfield" as the small primitive forms are invisible in "brightfield."

(See “Darkfield Microscopy or Live Blood Analysis” later in this chapter.)

Even Louis Pasteur said in the last minutes of his life: "Bernard is right; it is the soil and not the germ, that makes the plant grow."

The second major error originates from William Harvey who stated in 1651 (!!) that the cell is the smallest unit of life. This statement can be easily understood considering the very limited magnification and resolution of the microscopes of his time. Enderlein demonstrated and published in 1921 and 1925 that the smallest unit of life is not the cell but the protit, named microzyma by Bechamp and somatid by Gaston Naessens.

The third error came again from Pasteur, who claimed that the blood is sterile, a piece of nonsense still taught by modern bacteriologists. A look through a high power darkfield microscope quickly disproves this theory (provided one wants to see). Pasteur had the talent of teaching the biggest nonsense and of making people believe it. It is now well known that he even falsified the results of his research when it did not show the results he wanted. He was also quite ready to plagiarize the results of others. The vaccination fraud is based on his manipulated "research". Whole generations of researchers followed his example. Modern "scientific medicine" became a collection of long disproven theories (blood clot and obstruction theory of coronary heart disease, germ theory and infection theory, single cell theory of cancer, etc.).

Microbes follow the same basic urges as other living beings:

a) Urge for survival

The urge for survival shows in the urge to eat. Our "endobiont" eats protein. Naturally it also has a typical metabolism which produces lactic acid (Mucor racemosus) and citric acid (Aspergillus niger) as mentioned before.

b)Urge for sex and multiplication;

The urge for sexual multiplication can be seen in the strong attraction in all stages of development from the very first stages, even when they are within blood cells. This leads to the formation of "clots" (called symplasts) which can block our blood vessels with the relevant consequences. Symplasts can be made out of colloids or symprotids, thrombocytes, erythrocytes, leukocytes or a mixture of all.

c) Urge for power.

The urge for power is seen in the urge to combine with other cells to form a higher, more stable form. In this combination (systatogenesis), all stages of development can be involved as this is not a sexual combination. But it is strictly within the same kind. This combination stops all forms in further development. On the other hand those formations are a major obstacle for the circulation. (They can be impressively demonstrated by staining and are often misdiagnosed as fungus structures.)

All those structures can be easily observed in the living blood, and from the observed stages we can draw conclusions regarding the health of our patients.

We have to finally stop believing in long disproven theories and stick to the old principles of science: when reality shows results different from the theory, the theory is wrong, not reality. Medicine has to change from a religion with popes and dogmas into a real science.

The most important terms created by Prof. Enderlein

Ascit: Name for all phases of bacterial development. The nuclei are in a row (katatakt)
Chondrit: Name for the very first primitive phases
Cystit: a Mychit with polydynamic nucleus
Dioekothecit: a Colloidthecit, filled with very small nuclei
Filum: linear unification of several Protits
Kolloidthecit: a cell without nucleus
Mych: the symprotit in its function as nucleus in a cell
Mychit: the first bacterial cell; it has only one nucleus
Protit: the most primitive form of every microbe
Spermi: the sexual cell = 1 Filum and 1 Symprotit
Symplast: the unification of all different phases in order to copulate
Symprotit: the three-dimensional unification of several protits (spherical shape)
Synascit: name for all bacterial phases with multiple nuclei in all directions
Systatogenie: the desire of primitive units to get together and form a more stable form
Thecit: a Mychit with more than 8 nuclei
Thrombocyte: a Mychit with 2 to 8 nuclei

Enderlein could find the following errors in the official teachings:

Bacterium paracoli is not a "degenerated" Bacterium coli but the Phytit of the endobiont.

The cause for the infectivity of filtrates from tuberculous material is the chondrit of mycobacterium tuberculosum. This was already proven in 1910 by Fontes (Brasil) - (cf. Mem. Instit. Oswaldo Cruz, I, 2, 1910, pg. 186).

Dostal could demonstrate that it is easily possible to convert mycobacterium tuberculosum into a spherical form (Basit) - (Wien. Med. Wochenschr., 60 Jahrg., 1910, pg. 2098-2100 and 63. Jahrg. 1913)

Fibrin is not the result of precipitation of protein but Thecits of the endobiont.

Megacariocytes (Metschnikov) are not "normal" cell elements but a mass infestation with primitive forms of the endobiont which disabled the ability of the cell and nucleus to divide. They do not originate from a leukocyte but from an erythrocyte!

The megaloblasts in anaemia perniciosa are not erythrocytes with nuclei but erythrocytes which have a colony of endobiont chondrites (pseudonucleus) inside them which causes the abnormal size.

Normoblasts are erythrocytes that do not have a nucleus but a pseudonucleus made out of colonies of endobiont-chondrites.

Macrocytes are enlarged erythrocytes without nucleus. This is also caused by a massive invasion of endobiont-chondrites.

Reticulocytes (Heilmeyer) are not erythrocytes with special organellae but erythrocytes that have a little "tree" of endobiont-chondrites inside.

The Round and Spindlecells of sarcomas do not contain round and spindlecells of the host. They contain round cells and spindlecells of mycelias of the endobiont.

Royal R. Rife stated that there are only about ten different germs. All the various appearances that are classified in bacteriology are adaptations (pleomorphic changes) to the toxicity (or varying pH) of the medium they live in.

He describes the pleomorphic development of E. coli as follows:

E. coli
salmonella typhi
mycobacterium tuberculosum
yeast forms
BX (bacterium X)
BY (bacterium Y)

Rife could isolate BX from all cancerous tumors, the BY he found in sarcomas. The change from one form into another happens in about 36 hours. BX and BY pass readily through 000 ceramic filters and cannot be seen in an ordinary light microscope.

Antibiotics severely increase the toxicity of the host organism, especially when highly toxic halogenated antibiotics are used. The "disappearance" of a particular germ from the culture does not mean that the germ is dead; it only became invisible due to its transformation into an invisible form. That means, that the host organism is now in a cancerous state.

Above is adapted from http://curezone.com/forums/fm.asp?i=919966

****

Below is from < http://csn.cancer.org/node/222132>

Lemon (Citrus)

A Miraculous Product To Kill Cancer Cells

Institute of Health Sciences, 819 N. L.L.C. Charles Street Baltimore , MD 1201. Jul 09, 2011 - 6:35 pm

This is the latest in medicine, effective for cancer!

Read carefully & you be the judge.

Lemon (Citrus) is a miraculous product to kill cancer cells. It is 10,000 times stronger than chemotherapy.

Why do we not know about that? Because there are laboratories interested in making a synthetic version that will bring them huge profits. You can now help a friend in need by letting him/her know that lemon juice is beneficial in preventing the disease. Its taste is pleasant and it does not produce the horrific effects of chemotherapy. How many people will die while this closely guarded secret is kept, so as not to jeopardize the beneficial multimillionaires large corporations? As you know, the lemon tree is known for its varieties of lemons and limes. You can eat the fruit in different ways: you can eat the pulp, juice press, prepare drinks, sorbets, pastries, etc... It is credited with many virtues, but the most interesting is the effect it produces on cysts and tumors. This plant is a proven remedy against cancers of all types. Some say it is very useful in all variants of cancer. It is considered also as an anti microbial spectrum against bacterial infections and fungi, effective against internal parasites and worms, it regulates blood pressure which is too high and an antidepressant, combats stress and nervous disorders.

The source of this information is fascinating: it comes from one of the largest drug manufacturers in the world, says that after more than 20 laboratory tests since 1970, the extracts revealed that: It destroys the malignant cells in 12 cancers, including colon, breast, prostate, lung and pancreas ... The compounds of this tree showed 10,000 times better than the product Adriamycin, a drug normally used chemotherapeutic in the world, slowing the growth of cancer cells. And what is even more astonishing: this type of therapy with lemon extract only destroys malignant cancer cells and it does not affect healthy cells.

Above is from < http://csn.cancer.org/node/222132>

****

Below is adapted from <http://www.naturalhealth-solutions.net/healthy-eating/lemon-water-excellent-for-alkalizing-cleaning-strengthening-nourishing-your-body> (No longer available as of September 2016)

Many other web sites have similar information.

Alkalinize the body with lemon

Lemon Water: Excellent For Alkalizing & Cleaning, Strengthening & Nourishing Your Body

Drinking **lemon water** helps you to stay healthy. Lemons are one of the very few foods on this planet to have more negative than positive ions. That is why they help for alkalizing the body.

Many of the foods we crave — coffee, carbohydrates, meats and sugar — are acidic. Our bodies do not function nearly as well when they are acidic. They are more susceptible to sickness, disease, fatigue, wrinkles etc.

Within minutes of drinking warm lemon water it can re-hydrate you. (unlike coffee which is loaded with the diuretic caffeine)

Lemon water helps clean the toxins out of your body. It assists in "*cleansing* the system of impurities" and will help prevent disease.

Your skin can't look healthy if your body is holding onto toxins! When you get rid of toxic waste in your system, your skin will show it first!

If taken regularly, lemon water acts as a tonic to the liver to stimulate its daily digestive and cleansing functions. Lemon is also believed to help dissolve gallstones and is a superior body alkalizer. Lemon water helps to lower blood sugar and can lower the glycemic impact of any meal.

It has been studied that even a little lemon can help you lower the absorption of sugars from the food you eat simply because of its high acidic content.

You can go one step further and eat some lemon peels along with the juice, this acts like a double whammy on weight gain.

Why? Because the pectin present in the peels helps in weight loss by becoming a gel forming substance in your stomach which reduces the sugar absorption from the food you eat.

It is well proven that lemon water accentuates the acidity of the digestive system and this helps the body in the absorption of calcium from the foods you eat. Calcium is then stored up in the fat cells.

It has been studied that the more the calcium content in fat cell, the more its ability to burn fat. So this another benefit of lemon juice for weight loss.

One of the most important benefits of drinking lemon water regularly is its effect on the gastrointestinal tract. Lemon water assists in the process of *digestion* and elimination.

The digestive qualities of **lemon water** help to relieve symptoms of indigestion, such as heartburn, belching and bloating

Lemons have also been said to be good for the bones and fighting cancer; plus they have a great amount of vitamin C and potassium and is antioxidant-rich food. Limes are a great alternative if you have them more readily available.

Daily consumption of lemon water can make a huge difference in the appearance of your skin. It acts as an anti-aging remedy and can remove wrinkles and blackheads. Lemon water if applied on the areas of burns can fade the scars. As lemon is a cooling agent, it reduces the burning sensation on the skin.

Because of its high vitamin C content, it is used to prevent and treat many infections, hasten wound healing, and diminish allergies. Lemon water also relieves symptoms of asthma, tonsillitis, and sore throats.

Lemon is a diuretic. This means that lemon water is especially good for people with *urinary tract infections.*

And, lemon water is also used in *dental care*. If fresh lemon juice is applied on the areas of toothache, it can assist in getting rid of the pain. The massages of lemon water on gums can stop gum bleeding. It gives relief from bad smell and other problems related to gums.

How to make this magic drink: Squeeze the juice of two lemons — the heavier the better — into a glass of room-temperature water. Sip every morning and afternoon. Skip the sugar — it'll only cancel out all those amazing health benefits.

If you don't like lemons, use limes. To extract the most juice and pulp from the lemon, roll the lemon around on a table or the counter a few times.

Below is from <http://www.livestrong.com/article/500654-the-alkalizing-effect-of-lemons/>

Lemons are a refreshing addition to many foods and beverages and offer the nutritional benefits of vitamin C, vitamin A and potassium. Aside from their culinary and nutritional uses, lemons are thought to provide a variety of health benefits due to their alkalizing effects on the body. Consult your doctor before making any diet or lifestyle changes.

Digestion Effects

As a prime example of the wonders of chemistry, lemons, one of the most acidic foods we eat, become one of the most alkalizing foods once they are broken down in your body during the digestive process. Food scientists determine whether a food is alkalizing or acidifying by burning it in air to simulate the process of digestion, which, chemically achieves the same effects as combustion by flame, says naturopath and acupuncturist Michelle Schoffro Cook, D.N.M., D.Ac, author of the book "The Ultimate PH Solution: Balance Your Body Chemistry to Prevent Disease and Lose Weight."

Individual Variations

Lemons may be alkalizing or slightly acidifying, depending on your individual ability to break down, or metabolize, acidic foods, says Chirstopher Vasey, author of the book "The Acid-Alkaline Diet for Optimum Health: Restore Your Health by Creating PH Balance in Your Diet." Weak acids, including lemons and most fruits, whey protein, yogurt and vinegar are easier to metabolize and usually provide an alkalizing benefit. **<u>However, some people are less efficient at this digestive process and experience an acidifying effect from the same foods that are alkalizing for others</u>**. To determine which metabolic type you are, Vasey recommends using pH strips that you can purchase at a drug store to test your pH levels in response to different foods.

Kidney Stones

A study published in the August 2008 issue of the journal "Urological Research" found that supplementation with lime, a close citrus relative to lemon, had alkalizing effects that discouraged kidney stone formation, which occurs in an acid environment. In the study, participants with history of kidney stones consumed lime powder for three months. Results showed an increase in urinary pH, indicating an alkalizing effect of the lime extract and a decreased risk for kidney stone formation. Lime powder was as effective as potassium citrate solution at increasing alkalinity. Lime powder also decreased levels of oxidized lipids, while potassium citrate did not show this benefit. Researchers suggested that lemon consumption may also provide alkalizing effects for reducing kidney stone formation.

Low Sugar

Lemons, limes and grapefruit are low-sugar fruits that will provide alkalizing effects while not offsetting those benefits with the acidifying effects of sugar, says Robert O. Young, author of the book "The pH Miracle: Balance Your Diet, Reclaim Your Health." Lemon and lime contain about 3 percent sugar while a non-sweet grapefruit might contain 5 percent. Young recommends not taking lemon or lime half an hour before a meal or for 10 minutes after a meal.

Above is adapted from <http://www.naturalhealth-solutions.net/healthy-eating/lemon-water-excellent-for-alkalizing-cleaning-strengthening-nourishing-your-body> (No longer available as of September 2016)

Many other web sites have similar information.

****

Pleomorphic (Bion) Research

Below is from http://www.orgonelab.org/cart/xbions.htm

In the early 1940s in Norway, while on the run from the Nazis, Wilhelm Reich was observing, via high-magnification microscopy, the disintegration of organic materials into small energy vesicles, which he called *bions*. These bions, upon further observation and as documented with time-lapse movies, would organize themselves into basic life forms such as amoeba and paramecia. Various control procedures, involving high temperature and pressurized sterilization, demonstrated the reality of this "natural organization of protozoa". Reich came to believe that life did not originate only in some ancient, dark corner of history, but that life is being recreated every day, right under our noses, through the specific process of bionous disintegration and reorganization. He observed bions develop not only from *organic* materials, but also from *inorganic* materials as well. Before and since Reich, other scientists have also discovered what Reich called bions, giving them other names. However, Reich had one of the most comprehensive views as he was able to later connect the bions to cosmic life energy processes: what he called *orgone energy*. Presented here are works by many of the other scientists who have observed bionous processes, and the pleomorphic nature of cellular life. Unfortunately, none of the published materials by Reich on the bion question are in-print and available today from bookstores. Photocopies may be ordered from the Wilhelm Reich Museum Bookstore, PO Box 687, Rangeley, Maine 04970 USA, Telephone (207) 864-3443.

Above is from http://www.orgonelab.org/cart/xbions.htm

Pleomorphism - Sources of Information and Research

* **HIDDEN KILLERS: The Revolutionary Medical Discoveries of Professor Guenther Enderlein**, by DR. ERIK ENBY. This book focuses on Dr. Enderlein's live blood research and his development of "biological" medicines. Also includes the discovery and verification by others of bion-like microscopic vesicles at work in disease processes. More evidence on the pleomorphic nature of viruses, bacteria, and cells. 155 pp.

* **CELL WALL DEFICIENT FORMS: Stealth Pathogens (2nd Edition)**, by LIDA H. MATTMAN. A scholarly work outlining the development and persistence of unusual microscopical organisms (related to bionous decay?) in specific diseases, such as UTIs, meningitis, arthritis, leprosy, etc. Much new information; many photos. 404 pp.

* **THE BLOOD AND ITS THIRD ANATOMICAL ELEMENT**, by ANTOINE BECHAMP. The pioneer scientist's last work laying out in great detail the elements of his Microzymian theory of the organization of living organisms and organic materials. It shows that more than 100 years ago, the germ or microbian theory of disease was demonstrated by BŽchamp and those who worked with him to be without foundation and totally inadequate as an explanation of disease and its transmission. 217 pp.
* **BECHAMP, AN APPRECIATION**, by H. GRASSET. English translation of a 1912 publication reviewing the findings of Antoine Bechamp on microzymas, a bion-like microscopic particle. Import. 119 pages.

* **A NEW BACTERIOLOGY**, by S. SONEA & M. PANISSET. A controversial empirical work on bacterial symbiosis and pleomorphism; "... in nature, bacteria form a unified global entity in which all bacteria are linked, both genetically and by specific high-level functions." Fascinating work. 140 pp.

* **THE CANCER CURE THAT WORKED: Fifty Years of Suppression**, by BARRY LYNES. Documents the discoveries of Royal Rife and Arthur Kendall on the pleomorphism of bacteria, the powerful Rife microscope, and the effect of electromagnetic frequencies on cells and bacteria. Also details the repression experienced by Rife after the initial acceptance of his case studies on curing cancer. Again, the head of the AMA tried to buy the patent rights to Rife's discoveries, and when they weren't for sale, the AMA in collusion with the FDA, set out to destroy Rife. Import. 167 pp.

* **THE PERSECUTION & TRIAL OF GASTON NAESSENS, Galileo of the Microscope**, by CHRISTOPHER BIRD. Naessens' discovery of the somatid, a microscopic particle similar to Reich's bion, & the subsequent attack by the Canadian FDA. One of the more well-known researchers in the field of pleomorphism, he continues his research specializing in dark field microscopy. Import. 320 pp.

* **THE CANCER MICROBE**, by ALAN CANTWELL. JR. Outlines the author's extensive work, and the work of others such as Bechamp, Reich, and Livingston, on the discovery of a

specific cancer microbe, and the hostile reception of this discovery by an arrogant, power-hungry, and greedy cancer industry. 281 pp.

* **THE DREAM & LIE OF LOUIS PASTEUR**, by R.B. PEARSON. Critical look at how Pasteur built his reputation on the stolen discoveries of Antoine Bechamp. Reprint of the 1940s "Pasteur, Plagiarist, Imposter! The Germ theory Exploded". Provides a good historical background to the current controversy surrounding vaccination. 107 pp.

* **PASTEUR EXPOSED: The False Foundations of Modern Medicine: Germs, Genes, Vaccines**, by ETHEL D. HUME. A comparison of Pasteur's theories to Bechamp's more empirical discoveries on microzymas & pleomorphism. Import. 259 pp.

* **THE ORIGIN OF LIFE EXPERIMENTS OF ANDRIJA PUHARICH**, by THOMAS VALONE. Saltwater, under sterile conditions, can produce complex amino acid molecules, the building blocks of life according to the discoveries of medical researcher Puharich. This book examines his electrolysis process and research. 42 pp.

Darkfield Microscopy or Live Blood Analysis

Below is adapted from http://altered-states.net/barry/darkfield/index.htm

Blood analysis can reveal and pin-point many underlying issues which are contributing to a current health challenge and although not diagnostic in itself, Blood Analysis will highlight the factors compromising the ability to achieve balance and health.

Live blood analysis can play an important part in the process of tailoring any health plan.

The quality of the blood will be reflected in the way you feel.

(Live Blood Examination in the Darkfield according to Prof. Dr. G. Enderlein)

Darkfield Microscopy or Live Blood Analysis is a way of studying live whole blood cells under a specially adapted microscope. Digestive, eliminative and immune functions can be assessed as well as the presence of bacteria and other micro-organisms.

The darkfield microscopic examination of the freshly taken live blood is one of the most important examinations of the holistic medicine applied at the Tara Centre. It enables us to view the inner terrain (milieu) and to examine the functions of the red blood cells. It also shows the evolutionary stages of the smallest proteins (endobionts) which are found in every human body. We are also able to see any developed structures such as bacteria, virus and fungus. The darkfield examination shows the state of the blood cells, endobionts and the plasma in a functional and structural way, making bacterial processes and fungal pre-stages in the blood clearly visible.

The darkfield examination is most suitable for the evaluation of clients with chronic diseases; for children who are prone to infections; for recurrent bacterial problems; for candida and other fungal problems and also to answer questions concerning chronic problems of toxicity (e.g. amalgam disturbances).

The darkfield microscope is a vital instrument for the supervision of biological therapies. For example, therapy tests can be made by adding blood directly to the medication and by controlling its reaction. The examination is very motivating for the client because the results can be discussed and demonstrated live on the screen. It cannot be replaced by any other blood examination, neither by normal microscope examination, nor by blood tests sent to laboratories. The blood rapidly changes its function with changes of the inner terrain after taking a sample.

How is the examination carried out?

Using a very fine needle, a drop of blood is taken from the finger and directly placed on a glass slide. Without fixation or coloring, the blood is examined right after taking it through a special darkfield microscope with up to 1000x enlargement. The patient can follow the process via video transmission on a large screen if the microscope is set up to project. The examination lasts approximately 15 minutes. The blood can be examined again several hours after taking the sample. This procedure informs us about the speed of degeneration of the cells (shows cell resilience, the immune system and the degenerative tendency).

We recommend repeating this examination every 3 months during an isopathic and immune biological therapy.

This examination was developed and described by Prof. Dr. G. Enderlein. With this method he proved that co-relations exist between blood parasites, symbionts, bacteria and fungi. The main proven fact is that chronic diseases are created by increasing sickness tendencies of the endobionts and that bacteria, viruses and fungi developed in the human body, or are changed to pathogenic agents of diseases depending upon the inner terrain (determined by acid-base balance, protein content and level of trace elements). The existence of pre-stages which are not yet able to make one ill but that can endanger an illness can also be found in the darkfield examination. Therefore it is also an important preventative examination.

The isopathic remedies of the SANUM company (fungal and bacterial supplements) and the immune biological remedies significantly change the endobiontic system of the symbionts by reversing the ascending evolutionary cycles that could make one ill.

> Remedies developed by Dr. Enderlein and his associates consists of biological medications , some of which are homeopathically diluted to low concentrations , and suspensions of Mycobacteria or bacilli. Produced primarily today by SANUM-Kehlbeck GmbH in Hoya , Germany , the preparations work on the body on the whole (systemically) , although their effectiveness can be enhanced by local application. The biological medications contain benign protein particles , called protits , that fight disease-causing micro organisam (and assist antibodies produced by the immune system , according to research by Swiss biologist Haefeli). In addition , the bacterial medications stimulate the immune system response to disease.
>
> Unlike antibiotics and other drugs that often require strong doses to kill disease causing agents , Dr. Enderlein's SANUM medications work by changing the harmful microorganisam in the body fluids to non-aggressive forms, which permits gentle self-healing (isopathy). Harmful bacteria and their toxins are broken down and excreted through natural processes. Because these remedies promote healthy cell metabolism and

hormonal balance, the body's internal environment experiences profound changes that benefit the entire constitution. Therefore , when treating illness , combinations of different SANUM products , as well as natural medications produced by other companies , are often indicated to restore the internal symbiosis required for good health.

So what is Live Blood analysis by Darkfield Microscopy?

Some medical doctors, in Germany, refused to use the same method of microscopy as others in the mainstream in their profession.

They have developed the darkfield technique.

Under the darkfield microscope, which examines the blood live, rather than dead as is the accepted norm by main stream medicine, these researchers noticed that the human being was full of natural parasites.

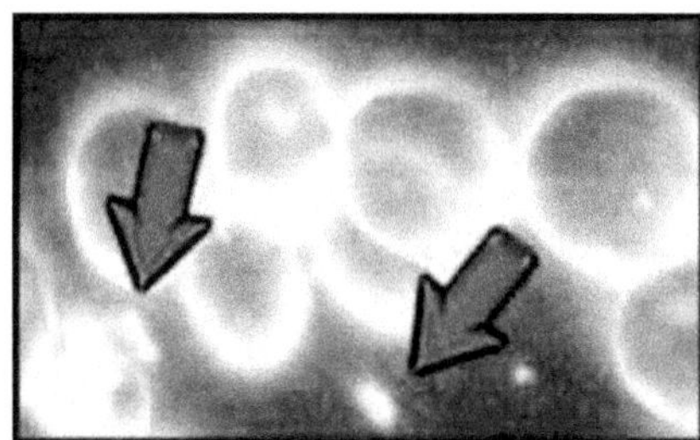

Parasites

These parasites, which live with the human being, are harmless in their early stages. But when they go into a higher cycle of development, they attack the red blood cells.

In AIDS for example, the parasites proliferate and the red blood cells are reduced to a jam-like consistency, prohibiting oxygenation and its transportation. Death ensues.

In essence, much research has been done now and with this darkfield microscopy technique, we know what a healthy blood picture looks like. Also we know what the very sick blood sample looks like. Most of us are somewhere in between.

A most impressive aspect of this darkfield technique is that when the right treatments, medicines and supplements are given, you can see, from visit to visit, the blood clearing before your eyes.

It is essential to be quite sure what medicines to give, so a tailored treatment plan is necessary. Each remedy is tested against your own body's resonance to ensure it is in tune with you. This identifies positively the correct blood cleansers required.

Other measures of course such as homoeopathic nosode therapy and high doses of vitamins, minerals and trace elements, may be required to get people well.

What exactly is a 'darkfield' microscope?

A darkfield microscope is simply a standard laboratory microscope, to which certain optical techniques are utilized to transform how light comes through the specimen being viewed. For example, let's say we are viewing live blood on a glass specimen slide. The normal mode of a microscope is called 'brightfield'. In this mode of viewing, light shines straight through the specimen. When light shines straight through a specimen, transparent objects are invisible. It's as if you were standing to the side of a sunny window gazing through dust. If there was a white wall between you and the dust, you'd never see the dust because it is transparent when trying to be seen against the white wall. However, if you put a black curtain where the white wall is, all of a sudden the dust pops into view. The darkfield microscope does the same thing. The specimen sits over a dark background (or field), and light is angled onto the specimen from the sides. Things that were once invisible now come into view.

What is a 'phase contrast' microscope? This is another way to view live blood for nutritional work. With this lighting technique, the light coming through the specimen is altered so that a portion of the light is shifted slightly out of phase with the original. The light now strikes the specimen and lights up invisible particles while also giving shades of gray. This is an excellent way of viewing blood for nutritional screening.

Live Blood Analysis: an alternative blood test

The microbe is nothing, the terrain is everything." **Claude Bernard, France 1813-1878**

Our blood is the vital fluid of life. Its condition is of paramount importance to the state of our health. Blood is responsible for transporting and delivering oxygen and nutrients to every cell in the body, and for picking up carbon dioxide and waste products for delivery to the organs of elimination. It also carries the immune system's white blood cells that are responsible for keeping us free of the pathogens that make us ill.

Conventional medical tests check the structure of the blood and can tell you a lot about the level of blood constituents and the status of certain diseases. Live blood analysis is not a replacement for medical blood tests, but these often don't reveal the causes of that feeling of 'unwellness', fatigue and chronic debilitation for which no medical reason can be found.

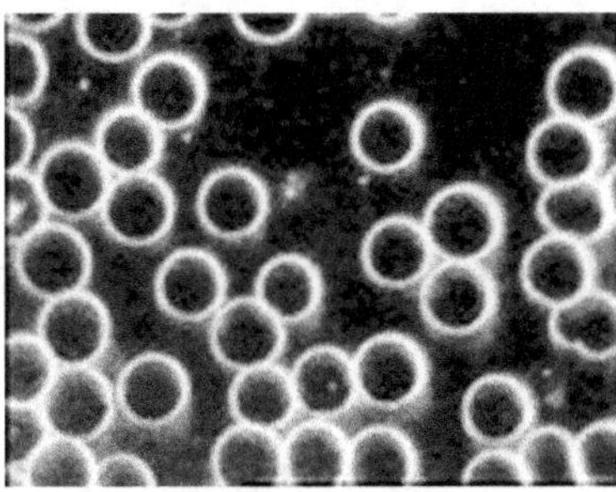

Healthy Blood

In live blood analysis a drop of blood taken from a finger prick is examined under a darkfield microscope. This illuminates the sample in a way that makes the minutest detail visible. The practitioner can see whether your blood is flowing like a river, or resembling a stagnant swamp - a sure indication of latent or undiagnosed problems. We all know that swamps are a breeding ground ....

Of paramount importance in achieving good health is the maintenance of a correct acid-alkali (pH) balance in every part of the body. Checking the blood pH visually under the darkfield microscope is the best indicator of what is going on in the rest of your system. An unhealthy pH balance will lead to problems. Most of us are too acidic due to the various stresses of life.

See the congested blood picture below.

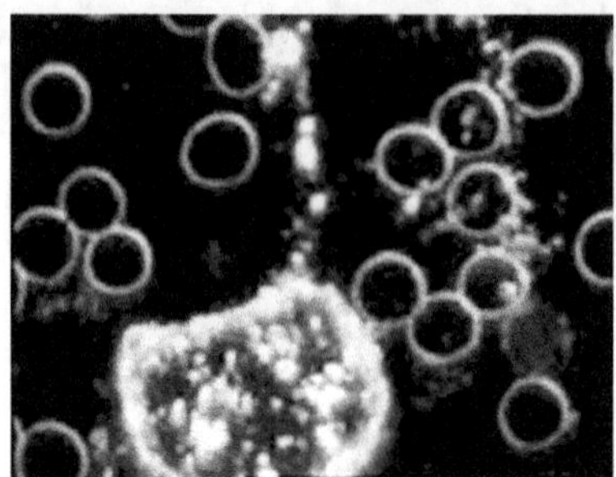

Chem-crystal
(consisting of fats, chemicals and other debris)

In the live blood picture the practitioner can see:

- The health and efficiency of the red and white blood cells
- Whether the red blood cells are free flowing or clumped together due to acid/alkali imbalance
- The health and clarity of the watery plasma that transports the cells
- Crystals consisting of fats, chemicals and other debris
- The quality of the terrain within your body in respect of the pH balance
- The health of your immune system

In the 21st century the world is a polluted place, our food is no longer natural and wholesome and we live under stress. These factors create disturbances in the delicate acid-alkali balance in our body fluid and tissue. This imbalance can create havoc within us leading to the unwellness that you may be experiencing. Your blood picture will reveal the degree of disturbance your body is having to cope with.

The main question to be answered is this:

Is your internal terrain a clean friendly environment for our helper organisms to thrive and the blood to flow, or is it a congested hostile environment beloved of toxic substances and pathogens?

A dry blood analysis as well as the live blood analysis may be done during the consultation.

Dry Blood Analysis

This is an additional test done during a consultation and provides a view of your health at a more general level. It can also reveal information about your health history, for example:

- Are there parasites still active in your system even though you may have had a 'tummy bug' many years ago?
- Is there toxicity in the digestive tract?
- Is there any heavy metals toxicity?
- Is your immune system supported sufficiently?
- Are there signs of weakness in any particular organs?

- Are there signs of free radical damage in your system?

Naturopathic Treatments

The basis of good health starts with what we put into our bodies. A tailor made treatment program and guidelines to help you make helpful changes to your lifestyle may include the following as well as additional modalities:

- Nutrition - how you should eat according to the results of your tests and condition being treated.
- Nutritional Supplements: Where there are chronic deficiencies or your condition could benefit from increasing certain nutrients, nutritional supplements will be recommended.
- Detoxification - if your condition has been brought about by your body storing up toxins due to over-exposure to chemicals, drugs, poor quality food or stress then a detox program will be recommended. This could involve following a detox diet for a period of time, undertaking an intestinal cleansing programme (not colonic irrigation) or a liver cleanse program or a short fast.
- Herbs - western herbal medicine is recommended to promote healing, relieve symptoms, support the organs and function and much more. Tinctures or capsules made up by a master herbalist to suit each patient and the specific condition being treated. Only the best, pure organic herbs are used.
- Specific remedies to deal with the disturbances in your system as seen in your blood picture.
- Acupuncture
- Manual Lymphatic Drainage
- Reiki
- Reflexology

Above is adapted from http://altered-states.net/barry/darkfield/index.htm

Below is adapted from http://www.explorepub.com/articles/darkfield.html (web page lo longer available as of September 2016)

Michael Coyle, Petaluma, California, USA (Explore Issue: Volume 8, Number 3)

Darkfield Microscopy - More Detailed

Fungus - The species specific understanding of, and difference between bacterial phase and fungal phase developments in blood pictures.

Diseases of the skin, digestive organs, urogenitary tract, mouth, etc. are caused by the multiplication and spread of fungal microorganisms known as mycelia. Mycoses (fungal infections) range in degree from unnoticed to fatal. They are directly related to asthma and allergic alveolitis reactions. They are dealt with by the immune system and competition from other microbes or earlier developmental phases of their own cyclogeny.

Fungal infections can be classified as;

Superficial - those that effect hair, skin, nostrils, genitals, and oral mucosa

Subcutaneous - those which occur beneath the skin

Deep - those which effect the internal organs, lungs, liver, bones, lymph, brain, heart, and urinary tract

These infections often occur in those on long-term antibiotic therapies, corticosteroids, and immunosuppressant drugs. This type of opportunistic infection is common in those with the acquired immunodeficiency syndrome, commonly known as AIDS, and also CFIDS (chronic fatigue syndrome.
(see http://www.dreddyclinic.com/findinformation/ff/chronicfatiguesyndrome.htm).

Primitive bacterial varlents (thecits)

Some of these fungal forms are received from the environment, are transmitted sexually, or are transmitted through mother's milk (see Candida albicans http://www.dreddyclinic.com/findinformation/oo/oralthrushandcandidaalbicans.htm). Candida remains in non-virulent phases of development until the terrain allows for its progression into more complex pathogenic forms. The efficacy of many of the SANUM fungal remedies is based on the sexual activity of the particular species of microorganisms (and/or the benign effect altogether, through competition, on the terrain) which is initiated through the process of reinstalling the microbial flora in the body in its apathogenic earlier phases of development. The flora that was installed then copulates with the pathogenic variety and shares the sexual information of the earlier phases, which, all things being equal (terrain modulation, removal of stressors, proper diet, lifestyle, etc.) causes the pathogenic form to convert or be reduced to the apathogenic variety. It is believed that the pathogens are also reduced in valence through the actual activity of the copulatory process.

The main causes of pathogenic albicans overgrowth are indiscriminate antibiotic application and dental inclusions from mercury tooth amalgams. Other factors include addictions to coffee, chocolate, drugs, unsafe sexual practices, immuncompromisation, stress, chemicals, radiation, improper diet, etc.

The fungal overgrowth occurs because its natural competitors have been removed in the case of antibiotic usage. In the case of dental amalgams or metals it is due to decreased immunity from immunocompromisation. The candida also adsorbs the mercury in the gut, thereby serving the function of keeping it from moving deeper in the system, to some degree. A good inclusion in a program of remedies for alleviation of mercury toxicity in the nervous system and brain is broken cell wall chlorella, because not only is it similar to the fungus in that it adsorbs the mercury, but also carries it away.

Primitive bacterial variants and cell wall deficient fungal species

I begin this section with a quote from "Cell Wall Deficient Forms: Stealth Pathogens" by Lida Mattman.

"Wall-deficient bacteria are called fungoidal as they produce **yeast-like** (emphasis added) budding spheres or simulate molds with elongated branching threads. (See chondrothecit and free chondrit plates, respectively). How, then, does one solve the dilemma of recognizing a wall-deficient fungus ? One can start with the vital activity in a fungal filtrate of Candida Albicans where the tiny 0.15-μm particles cannot possibly possess the wide hard wall of the parent. Colonies developing are usually comprised of twisted Gram-negative skeins so delicate that their course is interrupted by submicroscopic gaps. **These fine threads of growth have never been described as part of the classic growth of fungi**. (Emphasis added where bolded)."

The above description corroborates the findings of Dr. Günther Enderlein when he described such coccoidal manifestations as being either primitive bacterial variants or the most primitive mycelian strands.

Species of microorganisms which exhibit fungal variants in tissue (in vivo) are only microscopically visible in the blood as the most elementary and minute primitive spore forms, ranging in size up from approximately 0.15 microns. The notion that anyone is viewing fungus balls in phase contrast or darkfield is technically a complete misconception, as the forms which are being regarded as fungal developments are appearing in an alkaline milieu in the blood which will not support the fungal stages of development. This is not to say that the microorganisms may not be a species that can represent fungal developments elsewhere in the body. But this species specificity is indeterminable by viewing the fresh live blood, as there is no way to distinguish which species is being viewed without culturing it out through the use of a medium, or by aging or heating the sample, under some conditions. This process changes the phase of development into phases that do not appear, again, in the alkaline milieu of the blood. The forms that are being viewed (and mistaken for fungus stage) are actually colloid thecits, thrombocytes, chondrits, ascits, synascits, and mychits, all of which are part of the bacterial phase of development, which develops in an alkaline milieu. Also, the cell wall deficient forms, chondrits which are symplastic, are mistaken for fungal appearances. These chondrits do represent a fermentative process, but not at the level of a fungal appearance. They are even an earlier stage appearance than the most primitive cell wall mediated bacterial variants. The species, again, are unspecified upon appearance, as they are the same common stages that appear in many species of microorganism developmental cycles.

Some of these developments in polymorphic progressions are actually thrombocytes, and act as regulators, per Dr. Enderlein, and even (in some species) emerge from the red corpuscles in the serum. Some of these ball or balloon-like forms may become functionally pathogenic under certain specific terrain related conditions, and conversely, some of these devlopments certainly are an expression of the body's capacity to mount a defense. The possibility of making these determinations within this phase of bacterial cellular developments requires that the viewer be able to distinguish the number of nulei which appear within these delicate diaphonous bacterial cells. This microscopic imagery is only obtainable in a true, ultra illumination darkfield, employing superior plan achro or plan apo medical grade oil immersion iris diaphragm objectives and the proper condenser, which would be of the oil immersion variety also. This determination of the developmental progression of the bacterial variants is generally not able to be made in a phase contrast or differential interference field microscopically, because these fields generally do not provide adequate resolution to count the nuclei which appear within the ball-like cells that develop in conjunction with their primary nuclei (which are the cell wall deficient symprotits until they develope this cell wall mediated appearance). This is a crucial determination which must necessarily be made in order to distinguish the function which is related to the cell's very appearance.

It should also be noted that the pathogenicity of most microbes only exists in one stage of development, being either viral sized, bacterial or fungal. The exception to this is the Endobiont, Mucor racemosus Fresen, wherein any stage above the primitive stages is pathogenic.

Candida is never observed in its fungal phase in the blood because the blood's inherent alkalinity supports it's development only to a spore stage. These spores are extremely minute, and do not progress to visibility at the level where they can be distinguished from other similar microorganisms in the blood except possible through staining. The primitive bacterial phase microorganisms that are mistakenly called fungus may be part of the developmental phase of a species that has a fungal variant or may culminate as a fungus, but it is an error to call it a fungus in the blood. It is a species that has a fungal variant, and may also have a bacterial phase that occurs in the alkaline milieu of the blood. the ball-like appearances are bacterial phase developments.

These so-called 'fungal balls' appear very similar to each other, regardless of the number of nuclei, in phase contrast, but differ greatly in the higher resolution of Ultra darkfield. In the Ultra-darkfield the number and valence of the nuclei determines their status as potential regulators or pathogens, and it is a mistake to classify them all as the same thing, or as having the same function. Therefore, there may be a thecit (primitive bacterial) phase in the life cycle of the species Candida Albicans. It follows that if Candida appears in the blood, it may exhibit a bacterial phase rather than the fungal phase, or certainly will appear as cell wall deficient spores.

Virus is a primitive stage of development of all microorganisms share and this phase is virtually invisible in the present context of known light microscopy techniques. Microbes are ubiquitous and can rise to their pathogenic phase from any other phase, as their progression is not linear, and the progression is terrain dependent. One must know which stage is pathogenic in order to treat related conditions. For instance, acid-fast rods are not necessary for tuberculosis.

Candida Albicans

This may be one of the most controversial and misunderstood areas in natural health, especially as related to the correction of this fungal condition. I have observed more individuals with failed programs for this condition than any other. And by failed program, I am referring to ending up on what I call the "coping diet". Candida sufferers know this one well. It is the one where you live on this very weird, limited diet and supplementation regimen because you have been unable to determine and reverse the stressors that are causing and maintaining the problem. This problem of epidemic proportions is where great numbers of the victims of indiscriminate antibiotic use and amalgam dental fillings recipients have ended up.

Pathogenic albicans (chronic candidiasis, more commonly known as candida or thrush http://www.dreddyclinic.com/findinformation/oo/oralthrushandcandidaalbicans.htm) is generally caused by drug use, particularly antibiotic drug use, and poor diet, lowered immunity altogether, and metals, especially dental amalgams. Mercury will promote the growth of Candida, as it adsorbs the mercury and thereby protects the system. Candida cannot be effectively dealt with without dealing with the dental issues first. This is not an optional appraoch, but necessarily part of the primary approach.

The progressive decline which occurs as related to these mycotic conditions does so in this order. First the antibiotics (which are aimed at E-coli, strep, staph, etc, infections) wipe out the benign and necessary floras in the gut. The presence of these benign floras (L. acidophilus lactobacillus, bulgaris, B. longum, L.plantarium, L. salivarius, S. faecium, S. thermopilus) is necessary for the equilibrium in the flora system which keeps the competing (potentially pathogenic) yeast forms in check and allows these ever present yeast forms to be a natural occurrence which is apathogenic. The natural balance is maintained through competition of the multiple microbes which are present. It is interesting to note that many physicians treat this condition with additional antibiotics, causing tremendous problems. Many use Nystatin or other antifungals which can cause the creation of a resistant strain of fungus. They just mutate around it. The preferable remedies would be benign pro-biotic remedies such as SANUM Albicansan, Fortakehl and Pefrakehl which neither create nor further these harmful situations.

When their natural regulators and antagonists are wiped out through antibiotic drug use, the potentially harmless floras (colloids), which are generally kept in check, become more highly developed and propagate in massive numbers in the gut and tissues (and thereby contribute to a conversely high alkaline pH in the blood), while producing their own species specific acids which maintain the terrain that they require for their maintenance and propagation. In this environment they become more and more virulent and even penetrate and root into the intestinal walls and invade the cells. These fungal microorganisms become quite at home in the cell, and can be considered to be a third primary potential parasite, along with Mucor and Aspergillus, because of the advent of runaway antibiotic usage over the many years. The only difference is that there is no known symbiosis occurring from the presence of Candida Albicans in the body.

Certain vegetable species colloidal microorganisms produce particular acids to maintain their environment. Examples of this are:

Mucor lactic acid

Aspergillus citric acid

Penicillin penicillic acid

The **developmental life-cycle of microbes require differing pH conditions**. Some microorganism species find their culminant phase of development in the bacterial phase. The different phases of development of microorganisms require the following terrains for development:

virus, microbe, or primitive form strongly alkaline

bacterial phase weakly alkaline

fungal phase acidic

(Refer to section on lemon water which raises the body's pH into an alkaline state and flushes the kidneys)

This developmental process is related to leaky gut syndrome, as the tissues are weakened, even by the infection. The microorganisms continue to multiply and then invaginate the venous wall (in spore form) and are carried again out of the bloodstream and multiply in the tissues where they deposit their acids, thereby enhancing the acid pH which they require for propagation. This is why individuals with candida feel acidic. At this point in the total progression of the problem, it is not just because their diet is acidifying. An acidifying diet may be one of the original factors which contributed to this complex problem, though. At this stage it probably will not be possible to balance the pH through diet alone, because of the proliferation which is creating and maintaining its own environment, at that point, through the processes inherent to its upward development which are related to the production of acids. To achieve the necessary optimum pH balances, these individuals must use some combinations of Alkala (or other bicarbonate combinations), baking soda baths, **lemon water** and maple syrup combination (juices only where tolerated), fresh pineapple juice, and electrolyte solutions such as Cell Food, macro minerals, and all citrus fruits and their juices (again, if tolerated). At this point the reader may think, "Fruit juices are full of yeast and sugars. Doesn't this feed the yeast?". This is true, but the point should not be to try to create a dietary approach in order to cope forever with the problem, but rather to just create a diet which is tolerable and supportive to elimination and then to deal with the problem therapeutically with other means being the primary methods. The imbalance is not created strictly by dietary imbalances and is not eliminated in this fashion either. I will elaborate to some degree on these approaches further on in the article.

pH balancing and gut flora enhancement or replacement alone will not affect this condition, and most practitioners experience temporary results or failure if they attempt this in combination with an exclusively dietary approach. Most will find some relief with this approach (diet combined with flora replacement) but will then end up living off of the shelves of health food stores, on a continual supplementation regimen that addresses some percentage of the associated symptomology and pathology. The reason for this failure is that the candida has the upper hand in the gut and also systemically, and has to be weeded out first or simultaneously, through utilization of therapies that the yeast cannot mutate around (as in the case of Nystatin and other antifungals).

These therapies may include SANUM remedies (isopathic combinations), ozone, colloidal silver, Beck's box, and Rife type or other electromagnetic field generators. These therapies may be effective in numerous different ways and for varying reasons and must be recommended and guided by an experienced practitioner who will know how to combine all of the different elements. Often individuals expect immediate, symptomatic relief. In reality, one should expect to feel worse first, as a great deal of eliminative activity is in order. So it is important to understand that this condition was not created in all of its severity overnight, and it may take a fair amount of time in order to reestablish balance. For severe fungal infections a good approach is to utilize Utilin, Latensin, Pefrakehl, Notakehl, and Albicansan, w/ Alkala, colon cleansing, and kidney and liver drainage. Again, the stressors must be removed first or simultaneously.

The SANUM remedies reintroduce the original form of the microbe which appears in the body and is harmless, before it mutated. In a regulated pH environment this benign form copulates (exchanges information) with the pathogenic forms and they devolve into their original apathogenic forms and can be maintained in the range of development.

The mode d' employ of Rife generators is to disturb the microbe's progression through the application of electrical Herzian fields and also through the stimulation of interleukin II and other immune factors.

The Beck box emits pulsed micro-amps causing the blood and tissue cell membranes to oscillate, thereby interfering with the microorganisms ability to parasitize the cell by entering it and using its components for protection from the immune system. The cell membrane opens and closes rapidly, flushing the serum in and out, taking with it microorganisms which would otherwise be using the cell interior for its store of nutritional reserves and as an environment in which to replicate or develop into more advanced phases of manifestation. Simultaneously, nutrients are carried in and out, and feed the cell at a much more effective level.

Ozone stimulates interleukin II, alkalinizes the body through the production of ash, oxygenates the blood and tissues, and provides higher forms of oxygen (03 through 013?, or higher depending how it is produced) which share electrons with bacteria, virus, fungus, toxins, chemicals, and reduce all to ash or nonpathogenic forms.

Colloidal silver interferes with the enzyme system that the anaerobic microbes use for respiration. Therefore they cannot mutate around it or become resistant and are eliminated instead. Special care must be taken with colloidal silver to use one that is strong enough and simultaneously supplement the gut flora, as the silver can also interfere with aerobic microorganisms. Failing to supplement the flora, or using a product that only contains 3 to 5 parts per million of silver, appears to be the main limitations in terms of effectiveness. Naturally this approach, like any other, must be accompanied by a full regimen that includes cycles of purification, balancing, and rejuvenation. Contrary to popular gossip to the contrary by invested promoters, there appears to be some negative side effects to colloidal silver consumption, when used over long periods of time and in relatively high amounts. These include drainage problems and the destruction of intestinal floras. For some, the results of oral use have been complicated gastro intestinal dysbioses and Fortakehl, Albicansan and Pefrakehl and other SANUM preparations in combination may be a better approach as they do not tend to produce those negative results.

Many individuals have been known to exhibit extreme Herxheimer's (healing crisis) reactions with silver. This has particularly been a problem with chronic fatigue syndrome. Lymphatic drainage (homeopathic, herbal, or 714-X, which also regulates the immune system) along with juicing, consumption of a minimum of eight 8 oz. glasses of Crystal Energy water and/or other natural fluids such as juices and herbal teas, colonics or colemas, lymphatic massage, dry brush massage, bouncing exercises, and walking are all required in combination with colloidal silver as well as the other aforementioned approaches. It is not useful or necessary to load up the body with unnatural numbers of metals such as silver over extended periods of time in order to maintain good health. It is better to understand the overall biological terrain requirements and meet them through the adjustment of lifestyle. Nevertheless, it may be very useful to apply colloiddal silver for a measured period of time because of its ability to interfere with the repiratory enzymes of the microorganism. They also cannot mutate around this effect.

Ozone will cause less of a negative reaction than silver. The reaction will not as likely be a result of the breakdown of toxins, but rather congestion in the lymph and liver. This is because the ozone reduces toxins to ash, so they don't get recycled through your bloodstream as poisons on the way out (and by association, through the brain). The Rife and Beck therapies also require all of the same drainage requirements, and the lymphatic thumper (Beck's design) may be useful while the fungus is being reduced. The best approach, as always, is to combine elements based on the individual's tolerance and needs. Diet alone most likely will not correct this condition of candida overgrowth, but is certainly a necessary adjunct to any program. The dietary needs and reactions will be observed to change greatly after the problem has been addressed.

Many people have been misled through the wrongly held beliefs of most primarily dietarily oriented natural therapists on this subject. Therefore, I recommend that practitioners understand that the microbe must be reduced both in number and also to its apathogenic form, while adjusting the pH. Acidophilus replacement is not the answer, as the higher phase dominant yeast forms (which have overwhelmed the immune system's capacity to control them) are at such a high valence that they just feast on or suppress the installed lactobacillus strains when the subject is without proper therapeutic intervention. This mycotic condition was not generally created through dietary means alone, and although diet will be extremely necessary and instrumental in a program of complete recovery, it will not on its own be adequate therapeutically, which is the overwhelming and ongoing experience of the numerous masses who are led in the direction of this belief. The immune response is so overwhelmed that the body temporarily needs a "second immune system" in the form of the aforementioned therapeutic approaches, or other effective means.

All of the aforementioned therapeutic approaches (excepting Rife type generators, for some) also relate to how to deal with Chronic Fatigue Syndrome, although there are also many other factors, (especially sociological) which need to be dealt with. See *The Four Underlying Causes of Illness and What to Do About Them* by Michael Coyle, for a more complete explanation regarding these syndromes.

It may or may not be necessary for the client to eliminate all yeast containing products (breads, cakes, pastries, yeast related supplements), from the diet. The elimination of these foods is only necessary if they are reactive to them. There is no sound basis to the notion that yeast, such as brewer's yeast, feeds fungus. Yet individuals with fungal conditions can be reactive to almost anything, including yeast containing foods and food supplements. Metals are also an extreme deterrent to recovery.

Since microorganisms compete for terrain in the body, it is a necessary and useful corrective approach to supplement body floras once the proper therapeutic intervention has been established. The gut should contain a great deal of beneficial microorganisms, even measurable in pounds. Flora replacement is therapeutic in that the floras will compete with anaerobic microorganisms and thereby reduce their number, especially once therapeutic intervention has reduced the valence of the pathogens. This is why aerobic gut microorganisms are considered to be an indispensable aspect of the immune system, and should be present as at least 50%, and optimally 100%, of the flora content in the gut.

A good formula for gut flora supplementation, both after and during a program of correction of mycelium dysbiosis, is any flora product which contains:

L. acidophilus
B. longum
L.planaterium
L. rueteri
L. salivarius
L. bulgaricus
E. faecium
S. thermopilus
Fructo Oligo Sacharrides
Calcium ascorbate
Trace minerals

Albicansan and Pefrakehl are specifics for fungus, and Notakehl and Okubasan for reestablishing gut flora. The water drawn off of hulled barley, drunk, is also useful in reestablishing flora. Use one part barley to one part water, leave it overnight, and drink freely.

Many fungal disorders respond well to a series of courses of Latensin, Notakehl, Pefrakehl, Fortakehl and Albicansan. Reactions may accompany these remedies, and they should only be administered by a trained health professional. These remedies are not antibiotic, but probiotic, and work remarkably well. Because the type of fungal dysbiosis which is occurring will not be determinable in the blood picture, the remedies must be applied on the basis of other forms of testing such as point testing, Kinesiology, etc.

A strong empirical understanding of how the condition presents and what the primary stressors are in the subjects total life picture is likely the most important means of evaluation of both condition and remedy.

About the Author

Michael Coyle is a Natural Therapist, researcher and educator, and the author of the definitive "NuLife Sciences Applied Microscopy for Nutritional Evaluation and Correction" Workbook text. Michael generally conducts monthly or bimonthly training for health care practitioners in live-blood analysis.

Above is adapted from http://www.explorepub.com/articles/darkfield.html (web page lo longer available as of September 2016)
Michael Coyle, Petaluma, California, USA (Explore Issue: Volume 8, Number 3)

****

Below is adapted from:
<http://articles.mercola.com/sites/articles/archive/2014/05/08/heavy-metals-glyphosate-health-effects.aspx?e_cid=20140508Z1_DNL_art_1&utm_source=dnl&utm_medium=email&utm_content=art1&utm_campaign=20140508Z1&et_cid=DM45823&et_rid=514705428> 05/08/2014

Autism And The Connection To Vaccines, Heavy Metals, Glyphosate, Lack of Sleep, Lack of Sunlight, Lack of Sulfate

DETOXINGING THE BRAIN -Heparan Sulfate is needed to DETOX the brain

Heparan sulfate is needed to carry toxins out of the brain.

By Claire I. Viadro, MPH, PhD

Neurological disorders, autoimmune diseases—they seem to be everywhere these days. Scientists writing in *Neurology* in 2007 estimated that the burden of neurologic illness affects "many millions of people in the United States."

Autoimmune illness, too, is at epidemic proportions—nearly 24 million Americans as of 2012. These trends are disturbing enough in their own right, but even more disturbing is the general scientific apathy about *why* the surge in these diseases is occurring.

Why do the causes of these alarming epidemics remain "underrecognized and underaddressed?"

Stephanie Seneff is one of the all-too-rare scientists who *is* trying to ask the questions and connect the dots. Dr. Seneff is a senior research scientist at the MIT Computer Science and Artificial Intelligence Laboratory with an illustrious career and lengthy publication record.

Of late, she has been using computer science and natural language processing (NLP) techniques (NLP is a field of computer science, artificial intelligence, and linguistics) to delve into the impact of environmental toxins on human health.

She has developed some particularly convincing hypotheses relating to autism and, more recently, cancer. At the Third International Symposium on Vaccines presented in March 2014 as part of the 9th International Congress on Autoimmunity, Dr. Seneff was one of 15 speakers invited to present scientific research by the Children's Medical Safety Research Institute (CMSRI) on the adverse health effects of aluminum adjuvants and aluminum-adjuvented vaccines.

She discussed "a role for the pineal gland in neurological damage following aluminum-adjuvented vaccination." Along the way, she made many fascinating connections between various strands of her recent work, briefly summarized in this article.

The Critical Role of Sulfate

Dr. Seneff persuasively makes the case that neurological brain diseases have a common origin that begins with an insufficient supply of sulfate to the brain. Sulfate is the oxidized form of sulfur. Dr. Seneff has argued that systemic sulfate deficiency "may be the most important factor in many of the health issues facing us today."

I'll get to her thoughts on why so many people are deficient in sulfate in a moment, but suffice it to say that one of the consequences of insufficient sulfate in the brain is that the lack impairs the brain's ability to eliminate heavy metals and other toxins. To make matters worse, those same toxic metals also interfere with sulfate synthesis. The net result can be an accumulation of cellular debris.

How do our brains get rid of cellular debris? Dr. Seneff cited recent work showing that sleep is crucial in this regard Sleep is the brain's "housekeeper."

This housekeeping takes place in the lysosomes. (the cell's waste disposal system) are filled with enzymes that break down unwanted materials.) The lysosomes cannot perform their important clearing work without sulfate, specifically **heparan sulfate**.

Heparan sulfate belongs to the family of glycosaminoglycans or GAGs (complex polysaccharides that provide structural integrity to cells). Heparan sulfate regulates many different biological functions, including ion and nutrient transport as well as molecular signaling cascades for most of the body's cells.

It also plays an important role in fetal brain development The role of heparins and heparan sulfate as "endogenous antioxidants" protecting against damaging free radicals was recognized over 20 years ago.

Interesting evidence of what happens when heparan sulfate is deficient comes from human and mouse studies of autism. In one study, "designer" mice engineered to have impaired heparan sulfate synthesis in the brain displayed all the classic features of autism, including sociocommunicative deficits and stereotypies.

To understand this area of autism research, it is helpful to visualize the ventricles in the brain. The ventricles (a communicating network of cavities filled with cerebrospinal fluid) consist of two lateral ventricles, the third ventricle, the cerebral aqueduct, and the fourth ventricle.

A 2013 study in *Behavioural Brain Research* found heparan sulfate deficiency in the subventricular zone of the lateral ventricles of four autistic individuals. The authors posited that this "may be a biomarker for autism, *and potentially involved in the etiology of the disorder*" [emphasis added]. Other studies have identified heparan sulfate depletion in the third ventricle.

Enter the Pineal Gland

A notable feature of sulfate is that it is difficult to transport. Dr. Seneff's extensive work on sulfur deficiency has led her to consider the important but perhaps underestimated role of the pineal gland in the transport process. The pineal gland is a neuroendocrine organ of the brain that resides in close proximity to the ventricles (small chambers), as seen in the following illustration.

The Brain

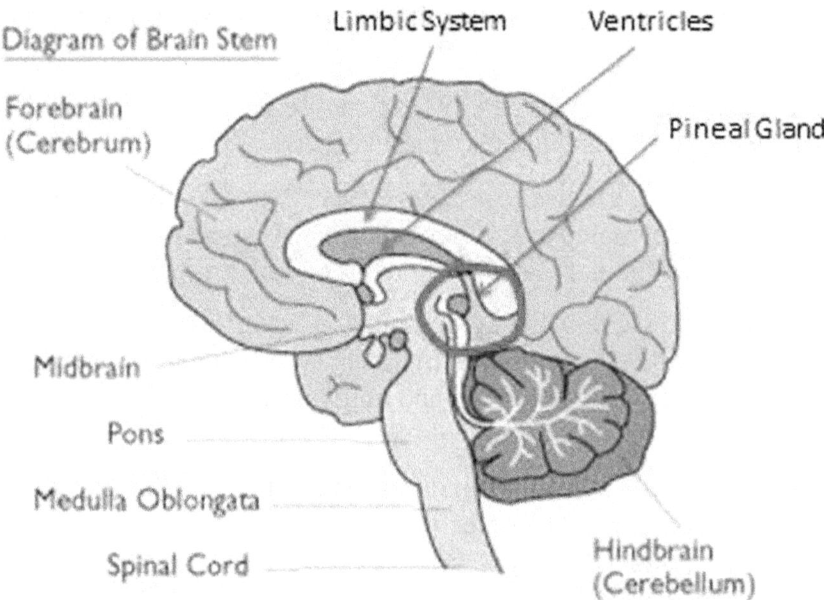

Figure 1: The Brain and The Pineal Gland

A key role of the pineal gland is to synthesize and secrete melatonin, which controls the sleep/wake cycle. Dr. Seneff suggests that one of the critical purposes of melatonin, in turn, is to deliver sulfate to the neurons at night during sleep. In her words, melatonin is clearly a "sulfate delivery system." Dr. Seneff outlined this intricate and elegant delivery system as follows:

1. With sunlight exposure serving as a catalyst, the pineal gland builds up supplies of sulfate by day, storing it in heparan sulfate molecules.
2. The pineal gland produces melatonin in the evening, transporting it as melatonin sulfate to various parts of the brain, including the third ventricle, where the melatonin releases the sulfate into the CSF.

The association of autism with heparan sulfate depletion in the lateral and third ventricles now gets more interesting, because the tip of the third ventricle is encased in the pineal gland. The pineal recess is in fact the "main site of penetration of melatonin into the CSF." In other words, under normal circumstances the pineal gland delivers melatonin sulfate to the third ventricle, which then diffuses the sulfate throughout the CSF. In addition, melatonin not only transports sulfate but also is an outstanding antioxidant and binds toxic metals to help dispose of them. It may come as no surprise, then, that melatonin impairment has been implicated in autism.

In healthy individuals, melatonin also plays an important role in inducing REM sleep, which may be the most important stage of sleep. Interestingly, Alzheimer's disease is associated with reduced REM sleep and a calcified pineal gland. Sleep disorders are also linked to autism as well as other neurological diseases, including depression, schizophrenia, ALS, Parkinson's disease, and others.

Your Pineal Gland and Heavy Metals

If one recognizes that heavy metals play a part in the modern-day epidemic of neurological diseases, then part of the explanation for the sleep disorders encountered in various neurological diseases may be that both aluminum and mercury (thimerosal) disrupt the pineal gland and its ability to make sulfate. When the pineal gland's ability to make sulfate is impaired, this, in turn, reduces production of melatonin, all-important for adequate and healthy sleep. The pineal gland is particularly susceptible to aluminum and other heavy metals because it is not protected by the blood-brain barrier and has a very high blood perfusion rate.

The pineal gland's vulnerability to aluminum is illustrated in a 1996 paper showing that the concentrations of aluminum in the pineal gland were "consistently observed" and "markedly higher" than in other brain tissues examined (pituitary, cortex, and cerebellum). Returning to the link between the pineal gland, heavy metals, and sleep, a telling fact gleaned by Dr. Seneff from the national Vaccine Adverse Event Reporting System (VAERS) is that insomnia occurs more often as an adverse reaction to aluminum-containing vaccines than to vaccines not containing aluminum.

Scientists are taking note of the fact that we live in an "age of aluminum," with aluminum exposure occurring through vaccines as well as multiple other channels. Moreover, although many experts would have us believe that the question of thimerosal and vaccine safety went away after federal agencies issued lukewarm recommendations to reduce its use as a vaccine preservative in the early 2000s, Dr. Seneff noted that thimerosal is still very much relevant.

Why Some Children May Be More Prone to Vaccine Damage

She called attention to a 2013 paper that reminds us that thimerosal not only is not found in nature but is a "designer" mercury compound created by humans that is the most toxic nonradioactive metal—"even more toxic than lead to human fetal and neuronal cells." Bringing things full circle back to sulfur/sulfate, Dr. Seneff pointed out that the article makes an important link between autism and sulfation, concluding that children with abnormal sulfation chemistry (among other factors) may be particularly susceptible to the toxic effects of the thimerosal in flu and other childhood vaccines.

In fact, due to expanded recommendations for flu shots in pregnant women and young children, exposure to thimerosal through vaccination has remained widespread in the US, and more than half of all flu vaccine doses are still thimerosal-preserved. Incredibly, the authors of the 2013 paper note the following:

"Estimates are that the maximum lifetime exposure to [thimerosal] a vaccinated person may receive is now ***more than double*** *what it would have been had the pre-2000 vaccination schedule been maintained."* (Emphasis added)

Dr. Seneff has done a lot of investigations using the VAERS database, which—despite its limitations—can be very informative. She notes that concurrent with the aggressive peddling of thimerosal-containing flu shots and other aluminum-containing vaccines, there has been a rise in reporting of both vaccine adverse events and autism spectrum disorders. She described one careful analysis of the VAERS database.

In a graph that speaks for itself (Figure 2 below), she plotted the number of VAERS reports mentioning three types of adverse events (autism, pervasive developmental disorders or

PDDs, and anxiety disorder) against the total burden of two heavy metals (aluminum and mercury) in vaccines according to the current vaccine schedule. One can immediately see that the adverse event and heavy metals lines are quite similar. Moreover, both lines show a sharp spike around the year 2000, which is when the burden of aluminum and thimerosal increased. Dr. Seneff commented that while aluminum and thimerosal are each bad enough on their own, they also work synergistically to cause harm.

Figure 2. Link between reports of vaccine adverse events (VAERS database) and aluminum (Al) and mercury (Hg) burden in current vaccine schedule (Figure kindly provided by Nancy Swanson)

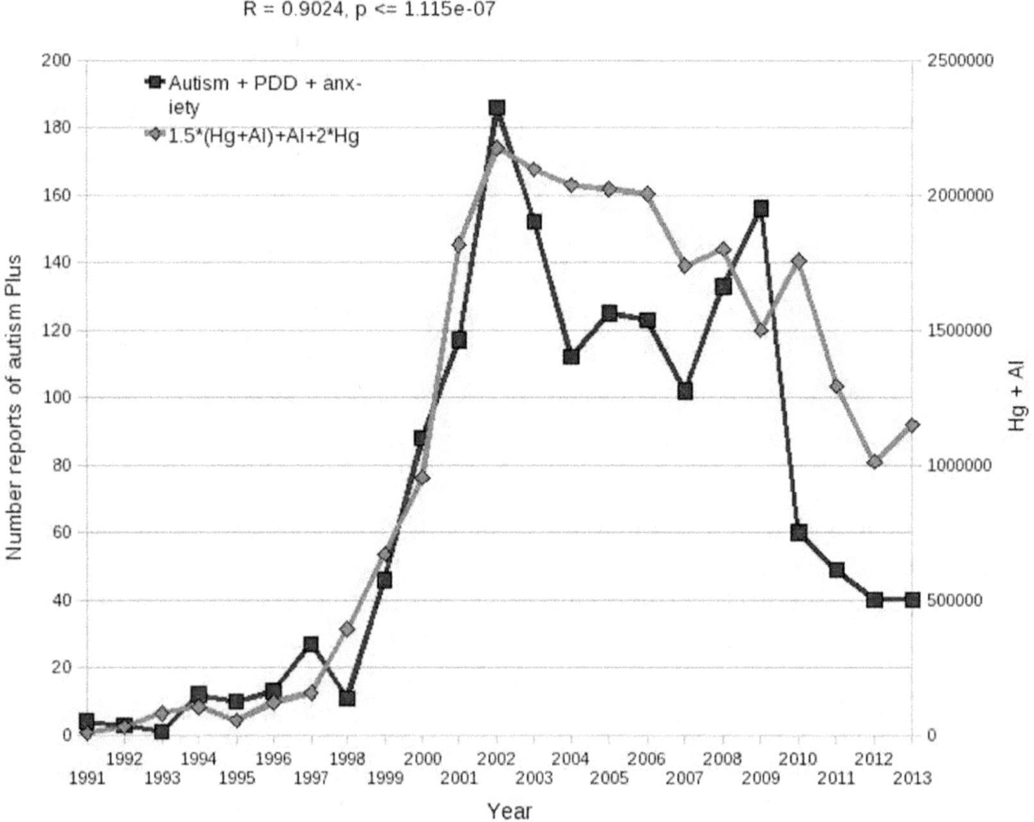

The Role of Sunlight

Returning once again to the topic of sulfate, Dr. Seneff underscored the important and neglected fact that sunlight is absolutely essential for human health because of its role in catalyzing sulfate production. We will be sulfate-deficient if we do not get enough sun. The pineal gland plays an important role in this process. Specifically, endothelial and neuronal nitric oxide synthase—both of which are present in the pineal gland—produce sulfate from reduced sulfur sources catalyzed by sunlight.

When this process is impaired through lack of sunlight exposure, the result is sulfate deficiency and—where a serum sulfate deficiency is present—an individual will also have an impaired ability to dispose of aluminum. Aluminum accumulation in the pineal gland over time will disrupt sulfate supplies to the brain by interfering with the pineal gland's ability to make sulfate. High-SPF sunscreens are one way in which the body can accumulate significant amounts of aluminum through skin absorption. Sunscreens contain aluminum nanoparticles, which are more dangerous than larger-sized aluminum particles and highly destructive in the brain.

A 2012 study found that nanoalumina destroyed mitochondria (thus severely depleting ATP, the body's energy source), induced autophagy and programmed cell death in brain endothelial cells, and decreased expression of tight-junction proteins, thereby contributing to elevated blood-brain barrier permeability. The nanoparticle effects were persistent and damaging. Thus, contrary to popular opinion, use of sunscreen is neither beneficial nor safe. (Dr. Seneff noted in passing that wearing sunglasses is also a terrible idea.)

Sunlight May Be Protective Against Autism

Dr. Seneff further assessed the importance of sunlight by compiling data from demographic studies in the 50 states (Table 1).

Table 1. Correlation of sunlight exposure and autism in public school students in 50 states (grades 1–6, 2007–2008)

Demographic	**Pearson Correlation Coefficient**	**Category**
Number of clear days	-0.40	Sunlight exposure
Rainfall and latitude	+0.34	Sunlight exposure
Vaccination rate	+0.38	Aluminum, mercury

Explanation of the table above is below.

Public schools in the US keep track of the number of students enrolled in each grade, and they also keep track of the number of students enrolled in programs specifically targeting autism. Using a ratio of these numbers, Dr. Seneff and co-investigators calculated a measure for autism in each state (using grades one to six for the 2007-2008 school year). They also obtained data for weather-related factors, using these as proxies for sun exposure (e.g., number of clear days and a combination variable capturing latitude and rainfall) and looked at states' vaccination rates as a proxy measure for aluminum and thimerosal exposure.

They then calculated Pearson's correlation coefficients as a way of understanding the strength of the relationship (or correlation) between sunlight exposure and autism. (Correlation coefficients range from -1.0 to 1.0, and a coefficient that is close to zero signals a weak relationship.) Bearing in mind that correlation does not necessarily mean causation, their analysis nonetheless produced correlations suggesting that sunlight is protective against autism, although other factors also clearly explain some of the variability.

One of the ways that the protective effect of sunlight exposure makes sense is recognizing the critical role that vitamin D plays in sulfate homeostasis. A study in mice found that activated vitamin D prevented sulfate wasting from the kidney in urine, and mice engineered to have defective vitamin D receptors (or with vitamin D deficiency) had significantly reduced serum sulfate levels, which were associated with sulfate depletion in the skeleton. Children with autism have high sulfate in their urine but low serum sulfate levels, which clearly indicates both generic sulfate deficiency and vitamin D deficiency.

Glyphosate: The Elephant in the Room

Dr. Seneff began paying attention to glyphosate after she had been intensely researching autism for five or six years. Glyphosate is a broad-spectrum systemic herbicide (known to the world under its trade name Roundup®). Among its many nefarious health effects, glyphosate disrupts the way the body manages sulfur.

In the process of examining all the known toxic chemicals in the environment and assessing which one(s) would be most likely to be causal for autism—given the specific comorbidities associated with autism—Dr. Seneff found that glyphosate matched up almost perfectly.

Both glyphosate and autism are associated with low melatonin, impaired sulfur metabolism (and low serum sulfate), low vitamin D, sleep disorders, disrupted gut bacteria, and more. Glyphosate—already a very dangerous chemical on its own—causes aluminum to be much more toxic. Glyphosate and aluminum can be viewed as "partners in crime," working synergistically with one another. This partnership plays out in several ways:

1. First, glyphosate preferentially kills beneficial bacteria in the gut, which allows pathogens such as C. difficile to overgrow. Not only does this lead to leaky gut syndrome, but C. difficile produces something called p-Cresol, a phenolic compound that is toxic to other microbes via its ability to interfere with metabolism. (C. difficile is one of only a few bacteria able to ferment tyrosine into p-Cresol.) As it happens, p-Cresol also promotes aluminum uptake by cells. P-Cresol is a known biomarker for autism and is also an important factor in kidney failure, which leads to aluminum retention in tissues and eventually to dementia.
2. Glyphosate also serves to increase aluminum toxicity by "caging" aluminum to promote its entry into the body. Glyphosate promotes calcium uptake by voltage-activated channels, which allow aluminum to gain entry as a calcium mimetic. Aluminum then promotes calcium loss from bones, contributing to pineal gland calcification.
3. Bringing melatonin back into the discussion, glyphosate interferes with what is known as the shikimate pathway. Although humans do not have the shikimate pathway, our gut flora do, and we depend on our gut flora to supply us with essential amino acids and many other things. Disruption of the shikimate pathway in our gut results in depletion of tryptophan, which is the <u>sole</u> precursor to melatonin. Besides needing melatonin to transport sulfate into the brain, we also need melatonin to reduce heavy metal toxicity. Where supplies of melatonin are adequate, melatonin will bind to

aluminum, cadmium, copper, iron, and lead, and reduce their toxicity. Where melatonin is low, a lot of damage can result.

Roundup® is the number one herbicide in use in the US and, increasingly, around the world. Unfortunately, its use has increased further in lockstep with "Roundup-Ready" genetically engineered crops, including genetically modified (GM) mainstay crops such as soy and corn.

Dr. Seneff believes that when children are overexposed to glyphosate, especially through consumption of the GM foods that are widely prevalent in the American diet, they are more likely to react badly to vaccination. To illustrate this point, Dr. Seneff and Nancy Swanson plotted a graph showing autism trends in the US (as measured by autism rates in the US school system), adverse vaccine reactions reported to the VAERS system, and glyphosate application to GM corn and soy crops in the US (Figure 3). As can be seen, the trends overlap almost entirely, presenting "tantalizing links" between these variables. Dr. Seneff infers from these findings that glyphosate is making vaccines far more toxic than they would otherwise be.

Figure 3. Autism, glyphosate, and vaccine reactions in the US (Figure kindly provided by Nancy Swanson)

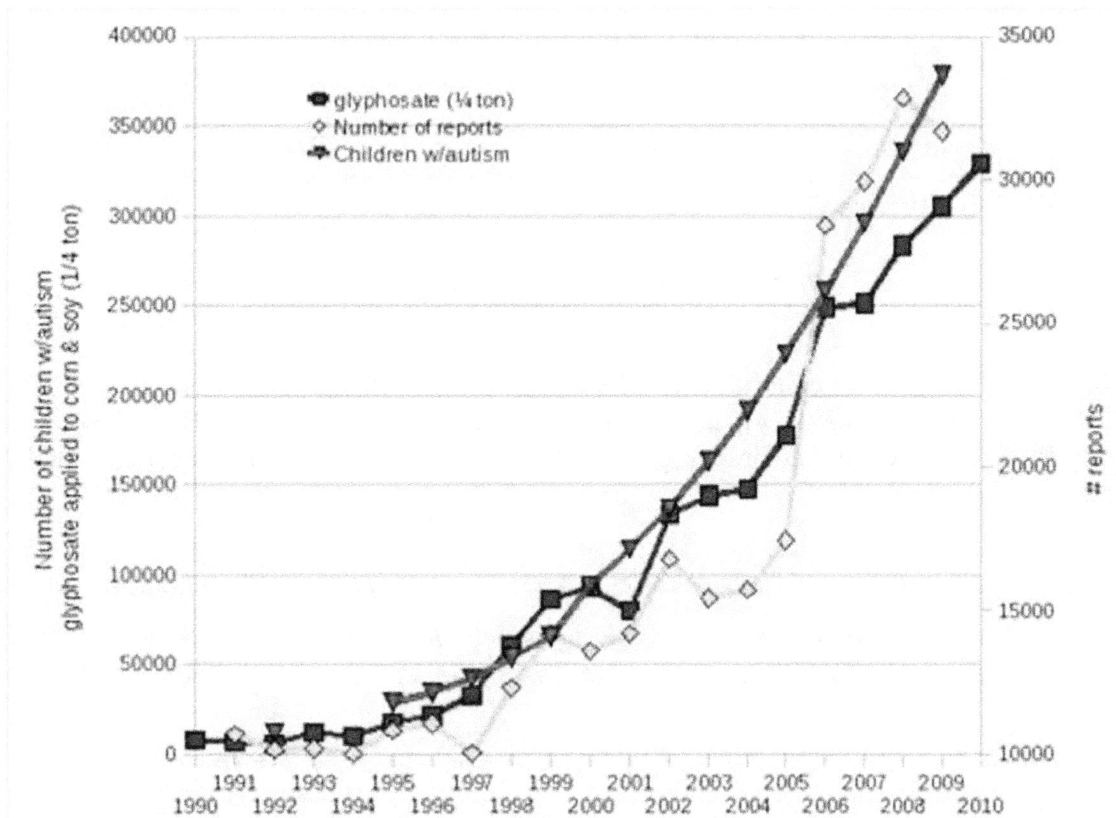

Summary

Taken together, the body of evidence elegantly assembled by Dr. Seneff supports her hypothesis that the epidemic levels of autism (and other diseases such as Alzheimer's disease) currently seen in the Western world are caused by a severe deficiency in sulfate supplies to the brain. Under optimal circumstances, the pineal gland can synthesize sulfate stimulated by sunlight and deliver it via melatonin sulfate to the brain. However, aluminum, mercury, and glyphosate are working synergistically to derail this process, and sunlight deficiency (exacerbated by the misguided use of sunscreens containing aluminum nanoparticles) is further contributing to the pathology.

About the Author of the above article

Claire Viadro, MPH, PhD, is a professional writer and editor with two advanced degrees in public health. Her work has included serving as past editor of Autism Science Digest *magazine; co-editing* Bugs, Bowels, and Behavior: The Groundbreaking Story of the Gut-Brain Connection*; and authoring or coauthoring over 20 peer-reviewed publications primarily focused on women's health.*

Above is adapted from <http://articles.mercola.com/sites/articles/archive/2014/05/08/heavy-metals-glyphosate-healtheffects.aspx?e_cid=20140508Z1_DNL_art_1&utm_source=dnl&utm_medium=email&utm_content=art1&utm_campaign=20140508Z1&et_cid=DM45823&et_rid=514705428> 05/08/2014
****

Below is from http://articles.mercola.com/sites/articles/archive/2014/04/29/children-vaccines.aspx?e_cid=20140429-remainder-z1_DNL_art_1&utm_source=dnl&utm_medium=email&utm_content=art1&utm_campaign=20140429-remainder-z1&et_cid=DM45200&et_rid=503112330

Dr Mercola on Vaccines

By Dr. Mercola

USA Today recently ran an editorial under the headline, "Vaccine opt-outs put public health at risk" and called for elimination of personal belief exemptions in state public health laws, including those that require children to get dozens of doses of up to 15 vaccines in order to attend daycare and school.

"When vaccination rates are very high, as they still are in the nation as a whole, everyone is protected. Diseases such as polio, smallpox and measles are wiped out," the editorial claims.

"This 'herd immunity' protects the most vulnerable, including those who can't be vaccinated for medical reasons, infants too young to get vaccinated and people on whom the vaccine doesn't work.

But herd immunity works only when nearly the whole herd joins in. When some refuse vaccinations and seek a free ride, immunity breaks down and everyone is more vulnerable."

Not Sharing the Risks of Vaccination = Selfish?

The editorial goes on to claim that outbreaks of infectious diseases such as measles are due to the "selfish decisions" of a few, who take vaccine exemptions and place everyone else in the "herd" at risk.

The answer, the editorial board says, is to eliminate personal belief vaccine exemptions from state public health laws and presumably force all children and adults to get every government recommended vaccine. The article finishes off with the curious statement:

*"Everyone enjoys the life-saving benefits vaccines provide, but they'll exist only as long as **everyone shares in the risks**."* [Emphasis mine]

I call it curious, because nowhere in the editorial did they actually address the issue of health risks associated with vaccines, which is one of the primary reasons for having *personal choice* in the first place. If safety and effectiveness of the product could be guaranteed, fewer people would have major objections.

Also noteworthy is the editorial board's statement that herd immunity protects "people on whom the vaccine doesn't work." Right there, they admit that vaccination isn't a foolproof disease prevention strategy. Vaccines can and often do fail to prevent disease.

What USA Today Didn't Tell You

What they *don't* spell out clearly is that the risk of vaccine failure must be weighed in along with the potential risk of harm from the vaccine. That inconvenient truth is cleverly hidden amid inflammatory rhetoric designed to get people to rally against those pesky free-thinkers who have the audacity to do their own risk-benefit analysis.

While the *USA Today* editorial board admits that *there are health risks associated with vaccines* and *vaccines don't always work,* they still insist that people should ***not** be free to make their own choices* when it comes to vaccination. Why?

Apparently, their reasoning goes like this: the only way to have any hope of success in eradicating disease is by forcing everyone to blindly accept the known and potential unknown risks of vaccination.

And since there *are* risks - even though the newspaper's editors only acknowledge risk briefly in their OpEd - the only way they say mass vaccination policies are "fair" is by mandatorily distributing the risk across the entire population.

The simpler argument is that it is done for "The Greater Good" and opting out is therefore proclaimed to be "selfish," which is an old utilitarian rationale that can be challenged on ethical grounds.

Sadly their reasoning is irrational. For starters, the premises of vaccine-induced immunity and herd immunity are both fundamentally flawed, and the medical literature is full of scientific evidence of this—none of which is ever mentioned in newspaper OpEds designed to make you fear and intensely dislike anyone who wants to make well informed, independent vaccine choices for themselves and their children.

The theory of vaccine-acquired herd immunity, which is regularly used as a justification for forced vaccination, is based on the premise that it will work the same way naturally-acquired herd immunity works. The only problem is that it *doesn't*. For a refresher on herd immunity, and the differences between vaccine-induced and naturally-acquired immunity, please refer to my previous article "Expert Pediatrician Exposes Vaccine Myths."

Leave Parents Free to Choose Vaccines

Barbara Loe Fisher, co-founder and president of the non-profit National Vaccine Information Center (NVIC) wrote an editorial opposing *USA Today's* call for an end to personal belief vaccine exemptions in state laws. She noted that US health officials now recommend twice as many vaccines compared to three decades ago.

If you follow the recommended vaccine schedule, your child will receive no less than 69 doses of 16 vaccines. Up to 15 of those vaccines are mandated by different states. Yet despite this cornucopia of "preventive medicine," American children are among the sickest in the developed world.

"With 95 percent of US kindergarteners fully vaccinated and one child in six learning disabled, one in 10 asthmatic and one in 50 living with autism, educated parents and health care professionals are asking legitimate questions about why so many highly vaccinated children are so sick," Fisher writes.

"They're examining vaccine science shortfalls and wondering why Americans are coerced and punished for declining to use every government-recommended vaccine while citizens in Canada, Japan and the European Union are free to make choices.

Vaccines carry two risks: a risk of harm and a risk of failure to prevent disease. The Centers for Disease Control and Prevention admit that US pertussis outbreaks are not due to a failure to vaccinate but failure of the vaccine to confer long-lasting immunity...

When doctors cannot predict who will be harmed by a vaccine and cannot guarantee that those who have been vaccinated won't get infected or transmit infection, the ethical principle of informed consent becomes a civil, human and parental right that must be safeguarded in US law. Non-medical vaccine exemptions immunize individuals and the community against unsafe, ineffective vaccines and tyranny."

Fortunately, judging by the newspaper's reader polls, few Americans agree with the *USA Today* editorial board. In fact, 82 percent of readers (as of this writing) "strongly disagree" with the editorial. In contrast, 85 percent of readers "strongly agree" with Fisher's "pro-vaccine choice" rebuttal. Clearly, most Americans who took the time to cast their vote expressed strong opposition to the newspaper's "anti-choice" stance and were not fooled by the same old emotion-based propaganda. And that's good news.

Is Mass Vaccination Causing Unforeseen Consequences?

When it comes to vaccination, there are a lot of unanswered questions. Some of these questions include:

> 1) Could injecting up to 69 doses of various vaccines into a child beginning on the day of birth and throughout childhood create immune system problems over the long term?
>
> 2) What are the multi-generational effects of forcing our immune systems to react to vaccines rather than naturally-occurring pathogens? One recent study found that women who received the Tdap vaccine during pregnancy had children whose immune responses to vaccination was far weaker compared to children whose mothers were not vaccinated.

Animals that are not yet weaned are typically not vaccinated as the mother's milk is known to interfere with antibody responses to vaccines. Many animals are titered to ensure they don't receive excessive vaccines, as the side effects are well known. As explained by veterinarian Dr. Jean Dodd

"A titer test is a simple blood test that measures a dog or cat's antibodies to vaccine viruses (or other infectious agents). For instance, your dog may be more resistant to a virus whereas your neighbor's dog may be more prone to it. Titers accurately assess protection to the so-called 'core' diseases (distemper, parvovirus, hepatitis in dogs, and panleukopenia in cats), enabling veterinarians to judge whether a booster vaccination is necessary. "

So, we're titering animals but not children? There are plenty of reasons not to accept a mandated one-size-fits-all vaccination policy: the right to self determination being first and foremost. The decision to participate in a medical intervention or experiment that carries serious risks, whether the risk is high or low, should belong to each individual person, including parents of minor children who are legally and morally responsible for protecting their children.

The Case for Reasonable Doubt

What is some of the evidence raising reasonable doubt about the "reasonableness" of forced vaccinations? How about the following:

- **Environmental toxins can reduce vaccine efficacy**. Research published in the *Journal of the American Medical Association* (JAMA) suggests that exposure to perfluorinated compounds (PFCs) prior to, and after birth, can significantly weaken the effectiveness of vaccines. PFCs are found in countless products, including non-stick cookware and food wrappings, personal care, and cleaning products, just to name a few. If poorly regulated environmental pollutants can dramatically decrease vaccine effectiveness, then that means your risk-to-benefit ratio of vaccination is automatically skewed toward higher risk and lower benefit. As reported by ABC News:

"The study found that higher levels of PFCs in both mothers and children meant lower numbers of disease-fighting antibodies in the children. Mothers who had twice the level of PFC in their blood had children with a 40 percent decrease in the number of antibodies formed after getting the diphtheria vaccine. The 7-year-old children who had doubled PFC levels had nearly a 50 percent reduction in their antibody levels."

- **Vaccinated people are asymptomatic carriers of disease, and can still both spread and contract the disease**. Mounting evidence shows that vaccinated people can actually unknowingly be infected with and spread diseases like pertussis (whooping cough) for which they were vaccinated. This was shown in an FDA baboon study last year, which concluded that while the pertussis vaccine can cut down on serious clinical disease symptoms, it does not eliminate *transmission* of the disease. As noted by the lead author of the research, when the baby baboons were newly vaccinated with either DPT or DTaP vaccines, they were asymptomatic carriers of pertussis and could infect others in their community.

Needless to say, if vaccinated people can be asymptomatic carriers of disease, this can place everyone at risk and really raises questions about the wisdom of vaccinating health care workers before permitting them to work with high-risk populations. Vaccinated people can still contract the disease because (a) most vaccine-acquired artificial immunity is *temporary* and (b) because microbes can evolve to evade the vaccines.

For example, 97 percent of those who contracted mumps during the outbreak in Ohio earlier this year were fully vaccinated against the disease. Some are quick to say that "sure, vaccinated people can contract the disease—*if exposed;* which is why no one should be allowed to opt out of vaccination." However, when a vaccinated person can contract the disease *from another vaccinated person*... this entire argument clearly falls apart.

- **Flu vaccination raises your risk of contracting more serious flu illness**. Research published in 2012 showed that the flu vaccine increases your risk of contracting more serious pandemic flu illness such as H1N1. This supported previous findings, such as that from a 2011 study which found that the seasonal flu vaccine actually weakened children's immune systems, thereby increasing their chances of getting sick from influenza viruses not included in the vaccine. Unvaccinated children actually built up *more* antibodies against a wider variety of influenza virus strains than the vaccinated children.
- **Vaccines promote disease mutations**. Vaccines have also been found to place pressure on microbes to develop mutated versions of the disease, and/or enhance the ability of other similar strains to become more dominant and cause disease. For example, a veterinary vaccine study at the University of Melbourne (Australia) found that using two different vaccine viruses to combat the same disease in an animal population quite rapidly caused the viruses to combine (referred to as recombination), creating brand new and more virulent viruses.

In Australia, dangerous new strains of whooping cough bacteria were reported in March 2012. The vaccine, researchers said, was responsible. The reason for this is because while whooping cough is primarily attributed to *Bordetella pertussis* infection, it is also caused by another closely related pathogen called *B. parapertussis,* which the vaccine does NOT protect against.

Two years earlier, scientists at Penn State had already reported that the pertussis vaccine significantly enhanced the colonization of *B. parapertussis*, thereby promoting vaccine-resistant whooping cough outbreaks. According to the authors, vaccination led to a *40-fold enhancement* of *B. parapertussis* colonization in the lungs of mice, and the data suggested that the vaccine may be contributing to the observed rise in whooping cough incidence over the last decade by promoting *B. parapertussis* infection instead.

Fraudulent Research Does Not Inspire Confidence

Please understand that efficacy of a vaccine relates to its ability to produce an antibody and this is NOT at all a good marker for whether or not immunity has been achieved, while effectiveness measures the ability of the vaccine to actually protect against infection. So let's look at the basic effectiveness of vaccines, and the reliability of the research backing up effectiveness claims. On a number of occasions, outright fraud has been revealed, raising serious doubts about whether or not the stated *benefit*—the ability of the vaccine to prevent disease—is even part of the risk-benefit equation. If not, you're taking on risk with very minimal, if any, benefit.

Case in point: in 2012, two former Merck virologists sued their former employer, claiming Merck overstated the effectiveness of the mumps vaccine in the company's combination MMR shot. A federal antitrust class action lawsuit was also filed that year, in which Merck was accused of falsifying test results and selling millions of doses of the vaccine that were of "questionable efficacy."

Clearly, vaccine effectiveness has a major bearing on disease outbreaks, and it would appear as though many vaccine failures are simply covered up by blaming outbreaks on the unvaccinated population. This way, ineffective vaccines can still be sold, while everyone's busy tarring and feathering those who have opted out of using every government recommended vaccine. You know, those who "selfishly" choose not to "share in the risks."

Another example: in 2012, a systematic review of pre- and post-licensure trials of the HPV vaccine showed that the vaccine's effectiveness is not only overstated (through the use of selective reporting or "cherry picking" data) but also *unproven*. According to the authors: *"[T]he widespread optimism regarding HPV vaccines long-term benefits appears to rest on a number of unproven assumptions (or such which are at odds with factual evidence) and significant misinterpretation of available data."*

A 2013 HPV vaccine effectiveness study also turned out to have significant discrepancies, raising doubts about the veracity of its conclusions. Upon closer scrutiny, the data actually revealed that *unvaccinated* girls had the best outcome. Furthermore, records obtained last year through a Freedom of Information Act (FOIA) lawsuit against the Department of Health and Human Services (DHHS) revealed that the National Vaccine Injury Compensation Program has so far awarded nearly $5.9 million to 49 victims for harm and/or death resulting from the HPV vaccine.

According to an April 7 report by WCPO News, the VAERS database has received more than 31,000 reports of adverse reactions to the HPV vaccine Gardasil. This is up from May 13, 2013, at which point VAERS had received 29,686 adverse event reports (including 136 deaths, 922 reports of disability, and 550 life-threatening adverse events). Is it reasonable to doubt the safety and efficacy of Gardasil? Ask Tracie Moorman, whose 15-year-old daughter Maddie became too chronically ill to attend school after receiving the HPV vaccine. *"If I ever could have a do-over, it absolutely would be this situation,"* Tracie told WCPO in a recent interview.

Vaccinated vs. Unvaccinated: Who's Healthier?

Large studies comparing the health outcomes of vaccinated versus unvaccinated children have not been a priority for vaccine researchers. This is a travesty, as this is the kind of research most desperately needed. Most vaccine studies are about developing more vaccines for children and adults to use.

Some claim that studies comparing the health of highly vaccinated and unvaccinated children cannot be done because it would be "unethical" to leave children participating in the study unvaccinated in order to do the comparison. But since some American parents are already delaying or avoiding vaccinating their children, this hardly seems like a reasonable excuse. It is more likely that comparing the health of vaccinated and unvaccinated children in appropriately designed studies are avoided because the results might upset the proverbial apple cart.

However, that doesn't mean there is a total absence of evidence about the health of vaccinated versus unvaccinated children to give us an indication of whether or not the use of many more vaccines by children in the U.S. is contributing to so many being chronically ill and disabled. In December 2010, a survey was initiated by VaccineInjury.info (www.VaccineInjury.info)to compare the health of vaccinated children with unvaccinated children. The survey is ongoing, so if you would like to participate, you can. Though this is obviously not a double-blind controlled study, and depends on the individuals submitting the data to give accurate information, it is still revealing. At the time of this writing, the results show:

Health Condition	**Prevalence in Vaccinated Children**	**Prevalence in Unvaccinated Children**
Allergies	36.71%	11.25%
Asthma	14.23%	2.26%
Hay fever	17.86% of German children	3%
Neurodermatitis (an autoimmune disorder)	23.90%	7.50%
Attention deficit disorder (ADD)	14.94%	1.28%
Middle ear infections	20.84%	7.50%
Sinusitis	12.14%	2.50%
Autism	7.43%	0.49%

Do You Want the Right to Choose Vaccination for Yourself and Your Child?

So, what do we know, and what can we be sure of? One thing that appears to be beyond dispute, based on overwhelming evidence that spans across decades, is that pharmaceutical companies have repeatedly demonstrated their willingness to bribe, lie, threaten and commit fraud in order to bring, and keep, their products on the market. This kind of behavior is so commonplace, it appears to be part and parcel of the accepted modus operandi of the drug industry, albeit unofficially.

So, based on what you know, do you think parents should have the legal right to choose whether or not to give their children every one of the dozens of doses of 15 vaccines that health officials mandate for infants and children attending school and daycare? Do you want that right to know and freedom to choose for yourself which vaccines you are going to get?

I cannot impress upon you strongly enough the importance of your active involvement when it comes to defending our legal right to make informed vaccine choices in America. In order to protect the health of as many children as possible, we cannot continue to ignore the signs that using vaccines as the nation's primary disease prevention strategy may have been taken *too far in the past three decades* - to the point that we're now seeing the health of too many children and adults being compromised..

When you follow the money, you realize that multi-national drug companies marketing vaccines and the organizations they fund are the ones pulling the political strings to eliminate non-medical vaccine exemptions in U.S. state laws. Eliminating the freedom to know and right to choose nationwide would be a major coup by a pharmaceutical industry already making huge profits from vaccine laws that require every person born in America to purchase and use their products. At the same time, the *safety* of vaccine policies are primarily based on the word of these very companies that not only have their products mandated but also enjoy a liability shield from vaccine injury lawsuits in civil court that was given to them by Congress and the Supreme Court!

Is any of this really wise?

No Time to Waste – Take Action Now

The non-profit National Vaccine Information Center (NVIC) has been working for 32 years to prevent vaccine injuries and deaths through public education and defend the informed consent ethic in vaccine policies and laws. NVIC is leading a grassroots movement to secure and protect broad medical, religious, and conscientious belief vaccine exemptions in state public health laws to prevent parents of minor children and adult workers from being discriminated against and harmed by "no exceptions" mandatory vaccination policies.

On NVIC's **"Cry for Vaccine Freedom Wall,"** you can read (and post) first-hand accounts of threats and coercion by pediatricians, government officials, and employers harassing and punishing Americans for refusing to get every government recommended and mandated vaccine. It is heartbreaking to read how many people are being bullied into using vaccines against their will - even individuals who have already suffered vaccine reactions and injuries!

In the past few years, states like Washington, Oregon and California have restricted the use of non-medical exemptions and the **Colorado legislature** is currently debating similar legislation. NVIC has testified and has educated families and helped them testify in **public hearings** in those states.

To become active in your state and make sure your community and elected officials are fully informed about the importance of protecting vaccine exemptions in state laws, sign up for the free online **NVIC Advocacy Portal (https://nvicadvocacy.org/members/Home.aspx)**. You will be notified by email when vaccine legislation is moving in your state to restrict or expand vaccine exemptions. You will also be put into direct electronic contact with your own elected officials and can let them know your views with a touch on your smart phone screen or a keystroke on your tablet or computer. If we all stand up for our right to know and freedom to choose the way we want to stay healthy – including whether or not we choose to use vaccines – we will be protecting a fundamental right we

Above is from http://articles.mercola.com/sites/articles/archive/2014/04/29/children-vaccines.aspx?e_cid=20140429-remainder-z1_DNL_art_1&utm_source=dnl&utm_medium=email&utm_content=art1&utm_campaign=20140429-remainder-z1&et_cid=DM45200&et_rid=503112330

****

Below is adapted from http://articles.mercola.com/sites/articles/archive/2014/05/05/oil-pulling-coconut-oil.aspx and http://articles.mercola.com/sites/articles/archive/2014/11/30/importance-oral-microbiome.aspx

How Your Oral Health Contributes to Your General Health and Wellbeing

By Dr. Mercola

Many people do not realize how their oral health can impact their total body health. But the truth is, it's very difficult to achieve high-level physical health if your dental health isn't effectively addressed.

Dr. Gerry Curatola, founder of Rejuvenation Dentistry, has over 30 years' experience in biological dentistry.

For Dr. Curatola, dentistry was a calling since childhood, but unlike most dentists, he really wanted to be "a physician of the mouth." So, after graduating from dental school in 1983, he enrolled in the country's first master's program in holistic health.

"My desire and my focus have always been to look at the mouth as the gateway to total body wellness," he says.

"Beyond that, I became very disturbed that I was a member of a profession—its organized component, the American Dental Association—that is still saying it's okay to put mercury in teeth.

In addition to that, all of the research that was emerging about fluoridation made it very clear that this wasn't the panacea for all dental problems. As a matter of fact, it's responsible for a lot of other problems that we're dealing with today."

How Your Oral Health Impacts Your Systemic Health

Thousands of studies have linked oral disease to systemic disease. Inflammation is well-known as a "ravaging" and disease-causing force, and gum disease and other oral diseases produce chronic low-grade inflammation in your body.

"This inflammation has very, very deleterious effects on just about every major organ system – from Alzheimer's to stroke, heart disease, and diabetes," Dr. Curatola explains.

Advanced periodontal disease or gum disease can raise your risk of a fatal heart attack up to 10 times. According to Dr. Curatola, if you get a heart attack related to periodontal or gum disease, nine times out of 10, it will actually kill you.

There's also a 700 percent higher incidence of type 2 diabetes among those with gum disease, courtesy of the inflammatory effects of unbalanced microflora in your mouth. But how does the microflora in your mouth cause inflammation, you might ask?

When the bacteria that cause tooth decay and gum disease enter into your circulatory system, it causes your liver to release C-reactive proteins, which has inflammatory effects in the entire circulatory system.

"There's a very, very close connection. As I said, the mouth is the gateway to total body wellness. That is an accurate statement that's well-accepted today," Dr. Curatola says.

Rejuvenation Dentistry, founded by Dr. Curatola in 2006, was created as a model for the future practice of dentistry. The model recognizes that dentists often see patients more frequently than most other healthcare practitioners, and can play a much more significant role in people's health than they do currently.

"[Patients] come in for regular checkups and cleanings. And we should be screening... In the mouth, we can diagnose a host of systemic problems.

There are some estimates that up to 80 percent of systemic disease have manifestations in the mouth – everything from blood problems, even leukemia, diabetes, other fungal and bacterial infections that have systemic components," he says.

The Importance of Your Oral Microbiome

Part and parcel of oral health is attending to your oral microbiome. Achieving oral health is really about promoting balance among the bacteria in your mouth. And contrary to popular belief, antimicrobial agents and alcohol mouthwashes designed to "kill bad bacteria" actually do far more harm than good.

The oral microbiome, while connected to the gut microbiome, is quite unique. Most importantly, it has a protective component that protects you from deadly viruses and bacteria in the environment. The second function of the oral microbiome is the beginning of digestion.

"When we look at the oral microbiome, it's an essential component of the salivary immune system; it aids in digestion, and it even makes vitamins. We are looking at ways to promote oral microbiome homeostasis.

When we do that, we see amazing things happen, so amazing that you might not get the flu this winter... immune competence is a very important first line of defense, and that immune competence starts in the mouth."

Interestingly, probiotics do not work in the mouth, so it's not as simple as adding more beneficial microbes. As an initial step, you need to *cease killing* microbes in your mouth.

"Pathogens have been redefined since the Human Microbiome Project (HMP) in 2002. Pathogens are now being recognized as resident microbes that are out of balance," Dr. Curatola explains.

"When they're under attack, they hunker down, they flick a switch... What we're recognizing is that the same bacteria that keep us alive can have a pathogenic expression when disturbed. I have been kind of tooting the horn about getting out of the 'pesticide business.' I'm also speaking about natural pesticides.

Not just triclosan, clorhexidine, and those synthetic types, but also tea tree oil, tulsi oil, oregano oil and other antimicrobial oils that, albeit they're herbal, they have a potent disturbing effect on the oral microbiome.

In the mouth, you don't want to have a 'scorched earth policy' or nuking all the bacteria and hoping the good bugs come back.

What we found in our research is that good bugs basically have a harder chance of setting up a healthy-balanced microbiome when you disturb them, denature them, or dehydrate them with alcohol-based products."

Why Fluoride Is Not Recommended for Dental Health

Calcium fluoride should not be confused with the chemical formulation of sodium fluoride, which is toxic. Sodium fluoride is the kind found in toothpaste, which carries a poison warning. This stems back to the 1980s with the introduction of a popular bubble gum flavored commercial toothpaste that led to a 280 percent increase in child fatalities from fluoride poisoning. As it turned out, there was more than enough chemical fluoride in a full-sized tube to kill a young child.

It took 10 years, but finally in 1998 the Food and Drug Administration (FDA) mandated a poison warning be placed on toothpaste, stating that children should be supervised, and to limit toothpaste to a pea-sized amount. If more than that is swallowed, you're advised to contact Poison Control Center immediately. Fluoride over-exposure from toothpaste, fluoridated water, and other sources, has led to a virtual epidemic of fluoride damage. At present, four out of 10 adolescents in the US have fluoride-damaged teeth—a condition known as dental fluorosis.

"Fluoride was promoted because it stimulates remineralization of teeth. What they didn't look at is what type of mineral is left in that tooth—it's a mineral known as fluorapatite. Fluorapatite is very hard. It's like a porcelain plate; I can't scratch it, but if I bang it on this counter, it would break in a million pieces... [Natural] teeth and bones are made of hydroxyapatite... We now have teeth and bones that are fluorapatite," Dr. Curatola explains.

"Skeletal fluorosis has also become a big concern. We have an exponential rate of hip fractures. A lot of doctors and scientists have been pointing to the fact that teeth and bones are less flexible as fluorapatite than hydroxyapatite. This is aside from all the controversy in terms of fluoridated water lowering IQ, kidney disease, and cancer..."

The Case for Oil Pulling

Dr. Curatola's clinical and experimental experience over the last 30 years suggests that most toothpastes should be avoided. As a substitute, you need to have a good nutritional program for systemic health, along with an oral rinse that specifically nourishes your oral microbiome. He also recommends oil pulling, using coconut oil, noting that: *"If you don't want to use toothpaste right now and you don't have a good nutritional that promotes oral microbiome homeostasis, coconut oil pulling is great."*

Coconut oil pulling has a lipophilic effect, helping to eliminate unhealthy biofilm from your teeth. And while it has a natural detergent effect, it doesn't do the damage that chemical detergents do. Coconut oil also contains a number of valuable nutrients that help promote oral health. Another tip: If you want a healthy oral care rinse, Dr. Curatola suggests rinsing with some Himalayan salt dissolved in water, as it contains more than 85 different microminerals. As I said earlier, I personally have stopped using coconut oil and now am using fermented vegetables for pulling.

Optimizing Your Nutrition Is Key for Oral Health

It's also worth noting that while probiotics do not have a direct effect on your oral microbiome, addressing your gut flora can indeed make a big difference in your oral health. I used to be severely challenged with plaque—so much so I required very frequent visits to the dental hygienist just to keep up with it. Once I started adding fermented vegetables regularly to my diet however, the plaque buildup was dramatically reduced.

"You have to think about promoting balance," Dr. Curatola reminds us. *"We've looked at organic gardening and the environment around us and even eating organic foods. I'd like everyone to think about doing 'organic gardening' in the mouth. The way you do that is through a strong, healthy, and balanced nutritional protocol. I call it triple-A nutrition – alkalizing, antioxidant-rich, and anti-inflammatory. People should know what nutritional factors are inflammatory. There are inflammatory triggers, whether it's gluten, dairy, and a number of others. They can vary for different individuals."*

In addition to an alkalizing, antioxidant-rich, and anti-inflammatory diet, he recommends eliminating detergent-based products such as toothpaste and antibacterial and alcohol-based mouthwashes. Again, it's important to remember that your mouth is an organ that protects your body from dangerous infections and disease—provided it's nourished enough to do its job. You can learn more about Dr. Curatola's New York City based practice, Rejuvenation Dentistry, on his website.

The following links can also help you find a mercury-free, biological dentist who can help you optimize your oral health:

- Consumers for Dental Choice
  <http://www.toxicteeth.org/dentistsDoctorsProducts.aspx>
- International Academy of Biological Dentistry & Medicine (IABDM)
  <https://iabdm.org/about-the-iabdm/>
- Dental Amalgam Mercury Solutions (DAMS).
  <http://www.dams.cc/>
  E-mail them at: dams@usfamily.net or call 651-644-4572 for an information packet
- International Academy of Oral Medicine and Toxicology (IAOMT)
  <https://iaomt.org/>
- Huggins Applied Healing.
  <http://www.hugginsappliedhealing.com/ >
  You'll need to fill out a form and they will connect with you to find a suitable dentist in your area
- Holistic Dental Association
  < http://holisticdental.org/>
- International Association of Mercury Safe Dentists <
  <http://www.dentalwellness4u.com/freeservices/find_dentists.html>

- Talk International
  < http://www.talkinternational.com/holistic-biological-mercury-free-dentists-directory/#!directory/map>

Oil Pulling To Improve Oral Health

Oil pulling is making headlines as it seems to becoming widely popular. It's actually an Ayurvedic Indian tradition that's been around for thousands of years.

To perform it, you simply swish an oil in your mouth, "pulling" it between your teeth for about 20 minutes. You can use a number of oils for this, but sesame, sunflower, and coconut oil are the most commonly used.

As for the benefits, this is one of the easiest ways to support your oral health naturally, especially if you use coconut oil, which is a powerful destroyer of all kinds of microbes, from viruses to bacteria to protozoa, many of which can be harmful.

Ancient Ayurveda texts claim that oil pulling may cure about 30 systemic diseases and even today, it's widely discussed as a tool for detoxification of your whole body. These uses are controversial and I can't vouch for their validity. However, in your *mouth*, oil pulling does have significant cleansing and healing effects, which are backed up by science.

Anecdotally as well, virtually everyone who tries it notices an improvement in their oral health. Personally, this technique has significantly reduced my plaque buildup, allowing me to go longer between visits to the dental hygienist. As reported by the *Indian Journal of Dental Research*

"Oil pulling has been used extensively as a traditional Indian folk remedy without scientific proof for many years for strengthening teeth, gums and jaws and to prevent decay, oral malodor, bleeding gums and dryness of throat and cracked lips."

If you take a look at the research, it's easy to understand why:

- Oil pulling reduced counts of *Streptococcus mutans* bacteria – a significant contributor to tooth decay – in the plaque and saliva of children Researchers concluded, *"Oil pulling can be used as an effective preventive adjunct in maintaining and improving oral health."*
- Oil pulling significantly reduced plaque, improved gum health and reduced aerobic microorganisms in plaque among adolescent boys with plaque-induced gingivitis
- Oil pulling is as effective as mouthwash at improving bad breath and reducing the microorganisms that may cause it
- Oil pulling benefits your mouth, in part, via its mechanical cleaning action Researchers noted, *"The myth that the effect of oil-pulling therapy on oral health was just a placebo effect has been broken and there are clear indications of possible saponification and emulsification process, which enhances its mechanical cleaning action."*

What Type of Oil Works Best for Oil Pulling?

It's worth noting that the above studies used sesame oil, which is traditionally recommended. However, it has relatively high concentration of omega-6 oils. Therefore, I believe *coconut oil* is far superior, as most of us get far too many omega-6 fats, which distorts the sensitive omega 3:6 ratio. And, in my mind, coconut oil tastes much better.

From a mechanical and biophysical perspective, it is likely that both work. However, coconut oil has antibacterial and anti-viral activity that makes it especially well suited for oral health. In fact, coconut oil mixed with baking soda makes for a very simple and inexpensive, yet effective, toothpaste and research suggests it may be a valuable tool for fighting tooth decay.

Researchers at the Athlone Institute of Technology's Bioscience Research Institute in Ireland tested the antibacterial action of coconut oil in its natural state and coconut oil that had been treated with enzymes, in a process similar to digestion.

The oils were tested against strains of *Streptococcus* bacteria, which are common inhabitants of your mouth. They found that enzyme-modified coconut oil strongly inhibits the growth of most strains of *Streptococcus* bacteria, including *Streptococcus mutans*, an acid-producing bacterium that is a major cause of tooth decay

It is thought that the breaking down of the fatty coconut oil by the enzymes turns it into acids, which are toxic to certain bacteria. Enzyme-modified coconut oil was also harmful to the yeast *Candida albicans*, which can cause thrush. So when oil pulling is combined with the antimicrobial power of coconut oil, I believe it can be a very powerful health tool.

Oil Pulling Is Simple

Oil pulling involves "rinsing" your mouth with the oil, much like you would with a mouthwash (except you shouldn't attempt to gargle with it). The oil (about 2 teaspoons) is "worked" around your mouth by pushing, pulling, and drawing it through your teeth for a period of about 20 minutes. Oil pulling will work your jaw muscles as another benefit. If yours become sore or tired you're probably "swishing" the oil too vigorously. Just relax and focus on moving the oil with your tongue as well as your jaw muscles.

> Glenn’s note: Some people may notice a detox reaction for the first few days of using oil pulling that may include mild congestion, headache, mucous drainage or other effects.

When you're first starting out, you may want to try it for just five minutes at a time, or, if you have more time and want even better results, you can go for 30-45 minutes. This process allows the oil to "pull out" bacteria, viruses, fungi, and other debris from your mouth. Once the oil turns thin and milky white, you'll know it's time to spit it out. The best time to do oil pulling is in the morning before eating breakfast, but it can be done at any time. I try to do it twice a day if my schedule allows. When you're done, spit out the oil (into the trash instead of the sink) and rinse your mouth with water or a combination of water and baking soda and spit it out too. Avoid swallowing the oil as it will be loaded with bacteria and whatever potential toxins and debris it has pulled out. Brush well.

Candida and *Streptococcus* are common residents in your mouth, and these germs and their toxic waste products can contribute to plaque accumulation and tooth decay. Oil pulling may help lessen the overall toxic burden on your immune system by preventing the spread of these organisms from your mouth to the rest of your body. Many people think oil pulling sounds strange ... until they try it. Then many become hooked. It's just one more way that you can use a natural, simple substance to significantly boost your oral health. People have been using this technique, and others like chewing sticks, for centuries because they *work*.

Above is adapted from http://articles.mercola.com/sites/articles/archive/2014/05/05/oil-pulling-coconut-oil.aspx and http://articles.mercola.com/sites/articles/archive/2014/11/30/importance-oral-microbiome.aspx >

****

Below is adapted from http://articles.mercola.com/sites/articles/archive/2014/05/03/root-canal-alternative.aspx?e_cid=20140503Z1_DNL_art_1&utm_source=dnl&utm_medium=email&utm_content=art1&utm_campaign=20140503Z1&et_cid=DM45438&et_rid=508895019 (5/3/2014)

Safer and Healthier Alternatives to Root Canals and Other Common, Yet Harmful, Tooth Restoration Techniques

By Carol Vander Stoep, RDH, BSDH, OMT

Viper venom is an efficient killer. Its swirls of toxic proteins multitask. Some paralyze the nervous system of the victim by blocking nerve-to-muscle messages. Others can misdirect messenger hormones, dissolve tissues, or make blood so sticky the resulting clots stop the heart, or thin it to the point that the victim quickly bleeds out.

Just as surely, dead or dying human teeth can harbor similarly lethal agents working on at least as many levels throughout your body. The sophisticated multi-level attack of oral microbes, their metabolic waste products, and their interaction with dental materials can similarly give rise to an immune system crash, which can manifest in a multitude of disguises. Is a root canal procedure a gamble you really want to take?

Economics versus Health: There Is Always a Price

The complexity of interactions and the time delay before oral toxins express noticeable symptoms, compared to fast-acting snake venom, work well for the institution of dentistry and dental insurance companies. It does not bode well for you.

Institutions are by nature invested in the status quo. The insurance industry's business model is no different from most other business models – it values their bottom line over your health. We are left on our own to tease out root causes of disease.

It is only after the scare of cancer, the exhaustion of chronic fatigue, a nervous system derailment causing Parkinson's tremors, Multiple Sclerosis (MS), or Bell's Palsy, or even autoimmune issues such as lupus or ALS (Lou Gehrig's disease), that some people make the difficult decision to consider a "dental revision" to help their body recover.

A dental revision is no less than removing all possible toxic stressors of oral origin – dead teeth, dead jawbone, heavy metals like mercury, nickel and chromium, gum disease therapy, and often, removing meridian blockers like implants.

A dental revision may seem like a drastic and expensive step, but what is the cost of poor health to which these contribute? You can escape to clean mountain air or the ocean's cleansing waves, but you can never escape your internal environment.

There are several examples of DNA sequenced microbial profiles found in the jawbone socket of an extracted root canal treated tooth, and in cavitations. The root canal treated tooth may show no clinical or physical signs of failing. These interesting lab reports also connect the pathogens with their waste products' target tissues.

What Is a Root Canal?

A root canal is an embalming procedure dentists perform on a tooth. Root canals are designed to keep a dead tooth mechanically functioning in a live body.

Teeth die as a result of trauma (sometimes including the trauma of a high speed drill creating too much heat or sucking the organic material from the microscopic tubules that assist in keeping it alive), or from microbial invasion from deep decay or gum disease into the pulp that nourishes each tooth.

It is no longer a huge secret that root canals crank out microbial metabolic toxins. Even some root canal specialists (endodontists) are starting to "own" it. For instance, they acknowledge that "condensing osteitis" around a root-canal treated tooth is common.

Condensing osteitis is a thickening of the bone around a dead tooth as your body tries to wall off the infective toxins seeping from it. On the other hand, the American Association of Endodontists (AAE) position statement on the matter (2012) states that:

"...the practice of recommending the extraction of endodontically treated teeth for the prevention of NICO [painful jawbone death due to poor blood supply], or any other disease, is unethical and should be reported immediately to the appropriate state board of dentistry."

And yet, according to a 2006 study published in the *Journal of Evidence Based Dental Practice*

"A recent evidence-based review of the outcomes of both treatment modalities noted that if evidence-based principles are applied to the data available for both treatment modalities, few implant or endodontic outcome studies can be classified as being high in the evidence hierarchy."

Is a Root Canal Right for Your Situation?

No doubt about it, losing a tooth can be emotionally charged. I think it is one reason dentists work so hard to perfect tooth embalming procedures. The decision tree for considering tooth replacement is complex, and the solutions all involve compromise. There are a lot of hop off places for people to enter into denial.

Examine your own health status, priorities and philosophies and go with *your* best solution. *"I have three root canals? What do I do now? Are all root canals toxic?"* Probably. Eventually. Yet people have varying abilities to sustain the stress of toxins – and of course that ability varies over time.

Some biological doctors may recommend a root canal if a patient has a strong immune system, great genetics, and superior lifestyle. They suggest if one's immune system crashes it can always be extracted later. Because we are besieged by so many unavoidable immune system challenges in today's world, I'm personally moving further and further away from the idea of assaulting my immune system with avoidable challenges.

Proper Diagnosis Is Key for Failing Root Canals and Cavitations

Since health effects of root canals and cavitations are similar, and one can arise from the other, I'll digress to talk about cavitations for a moment. The existence of cavitations, also known as ischemic osteonecrosis (death of bone due to lack of adequate blood supply) when there is no pain present, and NICO when there is pain, seems to equate to a religious belief. Do cavitations exist or don't they?

The preferred answer might depend on if you have skin in the game. Root canal specialists, state dental boards, and insurance companies cast aspersions on their existence, and (as noted above) even threaten to take away a dentist's credentials should they acknowledge cavitations and recommend surgically treating the dead bone or extracting a root canal treated tooth to prevent them. Like the huge disservice of the domestic cooking oil manufacturers' vilification of tropical fats decades ago, the stance of these special interests may equally hurt public health.

Part of the problem is that diagnosis is difficult. Typical dental x-rays can no more accurately diagnose cavitations than they can accurately diagnose subtle root canal pathology. They show only the most obvious cavitations. CT scans are excellent if all metals are absent from the mouth, but they are expensive and come with the added price tag of high radiation exposure.

There is no definitive way to judge how infected a root canal treated tooth or cavitation is, but a traditional camera-imaged thermogram, which many also use to detect early stage breast cancer, can offer some guidance. Thermographic images display infrared heat emissions, with each color gradation indicating different heat emissions. High-heat emissions are suggestive of inflammation, which may indicate root canal toxicity or a cavitation—even if you're asymptomatic. You can read more about the use of thermography on PositiveHealth.com's website

Regulation Thermometry

A new type of system, the AlfaSight™ 9000, offers a more comprehensive and precise thermograph than the more widely known digital-imaging camera thermography mentioned above. This more objective thermometry system delivers a functional physiologic assessment of your body's bio-regulation system and offers insights into underlying dysfunction that both precedes and provokes developing disease processes.

Infrared measurements of skin temperature at over 100 points on your body including your head, torso, and back, taken both before and after exposure to a cool ambient room temperature assess how your body regulates temperature stress via the autonomic nervous system. Connected organs, glands, and other tissues influence the capillary blood vessel bed beneath each skin point location. Changes indicate either clear or blocked channels.

Scientific evidence shows that internal physiological abnormalities and dysfunction affect skin surface temperatures and that, therefore, skin temperatures and behavioral responses can reveal information about associated organ function. Medical clinics worldwide have studied, correlated and validated over 40 temperature patterns that define regulation incapacities, called signature recognitions. Alfa Thermodiagnostics' AlfaSight™ 9000 captures these signature patterns and provides a vivid integrative, computerized summary report that illustrates a system-wide overview and detailed dental, breast, and prostate evaluations.

Other Diagnostic Tools

- **Cavitat.** Just as seismologists use acoustic energy to look for oil and obstetricians image fetuses with ultrasound, some dentists use a Cavitat to explore 3D images of cavitations in jawbone. As with first generation Thermography, it requires a skilled clinician and there is room for error. In the process of gaining FDA approval, tests using the Cavitat showed that 94 percent of old extraction sites were positive for bone lesions. Perhaps not surprisingly, Aetna Insurance discredited cavitations and the Cavitat. As Dr. Wes Shankland states in an open letter:

"Aetna Insurance Company contacted other insurance companies and reported that jaw bone cavitations did not exist. Aetna Insurance Company also informed others that the Cavitat was inaccurate and those who used this device were 'quacks.'"

Such negative and inaccurate publicity literally ruined Cavitat sales. With no other recourse, Cavitat Medical Technologies made a decision to file a federal lawsuit, in Denver, against Aetna Insurance Company. Aetna lost and was ordered to pay a serious judgment, but the damage was done.

Glenn's note: In 1971 I had my four wisdom teeth removed while I was in the Air Force. In 1998 I saw a dentist who first used panoramic x-rays and found one cavitation that was very hard to see on the x-ray and one that was almost impossible to see. They were both at my lower wisdom teeth sites. He repaired them and about 2 weeks later called me and told me Bob Jones who invented the cavitat as a way to find hidden cavitations was coming to his office to demonstrate it. He asked if I was interested. I went and met Bob Jones and he and the dentist found 2 more cavitations at the upper extraction sites. The right one looked worse. The dentist repaired the left first and was well into good bone on the right when he stopped and asked Bob how sure he was. Bob said he was sure, the dentist asked me if he should continue. He soon hit a pocket filled with really nasty stuff. The infection had eaten the bone away well up into the sinus. Many dentists and the American Dental Association say there is no such thing. There is.

EAV (Electro Acupuncture according to Voll). An EKG measures electrical flow through your heart. Expressed as a graph, it pinpoints heart damage, since current does not flow through dead tissues. EAV works the same way. The EAV test uses an ohmmeter to measure energy flow along meridians at acupuncture points. If you understand meridians and you've signed on to "Healing is Voltage," "The Body Electric" and understand the science behind "Earthing", you know low-functioning organs are low in negative ions.

This state hinders electron flow along your body's energy meridians. Dr. WA Tiller, Professor Emeritus of Materials Science at Stanford University, set out to discredit the EAV, but became an advocate as his research verified organ degeneration correlated with low conductance. In fact, it was Dr. Tiller who mapped the Meridian Tooth Chart which correlates each tooth with its associated organs, glands, and anatomical structures on the same meridian. Infected or diseased teeth, as well as dental implants, block electrical conductivity on meridians and so can alter the health of other organs located on the same meridian and vice versa.

The Dark Side of Dental Implants

Perhaps you have decided you must extract your root canal treated teeth to maintain or regain health—against the clear position stated by the American Association of Endodontists above. You chose a biological dentist who can help you avoid cavitations, and boosted your immune system. How should you replace the space? Interestingly, the more complex and biologically incompatible the option, the more costly it is. Costs vary widely, as do longevity estimates.

Implants are essentially an artificial root screwed into your jawbone, topped with an artificial tooth or used as an anchor for a bridge or partial denture. Implants are displacing root canals because they look, feel, and function very much like a natural tooth, and do not interfere with normal oral activities.

They help maintain bone that normally dissolves over time after a tooth is extracted. They can last a long time, and do not require grinding down adjacent teeth, as a fixed bridge would require. But you have to remember success is not measured only by tooth function, but function within your body as a whole.

Here are a few important aspects of dental implants you must seriously consider before making the decision to go forward with this major investment. Dead tissues do not conduct energy, implants therefore, whether titanium or zirconium, slow energy flow along meridians. Your body must constantly compensate for this. As with root canals, your associated organs, glands, or anatomical structures may functionally decline.

Most people with a dental implant have other metallic dental repairs present, which only exacerbates energetic chaos. In fact, the implant screw and replacement tooth are usually different metals. These two dissimilar metals within an electrolyte (saliva) effectively turn your mouth into a battery. Additionally, if you still have gold, mercury, copper, tin or silver filings, or nickel-based crowns in your mouth, these will also contribute to the galvanic currents being generated.

What You Need to Know About Titanium Implants

Most implants used today are made of titanium. So when your mouth is functioning as a battery due to the dissimilar metals present, there are resulting chaotic galvanic currents that continuously drive ions from the titanium or its alloys, which include small amounts of vanadium or aluminum. These metallic ions are then transported around your body, around the clock, where they bind to proteins and can wreak havoc with your health. Some people are more susceptible to the resulting inflammatory, allergy, and autoimmune problems than others. There is a blood test to help determine this sensitivity.

Though you're exposed to fluoride through many avenues, tap drinking water and dental products remain your most significant sources. If you drink tap water or use fluoridated toothpaste, it is important to know that fluoride accelerates titanium corrosion in the extreme (up to 500 microg/(cm2 x d)). Low pH values (acidity in the mouth or a dry mouth) accelerate this effect profoundly. Corrosion of the other metals also accelerates ion release.

Previous research has documented that:

"The amounts of tin released by the enhanced corrosion of amalgam [in the presence of titanium] might contribute measurably to the daily intake of this element; the corrosion current generated reached values known to cause taste sensations. If the buffer systems of

adjacent tissues... are not able to cope with the high pH generated around the titanium, local tissue damage may ensue; this relationship is liable to be overlooked, as it leaves no evidence in the form of corrosion products."

While most people do not notice galvanic currents, others experience unexplained nerve shocks, ulcerations, a salty or metallic taste or a burning sensation in their mouth. Noticeable or not, oral galvanic currents are commonly as high as 100 micro-amps, yet your brain operates on 7 to 9 nano-amps—a current more than 1,000 times weaker. Given your brain's proximity to your mouth, biological dentists are concerned the constant high and chaotic electrical activity may misdirect brain impulses. These currents can contribute to insomnia, brain fog, ear-ringing, epilepsy, and dizziness.

The possibility that titanium implants may act as antennas that direct microwaves from your cell phone and cellular transmission towers into your body also deserves study. As Dr. Douglas Swartzendruber, a professor at the University of Colorado has said: *"Anything implanted in bone will create an autoimmune response. The only difference is the length of time it takes."*

Titanium implants are certainly known to suppress important immune cells such as your T-cells, white blood cells critical to immune system function, and create oxidative stress as measured by rH2 values (a measurement of oxidation-reduction potential under a specific pH). Diseases associated with implants are not all that different from those associated with root canals, and include a number of different autoimmune and neurological disorders, such as:

Cancer	Multiple sclerosis (MS)	Alzheimer's disease
Parkinson's disease	Chronic fatigue	Fibromyalgia

Other complications of implanted titanium include occasional facial eczema as your skin tries to detoxify the titanium ions. Dental implants also have no fibrous "seal" to prevent microbial invasion. If you make the decision to get a dental implant, it's wise to use floss impregnated with ozonated oil around the neck of each implant daily.

Alternatives to Titanium Implants

Zirconium implants are a newer innovation in dentistry and many biological dentists now use them. These implants bypass some of the problems of titanium mentioned above. They still block energy flow, but at least they are electrically neutral, eliminating the potential to interfere with your brain impulses. The implant itself also does not contribute to electrical galvanic currents being generated in your mouth. But you still need to be careful as the artificial tooth that is ultimately screwed onto the zirconium implant may have a metal base. Zirconium implants also release ions, but at a much slower rate than titanium implants.

These implants seem to last quite a long time. One systematic review showed that over the 10-30 year period studied, there was only a 1.3 percent to five percent loss of implanted teeth in clinically well-maintained mouths. For those with less optimal maintenance, it was more like a 14-20 percent loss of implanted teeth over that time. Don't even think about smoking though! Endodontic literature has a very different slant on the benefits of implants, of course.

Traditional Bridges Can Be Costly and Relatively Impermanent

First off, bridges don't last all that long. The average bridge lasts eight years, with a range of five to 15 years. For this reason, "permanent bridges" are no longer considered "permanent." A traditional bridge is comprised of several units – the artificial teeth and the abutments. Abutments are the crowns (caps) made to cover the anchor teeth. The bridge is permanently bonded in place to span a gap that replaces at least one missing tooth. Whether thay are broken down or completely intact, the abutment teeth to each side of the gap are aggressively cut away to accept the covering crown.

Or should I say smothering crown? Think of a healthy tooth being like a fountain. A crown stifles the natural nutritive, cleansing, hydrating flow of lymph. It can no longer "breathe." Why do this to two good teeth that need no dental work for the sake of one (or two) missing teeth? Some biological doctors think these should be removed periodically so the underlying teeth can be cleaned up.

If one of the supporting crowned teeth breaks or develops decay or nerve damage, the bridge and its three or more crowns must be removed and replaced. As a hygienist, I can tell you that most people are terrible about cleaning around the abutment teeth and under the artificial tooth. Margins are very susceptible to decay. Again, I advise my clients to use ozonated oil around all crown margins as an extra degree of caution. Good personal care is one key to longevity. And once again, avoid smoking!

I am no fan of crowns as I explained in a previous interview with Dr. Mercola. The more a tooth is destroyed during restoration, the less able it is to withstand chewing forces. Also, forces which once could transfer through the organic, flexible bulk of the tooth to the root now must travel along the outside of a stiff crown to concentrate at the gum margin – hardly a recipe for longevity of either the underlying tooth or the crown itself.

Biomimetic Considerations to Take into Account

Biomimetic means mimicking nature. In choosing dental materials, a dentist must weigh the ability of the body's immune system to ignore dental materials after recognition, called biocompatibility, with the beauty and function patients demand. They must find materials that match the flexibility of teeth so they can absorb daily chewing and clenching stresses. Materials should expand and contract at the same rate as teeth do when exposed to oral temperature fluctuations and they must resist wear and fracture.

Porcelain crowns are about four times harder than natural teeth and accelerate wear on opposing teeth. They fracture far more easily than zirconia based ceramic crowns, which are biocompatible, beautiful, and strong. These benefits come at the cost of stiffness. Zirconia based ceramic crowns are poor shock absorbers, which can be hard on your jaw joint and the bones that anchor your teeth. A new material, poly-ceramic DiamondCrown, comes closer to meeting all these requirements, and is biocompatible for about 80 percent of people tested. More biocompatible and biomimetic dental materials will emerge as these principals are more widely recognized.

Other Points to Consider

Your cranial (head) bones rhythmically move. Their gentle movements are thought to help drain your sinuses, aid nasal breathing, and influence your nervous system via movement of cerebrospinal fluid, the fluid that bathes your brain and nerves in your spinal cord.

This rhythmic pumping of cranial bones is particularly important at night because it helps the glymphatic system (a functional waste clearance pathway for the vertebrate central nervous system) flush waste products from your brain that have built up during the day. Think of the glymphatic system as your brain's garbage truck; glial cells create high pressure channels for cerebrospinal fluid that dilate and flow during sleep as blood pumps through arteries and as cranial bones "breathe." They close during wakefulness. When movement is restricted, migraines or a build-up of the amyloid plaques associated with Alzheimers can occur. The glymphatic system may be one of the most important reasons you sleep.

TMJ (jaw joint) specialists, osteopaths and craniosacral therapists recognize the need to maintain cranial bone motion. These clinicians suggest that no fixed dentistry, whether "permanent" bridgework or metal partial, should cross the midline of the upper or lower jaw.

If you choose to have a permanent bridge, avoid porcelain fused to metal, since these metals contain nickel. Some dentists will assure you that they would never use a nickel-based metal; they use stainless steel! But stainless steel contains at least 10 percent chromium, vanadium, and nickel and/or manganese. I recommend going metal-free!

Fixed bridges were once considered premium care, since they, like implants, look, feel and function much like permanent teeth. In my experience, both require about the same amount of extra personal and clinical care. Incidentally, dentists will occasionally recommend a cantilever bridge, anchoring a false tooth to just one neighbor instead of two. These are less costly, but can certainly torque the anchor tooth, which it cannot always withstand.

Resin Bonded Bridge—A Less Costly Alternative, But Just as Impermanent

Resin bonded bridges (Maryland bridges) are a minimally invasive option for replacing missing teeth in certain situations. They are generally only considered for anterior tooth replacement. Design, materials, skill, and patient selection largely dictate longevity and satisfaction. Fortunately, design and materials have significantly evolved. Unlike traditional bridges, resin bonded bridges require much less reduction of supporting teeth. Instead, the dentist slightly reduces the backs of the neighboring teeth onto which "wings" attached to the artificial tooth are bonded.

Materials can be all resin, porcelain, porcelain bonded to metal, or zirconium. Most doctors still fabricate these bridges with a wing to either side of the artificial tooth, though the literature seems to suggest it is better to just have one – to cantilever the missing tooth off one supporting tooth. Interestingly, this is because it is recognized that cranial bones and teeth move and that the anchoring teeth do not move equally. This puts stress on the bonds, which can lead to failure. Also, since it is unlikely that both bonds would break at the same time, the debonding often goes unnoticed, allowing decay to set in under the debonded wing.

Resin bonded bridges are a good option for adolescents with missing teeth, when the bridge is well designed. Most replacement options cannot be considered until you have finished maturing physically. These bridges help maintain space and are fairly easy to care for.

If you have teeth that have loosened due to gum disease, some would add another advantage of resin bonded bridges – they help splint loosened teeth together. This is true, but unless your gums are disease-free and cleaned on a daily basis at home, it might be time to remove them because in this case, it might be extremely difficult to self-cleanse daily at home. We are not just looking at longevity of the teeth, but longevity of the host.

The downside of resin bonded bridges is that they're somewhat fragile. If made with metals, the usual caveats apply: mixed metals lead to galvanic currents and a panoply of problems already addressed. Again, 100 percent zirconium would avoid this. Remember, biological dentists try to be metal free and avoid metal-based crowns and bridges. It isn't just the galvanic currents these set up, but the release of nickel/chromium/manganese/vanadium ions. **A better restoration option might be the Carlson Bridge – a resin bonded bridge that requires no drilling into adjacent teeth. Placed in one appointment,** these economical, prefabricated, "winged" replacement teeth can last many years. An advantage is that the bond to adjacent teeth is less rigid, so cranial bones can shift as they should.

Partials—Your Least Expensive Option

Going back in time, removable partials were all dentistry offered to replace missing teeth. Our current culture values looking young, so partials – associated with our grandparents – are a difficult aesthetic choice. They may however be the choice that offers the best chance for aging *well*. Partials are designed based on how many teeth need replacing. Metal frameworks were once the norm, but the future lies in non-metal dental repairs. New materials:

1) Are less obvious.

2) Avoid the adverse properties of metal restorations already discussed.

3) Are able to distribute chewing forces over a greater area compared to metal framework partials, and are therefore more comfortable.

4) Relines are less frequent.

5) According to the Clifford Biocompatibility Test, Flexite and Valplast (light, flexible, yet strong nylon resins) are biocompatible for 99 percent of the population. Lucitone FRS is a very similar biocompatible nylon resin. None of these use a heavy metal (cadmium) as a pink colorant as some other dental materials do. Many patients choose a clear framework to avoid any possible reaction to the colorant. Nylon materials can draw in water and with it, odors and stain, though good hygiene can mitigate this problem.

6) VisiClear is another nylon-free biocompatible partial material.

For best aesthetics, biocompatibilit and biomimetic function, choose DiamondCrown or zirconia teeth in your partial rather than the default acrylic teeth most often used. If you must add another tooth to any of the above partials, that is possible, too. The lab simply reuses the artificial teeth, the most valuable component, and remakes the framework with the new tooth!

Biocomp Labs and the Clifford Consulting and Research Lab offer individualized dental materials testing, recommended especially for those with multiple chemical sensitivities or anyone who needs dental work and feels their health could be challenged by the wide range of dental materials available.

Most patients tell me they consider these newer partials to be comfortable and aesthetically unnoticeable, though they are annoyed that foods tend to trap under them. People with spider partials tell me they often take them out to eat, but wear them the rest of the time to maintain the space until dentistry offers them more biocompatible "fixed" choices.

At least one reader will likely comment that if only people adopted a certain lifestyle, these kinds of advanced dentistry would be unnecessary. I couldn't agree more.

The reality is that most people's mouths are in deplorable shape. I try not to spend much time thinking about the rescue dentistry presented here. Most of my advocacy work centers around changing how we approach dentistry so your children or their children can avoid these compromising options.

Ultimately, the answers to better oral and general health start in infancy and include a radically different model of dentistry and definition of health. The answers are out there now (see *Mouth Matters* book and <http://www.mouthmattersbook.com/>) along with a few clinicians who are well versed in these strategies. Seek them out, and if you can't find someone who does the kind of dentistry you want in your area, be ready to ask them to learn it.

Resources to Help You Find a Biological Dentist

If you are seriously considering any of the dental procedures done above, it is best to have them performed by a biological dentist. See the list earlier in this chapter

About the Author

Carol Vander Stoep, RDH, BSDH, OMT, is an advocate for change in dentistry. She believes mid-level providers – dental hygienists with expanded training – must be empowered to go beyond their serious limitations in the United States. Training a core of motivated hygienists at a clinic in Belize, her intent is to help bring an advanced model of Minimally Invasive Preventive Dentistry and posture-guided early facial development to India and China based on the model of "Barefoot Doctors." A clinical hygienist, orofacial myofunctional therapist, lecturer, and writer, she brought many of these concepts together in her book "Mouth Matters: How Your Mouth Ages Your Body and What YOU Can do About It."

Above is adapted from http://articles.mercola.com/sites/articles/archive/2014/05/03/root-canal-alternative.aspx?e_cid=20140503Z1_DNL_art_1&utm_source=dnl&utm_medium=email&utm_content=art1&utm_campaign=20140503Z1&et_cid=DM45438&et_rid=508895019 (5/3/2014)

****

Below is from http://articles.mercola.com/sites/articles/archive/2005/01/19/whole-food-supplements.aspx

Real or Synthetic
The Truth Behind Whole-Food Supplements

By Daniel H. Chong, ND

Americans are now spending more than $17 billion a year on supplements for health and wellness. Strangely enough, the rates of some forms of chronic disease have not changed, while the rates of others have actually increased. There are a number of reasons for these poor statistics and many things remain a mystery.

One thing seems fairly clear, however. Most supplements aren't helping very much.

I'm not saying there are no helpful supplements out there. There certainly are. What is becoming more apparent, however, is supplements will not help much if one does not first address the necessary basics of health and healing.

What is also clear is that not all supplements are created equal. The basics of health and healing were discussed in another of my articles, *The Six Foundations of Healing*. I believe these areas must be addressed for true healing to occur in any chronic disease. In this article, I will discuss some things you should consider if you need to or want to take some supplements. Specifically, I will address the differences between whole foods versus synthetic or isolated nutritional supplements.

Whole Food Nutrients Vs. Synthetic, Isolated Nutrients

Most people who read the eHealthy News You Can Use newsletter are at least somewhat familiar with the idea that whole foods are better for you than refined foods. Although there are numerous viewpoints on what kind of foods we should or should not be eating, as well as the ideal ratio of these foods, everyone from all corners of the diet and nutrition world seems to agree on one thing: No matter which foods we choose and in what ratios we eat them, whole foods are better for you than refined foods.

This fact has never really been argued. Everyone agrees raw honey is better for you than white sugar or that brown rice is better for you than white rice. Why should it be any different for vitamins?

Often, I have been puzzled by the average naturopath or nutritionist who goes on and on about the value of whole foods and how refined foods - having been robbed of all the extra nutrients they naturally come with - are not healthy for you. Then, they go on to prescribe a shopping bag full of isolated, refined vitamins for you to take!

Just like refined foods, these refined vitamins have been robbed of all of the extra accessory nutrients that they naturally come with as well. In turn, like refined foods, they can create numerous problems and imbalances in your body if taken at high levels for long periods of time. They can also act more like drugs in your body, forcing themselves down one pathway or another. At the very least, they won't help you as much as high quality food and food-based supplements.

Whole Food Supplements

Whole food supplements are what their name suggests: Supplements made from concentrated whole foods. The vitamins found within these supplements are not isolated. They are highly complex structures that combine a variety of enzymes, coenzymes, antioxidants, trace elements, activators and many other unknown or undiscovered factors all working together synergistically, to enable this vitamin complex to do its job in your body.

Nutrients from within this complex cannot be taken apart or isolated from the whole, and then be expected to do the same job in the body as the whole complex is designed to do.

The perfect example of this difference can be seen in an automobile. An automobile is a wonderfully designed complex machine that needs all of its parts to be present and in place to function properly. Wheels are certainly an important part of the whole, but you could never isolate them from the rest of the car, call them a car or expect them to function like a car. They need the engine, body and everything else.

The same analogy applies to the vitamin C (ascorbic acid) or vitamin E (delta tocopherol) you can find on most health food store shelves. They are parts of an entire complex that serve a purpose when part of the whole. However, they cannot do the job of the entire complex by themselves.

With similar logic in place, one can analyze what a typical multivitamin truly is. The automobile equivalent of creating a multivitamin would be going to a junk yard, finding all of the separate parts you would need to make up an entire automobile, throwing them together in a heap (or capsule in terms of the multivitamin) and expecting that heap to drive like a car!

Obviously, there is a difference. Science cannot create life. Only life can create life.

Synthetic or Isolated Nutritional Supplements

Isolated nutrients or synthetic nutrients are not natural, in that they are never found by themselves in nature. Taking these isolated nutrients, especially at the ultra-high doses found in formulas today, is more like taking a drug. Studies show the body treats these isolated and synthetic nutrients like xenobiotics (foreign substances).

By the same token, food-based supplements are never treated like this by your body. For example, your urine will never turn florescent yellow, no matter how much meat (a good source of B vitamins) you eat. This sort of rapid excretion happens only with foreign substances in your body.

Not only are isolated nutrients treated like drugs or other chemicals by your body. Like drugs, they can create problems for you too. Nature does not produce any nutrient in an isolated form. The nutrients in foods are blended together in a specific way and work best in that format. For an isolated nutrient to work properly in the body, it needs all the other parts that are naturally present in the food too.

If the parts are not all there from the start, they are taken from the body's stored supply. This is why isolated nutrients often work for a little while, then seem to stop working. Once your body's store of the extra nutrients is used up, the isolated nutrient you're taking doesn't work as well anymore. Worse yet, a deficiency in these extra nutrients can be created in your body.

And, because most nutrients are isolated from the foods they come in - using a wide array of potentially nasty solvents and other chemicals - taking high amounts of these products can also expose you to these potentially toxic chemicals, if care is not taken to remove them. With the burden we are already facing from the high number of chemicals in our environment, why would anyone want to add more?

Synergy and Potency

The various parts of a natural vitamin complex work together in a synergistic manner. Synergy means that the whole is greater than the sum of its parts. Nutritionist Judith DeCava puts it best: "Separating the group of compounds (in a vitamin complex) converts it from a physiological, biochemical, active micronutrient into a disabled, debilitated chemical of little or no value to living cells. The synergy is gone."

In other words, the automobile, in its original form, will drive better than a pile of its individual parts. Most people don't follow this logic when examining a nutritional supplement.

Supplement makers typically try to stuff as much as possible in a capsule, telling us that the more we take, the better it is for us. This is simply not the case. As you now know, it is not necessarily the amount of a nutrient you ingest that is important, but its form and how much is bioavailable that counts the most. In fact, remembering that ingesting single nutrients can actually create imbalances in the body, logic would dictate the higher the level of a single nutrient that you take in, the quicker this imbalance will occur.

What all of this means: **The potency of a supplement has much more to do with synergy than with actual nutrient levels**. It is a combined effect of all the parts of the food, rather than the chemical effect of a single part, that is most important.

Don't Forget the Basics

I fear all of this talk of supplements - food-based, isolated or synthetic - has detracted from the most important part of health and healing. The basics of proper diet; exercise, detoxification, structure, mental/emotional and spiritual health must all be in order for true healing to occur. No supplement will work on its own if these foundations are not in place.

However, even when these foundations are in place, or if the situation is acute enough to necessitate a more immediate treatment response, supplement support may still be needed for a while. You may also want to take one or more food-based supplements to ensure you are getting an adequate array of nutrients in your diet. When these situations arise, I strongly recommend food-based supplements be your first choice.

Keys to a Good Nutritional Supplement

How do you tell whether or not a supplement you're looking at is a good choice? For starters, make sure it has the following characteristics:

- It is as close as possible to its natural form.
- The utmost care has been taken in all phases of its production, from growing its ingredients, to manufacturing, testing for potency and quality control.

- It works! I always try to select from companies that have a long track record of providing high quality products that produce good clinical results.

Dr. Daniel Chong is a licensed naturopathic physician practicing in Portland, Ore. His practice focuses on chronic disease and pain management. Contact him at:

Chiropractic and Naturopathic Physicians Clinic
12195 SW Allen Blvd.
Beaverton, OR 97005
(503) 646-0697
www.danielchongnd.com

Above is from http://articles.mercola.com/sites/articles/archive/2005/01/19/whole-food-supplements.aspx

Below is from http://articles.mercola.com/sites/articles/archive/2011/11/18/dangers-of-vitamins.aspx and http://articles.mercola.com/sites/articles/archive/2005/01/19/whole-food-supplements.aspx

Experts Warn Vitamin E Can Trigger Cancer

They used synthetic vitamin E *in the study*

By Dr. Mercola

Over the past several weeks, the media has gone wild over studies allegedly showing that vitamins have lethal consequences.

Again and again, journalists who are clueless about health have misled readers while catering to the interests of Big Pharma and their hired lackey, the US Food and Drug Administration (FDA).

Will Vitamin E Increase Risk of Prostate Cancer?

Back in 2009, the initial report of the Selenium and Vitamin E Cancer Prevention Trial (SELECT) found "no reduction in risk of prostate cancer with either selenium or vitamin E supplements but a statistically non-significant increase in prostate cancer risk with vitamin E."

Then came the recently released update, which allegedly shows that high doses—400 IU's a day or more—of vitamin E may increase your risk of prostate cancer by 17 percent.

> According to CNN:
>
> *"Based on the results of this trial, [the researchers] suggested that men should have a serious conversation with their doctors about whether taking vitamin E supplements is a good idea."*

However, there's a glaring problem with this finding, which has been completely overlooked by conventional media, and the researchers of the study itself.

For some reason, many fail to appreciate that there are usually major differences between natural nutrients and their synthetic counterparts.

They simply do not have the same biological effects, and this appears particularly true when it comes to vitamin E.

Synthetic Vitamin E is Problematic, so Why Did they Use it?

In this case, the vitamin E used was *all rac*-α-tocopheryl acetate—a synthetic petrochemically-derived form of dl-alpha tocopherol, which has *known* toxic effects. GreenMedInfo.com has a listing of published research relating to the many ill health effects related to this compound. The Toxicology Data Network also lists numerous health problems related to synthetic vitamin E at various dosages.

Unfortunately, most studies investigating vitamins use synthetic versions. On the one hand this is good, as synthetic vitamins in general have overwhelmingly been shown to be largely harmless. However, studies such as this one—and the journalists reporting on the findings—can also do great disservice by failing to *specify* that the results pertain to *petrochemically-derived vitamin E.* The study says absolutely nothing about the health effects of *natural* vitamin E (d-alpha tocopherol).Part of the problem with synthetic alpha tocopherol is that it depletes gamma tocopherol.

> As explained in a recent article by Life Extension:
>
> *"In 1997, we announced that taking only the alpha tocopherol form of vitamin E displaces critically important gamma tocopherol in the body. By displacing gamma tocopherol, we feared that high doses of alpha tocopherol could increase cancer risks.*
>
> *In fact, three years after Life Extension's first warning, the Johns Hopkins School of Public Health released the results of a huge study (10,456 men). The findings showed that men with the highest gamma tocopherol blood levels had a fivefold reduction in prostate cancer risk. This same study showed that selenium and alpha tocopherol also reduced prostate cancer risk but only when gamma tocopherol levels were high. Confirmatory studies document higher levels of gamma tocopherol to be strongly associated with reduced cancer risks.*
>
> *While both alpha and gamma tocopherol are potent antioxidants, gamma tocopherol has a unique function. Because of its different chemical structure, gamma tocopherol scavenges reactive nitrogen species, which can damage proteins, lipids, and DNA.*
>
> *... The fact that supplementation with isolated, synthetic alpha tocopherol depletes plasma gamma tocopherol levels means that the researchers who designed the SELECT trial created a biological catastrophe... The fact that higher prostate cancer rates were observed in the group overloaded with synthetic alpha tocopherol in the SELECT trial was predictable and expected based upon fundamental facts Life Extension understood more than a decade ago."*

I believe Life Extension is correct in their evaluation of this study: it was designed to fail in order to protect the financial interests of the cancer industry, which thrives by providing very expensive toxic drugs, radiation, and surgery.

Did You Know? Some Vitamin E on Market May be Genetically Modified

Another risk factor of vitamin E supplements and foods fortified with vitamin E relates to the fact that it may be derived from genetically modified (GM) plants. The chemical name for vitamin E is "tocopherol." Tocopherol, which is the generic term for at least seven different types of vitamin E, are naturally formed in a variety of plants.

Tocopherol can be produced either by chemical synthesis, or by extraction from:

- Maize
- Soy beans
- Cotton seed
- Rice
- Wheat germ oil

The problem is that a large majority of these plants are now genetically modified—at least in the U.S. In Europe, foods and supplements containing GM-derived vitamin E must be labeled as such. The U.S. however, does not require genetically modified foods and products to be labeled, so there's no telling what you're getting. Unfortunately, verifying the non-GM status of tocopherols is particularly challenging as many companies that control the supply of vitamin E collect plant oils from commingled sources.

Are Dietary Supplements Risky for Older Women?

Another recent study is being reported as having found that dietary supplements are associated with an increased mortality in older women. However, this is yet another example of a flawed study being further misrepresented by poor journalism. First of all, this was an *observational study* based on *self-reported* use of supplements over a 22-year period—it was *not* a rigorous trial. Supplement use was reported three times, six years apart. Now, ask yourself, how accurately would your own recollection be of what supplements you've used over the past *six years?* Furthermore, the data collected was rather generic—there's no telling whether the supplements used were high or low quality; synthetic or whole-food based, for example.

> According to the Los Angeles Times:
>
> *"The research did not explore whether supplements contributed to the causes of death among the women ... It could reflect the possibility that the women who took ... supplements were more likely to be sick from other causes and died from their underlying disease."*

And there, in a nutshell, is the problem with the way this study is being reported in many places. That same Los Angeles Times article, for example, quotes a dietician arguing that the research "bolstered arguments against using supplements". Other articles have made similar claims.

But the study does no such thing.

It's quite possible that the people studied who were sick were trying to help themselves by taking supplements, and hence this group was biased towards being sicker. An almost identical study could be done associating frequency of visits to the doctor with increased risk of death. But you can bet that few in the media would jump the conclusion that doctor visits are deadly ... even though such a statement would not be entirely untrue.

Was the Data Manipulated with Preconceived Bias?

But there's more… Upon closer review, it seems the researchers went to great lengths massaging the data to reach their own preconceived conclusions. As explained in a recent article by Alliance for Natural Health:

"Dr. Robert Verkerk, our scientific director's… analysis reveals, among many other interesting points, that all of the data was "adjusted" by the authors using methods of their own choice. If you look at the study itself, the first thing you see is an adjustment for "age and energy"... After this adjustment, vitamins C, B complex, E, D, as well as calcium, magnesium, selenium and zinc all appear to add to years lived."

So, after that first adjustment, several supplements added to longevity. Next they "adjusted out" other lifestyle factors, which then resulted in most supplements contributing to earlier death. According to Robert Verkerk:

"It must be born in mind that this is an observational study where lifestyle factors, which are known to have a far greater influence on survival outcome than typical vitamin and mineral supplementation, have been 'adjusted out'. Before this data massage process has occurred, the findings are quite different, and appear to have been largely ignored by a mass media ever keen to find ways of damning supplements to appease their pharmaceutical industry advertisers...

This is what the study actually found before the data were adjusted... Supplement users were significantly (statistically) more likely than non-users to:

Be non-smokers	Be more educated (graduates)	Have lower risk of diabetes mellitus
Have a lower body mass index (BMI)	Have a lower mean hip-to-waist ratio	Be more physically active
Ingest fewer calories	Consume more protein	Consume less total fat
Consume more polyunsaturated fatty acids	Consume more fruit	Consume more vegetables
Consume more whole grain products		

Frustratingly, the authors don't tell us how these supplement users fared over the years. However, we can assume it's quite likely that they did rather better than the non-users, and that's why the researchers have left us only with adjusted data that's meant to have removed the influence of these all-important lifestyle factors."

Interestingly enough, and quite tellingly, the authors did NOT make any adjustments for drug use, despite the fact that many drugs are highly toxic and may contribute to premature death. And many who are sick take both drugs and supplements in an effort to maintain health and treat their disease.

As stated by Life Extension:

> *"The authors admit they did not factor in the increased intake of dietary supplements that occur in response to the development of symptoms or diagnosis of serious disease. Stated differently: If a woman was diagnosed with stage 4 breast cancer and began ingesting 40 supplements daily, but died six months later, she would have been counted as being a heavy supplement user who died prematurely."*

Smells Like a Ruse to Justify New FDA Safety Regulations...

If you ask me, the timing of these studies hitting the news couldn't possibly be more convenient. Last month, I wrote a couple of articles about the FDA's latest plan to effectively eliminate many commonly used supplements by amending the definitions for new dietary ingredients (NDI's) and retroactively applying them to products already on the market. You can read the FDA Draft Guidance on New Dietary Ingredients (NDI's) here. (A detailed analysis of the FDA Draft Guidance is also available.)

This proposed mandate goes hand-in-hand with S.1310: Dietary Supplement Labeling Act of 2011, introduced at the end of June by U.S. Senator Richard Durbin (D-Illinois). This legislation is, using the words of Byron J. Richards, "an alarming regulatory nightmare that is trying to **treat vitamins as if they are drugs**."

The open comment period on the FDA's proposed guidelines will expire on December 2nd, and I for one would not be the least surprised if the studies discussed above will be used as justification for driving through Durbin's legislation and the FDA's amended NDI definitions. After all, if they can sway public opinion once again into thinking that supplements can KILL you, then people will support the idea that we need to treat supplements like drugs and require them to undergo the same detailed and costly kind of testing.

This is ridiculous, as vitamins, minerals and herbal supplements have a *tremendously safe* track record. Meanwhile, drugs are known to cause well over 100,000 deaths per year when *taken as prescribed,* and two million more suffer serious side effects. For comparison, look at:

- Statistics available from the U.S. National Poison Data System, which covers acute poisonings: In 2007, 1,597 people reportedly died from drugs. Meanwhile there was *not one single fatality* caused by a vitamin or dietary mineral supplement that year
- CDC mortality data for 2005: Prescription drugs killed more than 33,500 people that year, second only to car accidents. That same year, the American Association of Poison Control Centers reported 27 deaths that were associated with dietary supplements (one of which was reportedly due to Ephedra; the herbal supplement banned the year before for being too dangerous. In 2005, low-dose Ephedra was also subsequently banned).

Yet, Durbin and the FDA want you to think that they're just acting in *your* best interest. Nothing could be further from the truth!

Up to this point, the FDA has had to prove a supplement unsafe in order to take action against it, but now they want the supplement industry to prove the safety of what in many cases amount to *food,* before they can reach the market. Now, since dietary supplements are not patented drugs with outrageous profit margins, very few supplement makers will be able to afford the required safety studies, which could run in the tens or even hundreds of millions of dollars per ingredient. Furthermore, the manufacturer is not the only one that would have to seek approval—every distributor that wants to use the NDI would have to file a separate NDI application.

By adding this extremely costly testing and approval process, small and medium sized supplement companies will be eliminated, which in turn will drive up costs while at the same time reduce your access to historically safe nutritional products. The end result is that fewer people will use supplements to improve their health; driving them back into the extremely profitable fold of conventional medicine and drugs.

So, Will Your Supplements Kill You?

Vitamins and minerals are essential for life. However, never in the history of man has the human body ever needed synthetic chemicals. And therein lies the crux of the matter. **Most studies evaluating the health effects of vitamins investigate the synthetic versions, which in many cases are more similar to drugs than they are to food.** And secondly, studies can be manipulated in any number of ways to come up with an end result that serves a particular agenda. The two studies discussed above are perfect examples of both of these problems.

Making matters worse, the media conveniently and consistently fails to report on rebuttals explaining the technical and statistical reasons why a study is invalid.

Common sense however will tell you that you cannot kill yourself with *nutrition*, per se.

That said, it's certainly possible to go overboard with supplements and push your health in the wrong direction by creating nutritional imbalances. It's important to understand that taking *mega-doses* of vitamins or minerals over extended periods of time, *especially synthetic ones*, can have serious health consequences.

Ideally, you'll want to get the majority of the nutrients you need from your food, which means you have to eat whole, preferably organic foods—*not* processed foods fortified with synthetic vitamins and minerals! Depending on your health status, you would then evaluate whether or not you might need to take a supplement to help address a particular health problem or counter any particular deficiency in your diet.

Examples of supplements I believe *most* people can benefit from, simply because it's very difficult to get enough of them from your diet, include high-quality omega-3 and probiotics. If you cannot get sufficient amounts of sunshine and don't have access to a safe tanning bed then an oral vitamin D3 supplement would also be in order.

In conclusion, Michael Long, ND sums this whole issue up rather nicely:

"Even with totally irresponsible use, you would be hard pressed to be killed by your vitamins... In truth, studies are published every day showing the safety and health promoting effects of vitamins, especially when used responsibly (i.e. used for a specific purpose, after objective testing showed a deficiency), and according to the evidence.

If you want to focus on something that will actually kill you, open your medicine cabinet and look at the drugs that stare back at you. Close to 1 million people die in North America every year as a direct result of adverse effects from prescription drugs. The safety record of pharmaceutical drugs is not even comparable to vitamins."

Above is from http://articles.mercola.com/sites/articles/archive/2011/11/18/dangers-of-vitamins.aspx and http://articles.mercola.com/sites/articles/archive/2005/01/19/whole-food-supplements.aspx

****

Below is adapted from <http://curezone.org/foods/saltcure.asp

Salts That Heal and Salts That Kill

Unrefined Ocean Sea Salt - NaCl (98%) + 80 elements(2%) versus Refined Salt - Table Salt - pure NaCl (99.9%)

Ocean water is currently an average of 3.5% (by weight) percent dry matter. Dry ocean salt is composed of 80 elements - minerals.

Salt is an essence of Life.

Natural Salt is an essential element in the diet of not only humans but of animals, and even of many plants.

Use of natural salt is as old as human history. Natural Salt is one of the most effective and most widely used of all food seasonings and natural preservatives.

Natural salt is a source of 21 essential and 30 accessory minerals that are essential to our health.

According to some sources, other elements are up to 5% of dry ocean salt.

Refined salt contain only 0.1 - 0.5% other elements.

Unrefined sea salt contain 98.0 % NaCl (sodium-chloride) and up to 2.0% other minerals (salts): Epsom salts and other Magnesium salts, Calcium salts, Potassium (Kalium) salts, Manganese salts, Phosphorus salts, Iodine salts, .. all together **over 100 minerals composed of 80 chemical elements**.

Composition of crystal of ocean salt is so complicated that no laboratory in the world can produce it from its basic 80 chemical elements.

Nature is still better chemist than people.

This salt has been used since beginning of life, by ocean plants, by animals and by people

(Percentage is referring to the percentage of dry matter. Salt can contain high percentage of water.)

Refined salt (Table Salt) is 99.9% NaCl (sodium-chloride), (chemical as clean as Heroin or White Sugar). It almost always contain additives, like 0.01% of Potassium-Iodide (added to the salt to avoid Iodine deficiency disease of thyroid gland), Sugar (added to stabilize Iodine and as anti-caking chemical) and Aluminum silicate.

Beware of "Sea salt" Labels

On the labels of many packaged food, in supermarkets as well as health food stores the name "sea salt" appears often. Reading this, we feel safe and reassured, thinking that when it comes to the salt part of the ingredients, all is fine...

But All Is Not Fine!

This supermarket or health food store "sea salt" has been totally refined. At its origin, it may have come from the sea, but:

It has been harvested mechanically from dirt or concrete basins with bulldozers and piped through metal conduits;

put through many degrading artificial processes;

heated under extreme heat levels in order to crack its molecular structure;

robbed of all of its essential minerals that are essential to our physiology;

further adulterated by chemical additives to make it free- flowing, bleached, and iodized.

These elements are extracted and sold separately to industry. Precious and highly prized by the salt refiners, these bring more profits than the salt itself.

To call what remains "sea salt" would be quite misleading.

In addition, harmful chemicals have been added to the processed, altered unnatural substance to mask and cover up all of the impurities it has. These added chemicals include free flowing agents, inorganic iodine, dextrose and bleaching agents.

Standard salt additives: Potassium-Iodide (added to the salt to avoid Iodine deficiency disease of thyroid gland), Sugar (added to stabilize Iodine and as anti-caking chemical), Aluminum silicate.

Use of salt is as old as human history. The oldest records come from China. Some 2,700 years B.C.-about 4,700 years ago. There was published in China the PENG-TZAO-KAN-MU. A major portion of this writing discussed more than 40 kinds of salt, including descriptions of two methods of extracting salt and putting it in usable form that are amazingly similar to processes used today.

How is Ocean Sea Salt Produced?

The ocean is allowed to flood huge, flat, shallow, beds and then the dam is closed to trap the water. The water is then naturally evaporated by the sun & this leaves a layer of sea salt. Dirty brown salt is on the bottom and pretty white salt at the top.

Since most people are used to white salt, they just skim off the top white salt & call it "sea salt". UNFORTUNATELY, the trace minerals are mostly in the brown stuff at the bottom.

Real **Ocean Sea Salt is produced from unseparated salt. That is why it is slightly darker.**

Celtic Salt, Muramoto Salt and Lima Salt also contain darker salt.

When producing table salt, other mineral salts are used for the chemical industry, or are washed back into the sea, or are used for animals. If we humans just could eat as good as animals!?

Natural salt is not white and it is not dry. It is a little gray with minerals and feels damp or clumps in humidity.

How is Mineral Salt Produced?

Mineral salt is mined from thousands of feet below the ground surface in areas where there is a layer of mineral salts.

Mineral salt can also be harvested by pumping water deep underground in areas where a layer of salt is discovered. Salty water that comes out is then used in salt production. This process is called vacuum pan salt refining.

Origin of Salt Layers

There are two theories. One says that mineral salt is a layer of salt created after evaporation of old seas. According to the other theory, the layer of mineral salt was created by chemical reaction.

Mineral salt is often in crystal form. It is transparent crystal, or light tan in color with little darker flecks. But, it can also be of many different colors. Not all mineral salts are rich in trace elements. Some are similar to ocean salt, others are not.

If you ask me, I prefer Ocean salt.

Salt Intake is Vital

Salt is a vital substance for the survival of all living creatures, particularly humans. Water and salt regulate the water content of the body. Water itself regulates the water content of the interior of the cell by working its way into all of the cells it reaches. It has to get there to cleanse and extract the toxic wastes of cell metabolisms. Salt forces some water to stay outside the cells. It balances the amount of water that stays outside the cells. There are two oceans of water in the body; one ocean is held inside the cells of the body, and the other ocean is held outside the cells. Good health depends on a most delicate balance between the volume of these oceans, and this balance is achieved by salt - unrefined salt.

When water is available to get inside the cells freely, it is filtered from the outside salty ocean and injected into the cells that are being overworked despite their water shortage. This is the reason why in severe dehydration we develop an edema and retain water. The design of our bodies is such that the extent of the ocean of water outside the cells is expanded to have the extra water available for filtration and emergency injection into vital cells. The brain commands an increase in salt and water retention by the kidneys. This is how we get an edema when we don't drink enough water.

Initially, the process of water filtration and its delivery into the cells is more efficient at night when the body is horizontal. The collected water, that mostly pools in the legs, does not have to fight the force of gravity to get onto the blood circulation. If reliance of this process of emergency hydration of some cells continues for long, the lungs begin to get waterlogged at night, and breathing becomes difficult. The person needs more pillows to sit upright to sleep.

This condition is the consequence of dehydration. However, you might overload the system by drinking too much water at the beginning. Increases in water intake must be slow and spread out until urine production begins to increase at the same rate that you drink water.

When we drink enough water to pass clear urine, we also pass out a lot of the salt that was held back. This is how we can get rid of edema fluid in the body; by drinking more water. Not diuretics, but more water!! In people who have an extensive edema and show signs of their heart beginning to have irregular or very rapid beats with least effort, the increase in water intake should be gradual and spaced out, but not withheld from the body. Naturally, salt intake should be limited for two or three days because the body is still in an overdrive mode to retain it. Once the edema has cleared up, salt should not be withheld from the body.

Salt has many other functions than just regulating the water content of the body.

The following information is from *Seasalt's Hidden Powers* . You should get your hands on this book and the entire family should be educated on the facts of life.

The late French scientist Dr. Alexis Carrel kept a chicken heart alive for over 27 years by having the pulsating heart **IN A SOLUTION OF SEA SALT, i.e. isotonic seawater**. Dr. Carrel voluntarily ended the experiment after a third of a century, having proven that living cells can have physical immortality.

Professor C. Louis Kervran with his scientific research and formulas has been an asset to the scientific establishment and he was a candidate for the Noble Prize. Professor Kervran links us to the secret of immortality and reveals its prime source is trace minerals from seawater [and used in] remedies. Other physicians continued research and found fermentations of briny salt pickles, salted sour plums and other salty fermentations to be powerful and effective medicines.

Dr. Jacques de Langre, Ph.D., who wrote the book "Seasalt's Hidden Powers", states that naturally and properly **sunshine-preserved** sea salt is the difference between life and death, health and illness, social sanity and planetary panic and its elements are vital for proper body functions. That natural hand-harvested Celtic ocean salt alone helps to maintain life, neutralizes toxins and detrimental bacteria, and enhances all our organic function.

Sea salt contain 92 essential minerals and most all refined adulterated sea salts contain only 2 elements (Na and Cl. Biologically, 24 of these elements in real sea salt have already been proven necessary and essential to maintain and recover health. See Scientific American, July 1972: "The Chemical Elements of Life," by Earl Friden.

When dietary deficiency of trace elements occurs, cells lose the ability to control their ions—with dire consequences for humans. Even a minute loss of ion equilibrium causes cells to burst, nervous disorder, brain damage, or muscle spasms, as well as a breakdown of the cell-regenerating process and growth.

In the theory of acid and alkaline balance, chronic disease such as cancer is caused by the acidification of the blood, lymph and all cellular tissues. Real sea salt is one of the basic elements necessary to correct this problem.

Natural sea salt [reconstituted seawater] allows liquids to freely cross body membranes, the kidney's glomerulus's and blood vessels walls. Whenever the sodium chloride concentration rises in the blood, the water in the neighboring tissues is attracted to that salt-rich blood, and the cells then re-absorb the enriched intra-cellular fluid. If they are functioning properly, the kidneys remove the saline fluids easily. Refined salt does not allow this free-crossing of liquids and minerals, and causes accumulated fluids to stagnate in joints, producing edema and chronic kidney problems.

Salt is the single element required for the proper breakdown of plant carbohydrates into useable and assimilable human food. Only when salt is added to fruits and vegetables can saliva and gastric secretions readily break down the fibrous store of carbohydrates, etc.

Once salt is dissolved and ionized, the salt possesses a definite reactivity, has full electromagnetic capabilities, and passes more easily into the large colon where it will have a sanitizing effect.

Table Salt: To further prevent any moisture from being reabsorbed, the salt refiners add aluminosilicate of sodium or yellow prussiate of soda as desiccants plus different bleaches to the final salt formula. After these processes, the table salt will no longer combine with human body fluids, it invariably causes severe problems of edema (water retention) and several other health disturbances.

In ancient Celts times, salt was used to treat major physical and mental disturbances, severe burns, and other ailments. Today biologists attest that seawater (also called 'mother liquor') restores hydro-electrolytic imbalances, a disorder that causes loss of immune response, creates allergies, and causes many health problems. Also the therapeutic effect of seawater is recognized and used by the best European medical professionals because of its effectiveness in so many situations.

Today people fear salt and we are witnessing a virtual ban on consuming products with high sodium contents and this is a major concern of biologists. The use of real sea salt-free diets are showing up in the reality of our modern world as society is coming apart. It is basically a starvation of macro- and trace minerals and biological deficiencies cannot be corrected by refined sodium chloride alone.

Celtic salt is a good product because it is naturally extracted by the use of sunshine. If one would re-dissolve salt in water in the proper ratio or combine it in the moisture of foods, its properties re-create the amazing powers of the "ocean" and bears an astonishing likeness to human blood and body fluids. During World War II, Navy doctors would use sea salt water for blood transfusions when blood supplies ran out and many lives were saved.

History

Dr. Langre mentions in his book that, "The Belgian historian Henri Pirenne observed that during the High Middle ages, the entire coast of the Atlantic was deserted and the entire continent was thrown into a Dark Age of human under-development. Historians tell us that it was caused to a great extent by the lack of salt in the human diet, the flooding of all salt flats having disabled every salt farm along the coastlines of the Atlantic Ocean and the Mediterranean Sea. The whole of Europe, therefore, suffered from a salt famine that was to last almost 500 years. The daily average ration fell to less than 2 grams per person and caused may to die from dehydration and madness. The extent of the salt famine reported by Henri Pirenne caused human flesh to be sold on the open-air markets and created an epidemic of crazed people who, to replenish their salt, drank blood from the neck artery of the person they had just slain. Quick to exploit this desperate situation for their own gain, the rulers of Europe grabbed the remnants of the salt stock and exacted exorbitant salt taxes. Heavily burdened by tariffs and gabelles, common salt became a luxury but also caused mass population shifts and exodus, lured invaders and caused wars. Mined salt from the depths of the earth was substituted, but the lack of live and balanced trace elements in rock salt lowered the mental equilibrium and intellect level almost as much as the sheer absence of salt."

Sea Salt Directions

Dr. Langre, Ph.D. writes that, "Rare gases are locked within real sea crystals and begin to release in contact of additional moisture and are effective in maintaining and restoring human energy. Note that Celtic salt should not be ground until used because as it is milled the salt releases a subtle fragrance reminiscent of violets, another telltale sign that gases, floral-like vital essences, are being released. Note that these elements are easily trapped and stored in a preparation called sesame salt and a recipe is given in the Seasalt's Hidden Powers. Real sea salt needs to be stored in an air tight container and kept in a dark cool place. The moisture has a tendency to settle to the bottom of the salt and the salt should be mixed before removing the salt.

Real sea salt needs to penetrate foods allowing the moisture of the fruits, vegetables, grains, etc. to liquefy the salt which activates it. If dry salt is used it enters the body in a non-ionized form and can create thirst (a sign of being poisoned) and lessens salts abilities because it is not being assimilated and utilized properly.

Sea water losses its properties of destroying bacilli if stored in bottles and when it dries out.

A pinch of salt can be added to a small amount of water to dissolve to activate its powers and added to fruits, vegetables, grains to aid in better digestion of those items while helping to alkalize the body. Adding a pinch to water supplies adds alkaline properties and the mineral content. The minerals it contains are too valuable to ignore.

Vital Functions of Salt in the Body

1. Salt is most effective in stabilizing irregular heartbeats and, contrary to the misconception that it causes high blood pressure, it is actually essential for the regulation of blood pressure - in conjunction with water. Naturally the proportions are critical.

2. Salt is vital to the extraction of excess acidity from the cells in the body, particularly the brain cells.

3. Salt is vital for balancing the sugar levels in the blood; a needed element in diabetics.

4. Salt is vital for the generation of hydroelectric energy in cells in the body. It is used for local power generation at the sites of energy need by the cells.

5. Salt is vital to the nerve cells' communication and information processing all the time that the brain cells work, from the moment of conception to death.

6. Salt is vital for absorption of food particles through the intestinal tract.

7. Salt is vital for the clearance of the lungs of mucus plugs and sticky phlegm, particularly in asthma and cystic fibrosis.

8. Salt is vital for clearing up catarrh and congestion of the sinuses.

9. Salt is a strong natural antihistamine.

10. Salt is essential for the prevention of muscle cramps.

11. Salt is vital to prevent excess saliva production to the point that it flows out of the mouth during sleep. **Needing to constantly mop up excess saliva indicates salt shortag**e.

12. Salt is absolutely vital to making the structure of bones firm. Osteoporosis, in a major way, is a result of salt and water shortage in the body.

13. Salt is vital for sleep regulation. It is a natural hypnotic.

14. Salt is a vitally needed element in the treatment of diabetics.

15. Salt on the tongue will stop persistent dry coughs.

16. Salt is vital for the prevention of gout and gouty arthritis.

17. Salt is vital for maintaining sexuality and libido.

18. Salt is vital for preventing varicose veins and spider veins on the legs and thighs.

19. Salt is vital to the communication and information processing nerve cells the entire time that the brain cells work - from the moment of conception to death.

20. Salt is vital for reducing a double chin. When the body is short of salt, it means the body really is short of water. The salivary glands sense the salt shortage and are obliged to produce more saliva to lubricate the act of chewing and swallowing and also to supply the stomach with water that it needs for breaking down foods. Circulation to the salivary glands increases and the blood vessels become "leaky" in order to supply the glands with water to manufacture saliva. The "leakiness" spills beyond the area of the glands themselves, causing increased bulk under the skin of the chin, the cheeks and into the neck.

21. Sea salt contains about 80 mineral elements that the body needs. Some of these elements are needed in trace amounts. Unrefined sea salt is a better choice of salt than other types of salt on the market. Ordinary table salt that is bought in the super markets has been stripped of its companion elements and contains additive elements such as aluminum silicate to keep it powdery and porous. Aluminum is a very toxic element in our nervous system. It is implicated as one of the primary causes of Alzheimer's disease.

22. Twenty-seven percent of the body's salt is in the bones. Osteoporosis results when the body needs more salt and takes it from the bones. Bones are twenty-two percent water. Is it not obvious what happens to the bones when we're deficient in salt or water or both.

* The information on salt intake is taken from Dr. Batmanghelidj's book, *Water: Rx for a Healthier Pain-Free Life*.

People who eat Refined salt develop craving for salt, because, salt that they eat is not satisfying their needs. Then they use more and more salt, in the desperate try to get what they need. Taking big amounts of refined salt (chemical) burdens kidneys and adrenal glands that are very important for calcium utilization. Modern physiology has demonstrated that an excess of salt interferes with the absorption of nutrients and depletes calcium, while if used in a moderate doses, salt enhances calcium absorption and nutrient utilization in general.

It is known that absorption of calcium depends on the health of the kidney-adrenal function and that calcium metabolism is of essential importance for the health of the nerves, muscles, heart, vascular system, and bones. Simply, the whole body is dependent on Calcium uptake.

Is a Low-Salt Diet a Risk?

London, March 12 - A low-salt diet may not be so healthy after all. Defying a generation of health advice, a controversial new study concludes that the less salt people eat, the higher their risk of untimely death. The study, led by Dr. Michael Alderman, chairman of epidemiology at Albert Einstein School; of Medicine in New York and president of the American Society of Hypertension, suggests the government should consider suspending its recommendation that people restrict the amount of salt they eat.

"The lower the sodium, the worse off you are," Alderman said. "There's an association. Is it the cause? I don't know. Any way you slice it, that's not an argument for eating a low sodium diet.

TOP ESSENTIALS of LIFE

1. Oxygen 2. Water 3. Salt 4. Potassium 5. Exercise 6. Oils

FACT - No one can live without these. Mainstream medicine too often ignores 2 & 3 in favor of selling drugs and procedures to treat the symptoms of dehydration.

FACT - The people with the worst health drink the least water and use the most deadly diuretic drought causing drugs - caffeine and/or alcohol.

FACT - The salinity of the water outside the cells in our bodies is similar to the ocean.

FACT - In the middle ages people were put to a horrible death by salt deprivation.

FACT - Health care makes big bucks by selling a quart of water with salt in it (Saline 4) for up to $350.00 installed, but won't tell the patients they do indeed need more water and salt in their diets.

FACT - How can you expect drug companies to do research on the importance of water in our daily lives when they can't make money on it? Who does research to put themselves out of business?

FACT - The environment of an unborn baby is water and salt.

Above is adapted from <http://curezone.org/foods/saltcure.asp

****

Below is adapted from <http://www.rowlandpub.com/> several years ago. I could not find the web site or page in Dec 2014

The Heart - Calcium, Magnesium and Potassium And The Importance Of Proper Ratios

Calcium, magnesium and potassium are electrolyte minerals that the body requires in balance. Together these minerals work throughout the body to help regulate fluid pressures, the transmission of nerve impulses, and muscular contraction. An imbalance in the ratio of these minerals may cause high blood pressure, insomnia, irregular heartbeat, irritability, muscle cramps/spasms, nervous tics and twitches, or unusual sensitivity to noise.

Interrelationships

1) Magnesium keeps calcium soluble, to prevent it from precipitating out. Calcification and bone spurs often indicate magnesium deficiency.

2) A calcium to magnesium ratio that is too high tends to constrict blood vessels and make the blood coagulate too easily, thus increasing the risk for coronary thrombosis.

3) Potassium and magnesium work closely together at the cellular level. Magnesium losses can induce a potassium deficiency. Potassium loss can be reduced by magnesium supplementation

4) Magnesium deficiency is associated with loss of cellular potassium. Potassium supplementation helps to reduce magnesium excretion

High Blood Pressure

Calcium supplementation lowers blood pressure; about one-third of people can be expected to respond well to calcium supplementation alone. Magnesium supplementation has repeatedly been shown to lower blood pressure in hypertensives under double blind conditions. Potassium supplementation lowers blood pressure, partly by increasing the dietary sodium/potassium ratio and partly by reducing calcium excretion.

Muscle Cramps

Calcium deficiency causes neuromuscular irritability. Magnesium deficiency causes muscular cramps and spasms. Muscle cramps may be associated with low potassium and usually respond to potassium supplementation.

Osteoporosis

There is a growing body of controlled trials which strongly suggest that some of the age-related bone loss in elderly women could be prevented by higher intake of calcium. Magnesium has been shown to increase bone density. Dietary potassium promotes calcium retention and may protect bone from osteoporotic changes.

Irregular Heartbeat

Magnesium helps to regulate the electrical activity of the heart. Magnesium deficiency increases the danger of cardiac arrhythmias. Magnesium supplementation may prevent and correct a wide variety of arrhythmias. Potassium deficiency is associated with arrhythymias. The heart muscle is unable to hold onto potassium in the absence of magnesium.

Absorption

Which mineral supplements are the easiest for the body to absorb depends more on how they are taken than which ones are taken.

In one study, fasting subjects were given 500 mg. of calcium from each of five calcium compounds and milk. No significant differences in absorption were found among the various sources of calcium. The mean net calcium absorption in each case was 39% from calcium carbonate, 32% from calcium acetate, 32% from calcium lactate, 31% from milk, 30% from calcium citrate, and 27% from calcium gluconate. "Fasting subjects" means that these people were given the various forms of calcium on an empty stomach. That is not the most efficient way to take mineral supplements, however.

Glenn's note: The form of calcium, as well as other minerals, is critical. See sections later in this chapter.

Mineral compounds require the presence of stomach acid for adequate absorption. (Hydrochloric acid levels usually decline as we get older.) One study found that calcium from calcium carbonate is well absorbed if this supplement is taken with a meal – even if stomach acid is otherwise too low

Chelated minerals do not require stomach acid and are ready to be transported through the intestinal wall. If taken on an empty stomach, chelated minerals may be better absorbed than their non-chelated counterparts. ***If taken with food,*** *however,* ***there is no significant difference in absorption rate from one mineral supplement to another.***

Calcium carbonate provides the highest amount of calcium (40%) of all supplementary sources (e.g., calcium citrate provides 24% and calcium gluconate 9%). Similarly, magnesium oxide provides the highest amount of magnesium (60%) and potassium chloride has the highest amount of potassium (52%). The chelates provide 5% or less of the minerals in question.

Ratios

The ideal ratio of calcium to magnesium to potassium varies from person to person, depending on each individual's unique biochemical requirements. There are no scientific studies to suggest what an average ideal ratio might be for the population at large. Recommended ratios are usually based on educated opinions.

There is some general agreement that a ratio of calcium to magnesium of 2:1 in supplements may be desirable. A few experts recommend a 1:1 ratio. Supplementary potassium is usually ignored, because it is assumed that most diets provide enough of this mineral without the need for supplements. Technically, this is true. But there is benefit to adding potassium to mineral supplements because the potassium helps the body to make better utilization of the calcium and magnesium in those supplements.

When all factors are considered, for most adults the ideal ratio of calcium to magnesium to potassium in a broad spectrum vitamin-mineral supplement is probably about 8:5:4. This needs to be changed to 4:5:4 in supplements whose primary purpose is the dissolving of arterial plaque – the relatively higher magnesium in that case is needed to dissolve the calcium that is released from the arterial deposits.

For a supplement containing only calcium, magnesium and potassium the ideal ratio is probably about 1:1:1. That is because this kind of supplement is used for individuals whose need for these electrolyte minerals is higher than can be met from other supplements. Since there is more variability in magnesium and potassium requirements than for calcium, the 1:1:1 ratio may be effectively utilized by the greatest number of people.

Supplementation

The following is a dietary supplement that provides an equal balance of calcium, magnesium and potassium. Its purpose is to increase the intake of these minerals, for an individual who has higher needs for them than can be met from diet or other supplements.

The amounts suggested below are for each tablet. The number of tablets per day can be adjusted to suit individual requirements. For optimal absorption, this formula needs to be taken with meals – together with any other vitamin-mineral supplements the individual may require, and especially those providing vitamins A and D.

Calcium (carbonate)	200 mg.
Magnesium (oxide)	200 mg.
Potassium (chloride)	200 mg.

Above is adapted from <http://www.rowlandpub.com/> several years ago. I could not find the web site or page in Dec 2014

Below is adapted from http://www.enerex.ca/en/articles/calcium-to-magnesium-ratio (web page no longer available as of 2016) and http://www.rowlandpub (web site is gone as of 2016)

Calcium to Magnesium Ratio

Calcium to Magnesium Ratio by Dr. K. Sharma (Ph.D.)

Both calcium and magnesium are involved in numerous metabolic functions and are absolutely essential for the maintenance of a healthy body.

Calcium is considered the **backbone mineral** because of its role in the formation of skeleton and teeth. Magnesium is called the **natural tranquilizer** due to its relaxing action on nerves and muscles. The biological functions and the therapeutic uses of these minerals are shown below:

FUNCTION	
CALCIUM	**MAGNESIUM**
Development and maintenance of bones and teeth (about 99% of body calcium is in bones and teeth)	Development of bones (about 70% of body magnesium is in bones)
Blood clotting	Crucial part of many enzymes involved in energy production and respiration
Muscle contraction and relaxation	Muscle **relaxation**
Transmission of nerve impulses	Transmission of nerve impulses
Enzyme activation for production of gastric juices	Regulation of body temperature
Fat, protein and carbohydrate metabolism	Absorption and utilization of calcium, phosphorus, sodium, potassium, vitamins C, E, & D.
pH balance	pH balance
etc.	Release of nerve tension
	etc.

THERAPEUTIC USE	
CALCIUM	**MAGNESIUM**
Arthritis, osteoporosis, rheumatism, other bone disorders, dental decay, epilepsy, insomnia, nephritis, pre-menstrual cramps, stress, constipation, muscle pains, high blood cholesterol, regulation of heart beat.	Arteriosclerosis, heart attacks, Infant death syndrome (SIDS), hypertension, bone fractures, epilepsy, diabetes, alcoholism, kidney stones, leg cramps, nervousness.

Both minerals require each other for their absorption and utilization and must be provided in adequate amounts. Depending upon the physiological environment, there are cases in which the roles of these two minerals are antagonistic to each other. Magnesium is located inside the cell (intracellular) while calcium is predominantly located outside the cell (extracellular). Consequently, the role of magnesium in intracellular metabolic functions, such as energy production, respiration, and muscle contraction-relaxation is antagonistic to calcium.

Let us briefly examine the role and relationship of these two minerals in known clinical studies:

REGULATION OF HEART BEAT

The heart is a muscle and its primary function is to pump blood throughout the body. The heart is composed of billions of cells, each of which works as an electrochemical generator, and contains both calcium and magnesium. On the outer surface of the heart cells, thin fibers made of a substance called "actin", continually expand and contract in unison with the heartbeat. The actin fibers are stimulated by calcium, and then relaxed by magnesium. An electrical charge produced by magnesium then pushes the calcium to the opposite side of the cell. Thus, calcium helps to produce the heartbeat, and magnesium regulates it.

MYOCARDICAL INFARCTION (Heart Attack)

Several researchers have shown that a heart failure involves drastic changes in the concentration of cardiac electrolytes.

1)During cardiac stress, some of the magnesium is moved out of the cell accompanied by an influx of calcium into the cell. Thus, the cardiac muscle shows a 20% decrease in magnesium and a 4 1/2 fold increase in myocardial calcium.

(2). The loss of magnesium and an influx of calcium seriously disrupts the energy potential of the affected muscle.

3). The situation can be prevented by increasing the level of magnesium. In clinical practice, intravenous or intramuscular administration of magnesium salts has proven very useful and is highly regarded.

4). It is known that magnesium therapy is the most effective to protect myocardial integrity during cardiac arrest.

5). It is interesting to note that in Canadian surveys of post-mortem tissue composition, about 24% less magnesium was found in ischemic hearts than in non-cardiac cases (6).

ATHEROSCLEROSIS (Heart Disease)

A high dietary intake of magnesium has been attributed to why heart disease is virtually unknown among Bantu tribesman of South Africa while the disease is prevalent among white South Africans. Clinical studies have revealed that the Bantu's serum magnesium level is about 11% higher than in the white South Africans. The Bantu's high dietary intake of magnesium is largely attributable to intake of unrefined cereals such as maize meal, which has a high magnesium content and also has a high fiber content. Also, it has been shown that the ability of high-fat diets to induce atherclerosis is prevented by a high magnesium dietary regime.

HYPERTENSION (High Blood Pressure)

For many years, hypertension has been associated with sodium. Consequently, the disorder is treated by substituting potassium in the diet. However, most of us do not realize that magnesium is also considered a well-known vasodilator. The anti-hypertensive effect of magnesium is achieved by a direct effect on the vascular wall or is mediated through the central nervous system. Magnesium competes with calcium for binding sites and the net result is that magnesium reduces the calcium-induced contractions. It is well established that magnesium infusions can cause vasodilatation and reduce hypertension in humans.

Glenn's note: "Salts That Heal and Salts That Kill" earlier in this chapter)

UROLITHIASIS (Kidney Stones)

Canadians appear to have a very high incident of kidney stones and the occurrence is particularly high in Newfoundland. In the U.S., South Carolina has the highest urolithiasis rate. South Carolina also has the highest U.S. rate for cardiovascular deaths. Both Newfoundland and South Carolina regions have "very soft" drinking waters with little magnesium.

In Canada, calcium urolithiasis accounts for 70 to 80% of the total kidney-stone problems. In the U.S., about 67% of all kidney stones are composed of calcium oxalate or calcium hydroxyapatite.

Several researchers have used the magnesium/calcium ratio as an index of susceptibility of urine to form kidney-stones in patients. In general, patients with a urinary magnesium/calcium ratio of 0.7 is **normal**, whereas a value lower than 0.7 may be considered as **stone-forming**. The ratio is especially low in the Canadian "Kidney Stone Patients", indicating inadequate magnesium intake.

Oral magnesium supplementation has proven very effective in the prevention of kidney-stone formation.

INFANT DEATH SYNDROME (Sids of Crib Death)

Magnesium deficiency has a primary role in sudden unexpected infant-death syndrome. The sequence-of-events are as follows:

Magnesium deficiency causes calcium-dependant release of histamine which, in turn, induces increased release of acetylcholine (especially at high calcium/magnesium ratio). The increased amount of acetylcholine leads to symptoms of neuromuscular hyperirritability and convulsions that can lead to reduced heart rate.

The sudden-death syndrome is puzzling since no recognizable allergens are involved. The symptoms are acute respiratory distress, and includes bronchospasm, shortness of breath, and eventual circulatory collapse. Hypomagnesemia is observed throughout this syndrome. Therefore, the role of magnesium in the infant-death syndrome is very significant.

NUTRITIONAL STATUS OF MAGNESIUM

The recommended dietary allowance for magnesium is 300 to 450 mg/day. There are several factors including pregnancy, rapid growth, or a high intake of protein, vitamin D, calcium, fat, carbohydrates or alcohol, that will increase the requirement for magnesium.

Surveys of dietary magnesium intake from different countries show a prevalence of lower magnesium intake than the desired levels. In Newfoundland, the intake is only 50% of the recommended amount. Other reports show that hospital and institutional diets contain only 61to 68% of the recommended intake, respectively. In other studies, it was found that the intake for pregnant women was only 45 to 60% of the recommended allowances. There is definite evidence that magnesium intake is suboptimal or marginally inadequate in regions of the Western World. The occurrence of hypomagnesemia in humans, due to low magnesium intake and due in part to factors such as, prolonged use of diuretics, alcoholism, pregnancy etc., have been shown to be more prevalent than generally believed.

CONTRIBUTION OF DRINKING WATER

Drinking water can significantly contribute to magnesium intake and hard waters can supply 9 to 29% of the daily magnesium intake. Because of the metabolic antagonism between magnesium and calcium, the ratio between these two minerals in the drinking water is of considerable significance. In a survey of 25 U.S. cities, the lowest death rates from coronary disease were found in areas where the drinking waters supplied more magnesium and less calcium than the U.S. average.

Australia has the highest cardiovascular death-rate in the world and also consumes some of the worlds softest drinking waters. On the other hand, the Western region of Texas has the hardest drinking waters and the lowest cardiovascular mortality rates in the United States.

The high mortality rate in Finland is associated with a high calcium/magnesium ratio, while the low mortality rate in Japan is related to a low calcium/magnesium ratio as well as to the "protective" effect conferred by the alkalinity (carbonate-bicarbonate content) of water.

CALCIUM TO MAGNESIUM RATIO

From the information presented here it is apparent that the ratio between calcium to magnesium is very important in dealing with the causes and prevention of a number of disorders including myocardial infarction or arrhythmia, atherosclerosis, hypertension, urolithiasis, and infant-death syndrome. In all cases, a lower calcium/magnesium ratio or a higher magnesium/calcium ratio is desirable. This need is further underscored by the fact that magnesium intake is generally suboptimal and that hypomagnesmia is more prevalent than generally believed.

The recommended dietary allowance (RDA) for calcium is 800 mg/day, whereas for magnesium it is 400 to 450 mg/day. Only about one-third of magnesium is absorbed from dietary sources. Therefore, a daily magnesium intake of 1200 mg/day has been recommended by some researchers. The traditional ratio of approximately 2 parts calcium to 1 part magnesium needs to be upgraded to increase magnesium intake in view of the overwhelming beneficial role of magnesium. The ideal ratio for most people's needs is an equal ratio of calcium and magnesium.

The absorption and metabolism of calcium and magnesium is one of mutual dependence, and therefore, the balance between these two minerals is especially important. If calcium consumption is high, magnesium intake needs to be high also.

VITAMIN D

Vitamin D is necessary to enhance calcium absorption. Vitamin D works with the parathyroid hormone "PTH" to regulate the amount of calcium in the blood. It also stimulates the production of a calcium binding protein (CABP) in the intestinal wall which helps absorption.

Above is adapted from http://www.enerex.ca/en/articles/calcium-to-magnesium-ratio (web page no longer available as of 2016) and http://www.rowlandpub (web site is gone as of 2016)

****

Below is adapted from < http://www.chiro.org/nutrition/ABSTRACTS/minerals.shtml (web site no longer available as of 2016)

I found the article on Sept 24, 2016 at
http://www.life-enthusiast.com/minerals-tim-oshea-a-68.html

Minerals And Their Different Forms And Functions

By Tim O'Shea, D.C.

Minerals is one confusing topic. Inorganic, chelated, elemental, ionic, colloidal, essential, trace - all these claims! What do we really need? Credentials in nutrition apparently mean very little when it comes to minerals. Much of what is written about minerals is speculative, market-oriented, or dead wrong.

A net search on minerals is an overwhelming assault on one's patience, time and credulity. How could all this stuff be right?

Minerals come from mines. Except when you're talking about nutrition. Then they come from food. At least they used to. When we still had some viable topsoil. Four elements compose 96% of the body's makeup: carbon, hydrogen, oxygen, and nitrogen. The remaining 4% of the body's composition is mineral. There are several opinions about how many minerals are essential. The following table shows the ones that are not in dispute, in the first column. Macro means more than 100mg per day. Trace usually means we don't know how much we need.

Essential Minerals

MACROMINERALS	TRACE MINERALS
Calcium	Selenium
Chlorine	Cobalt
Sodium	Chromium
Potassium	Tin
Phosphorus	Zinc
Magnesium	Vanadium
Sulfur	Copper
	Silicon
	Manganese
	Nickel
	Iron
	Molybdenum
	Fluorine
	Iodine
U.S. Dept. of Agriculture	**National Research Council**

The controversy primarily involves the second column - trace minerals.

Glenn's comment: There are at least 84 widely recognized trace minerals in total. Only about 13 to 17 are considered essential by most "experts". I believe the human body needs more than the 17. Do your own research.

Of the 14 trace minerals listed above, three or four may not have universal agreement as essential, but a majority of creditable sources admit that most of them are essential. Deficiency amounts have never been determined for most trace minerals, although several diseases have been linked with deficiencies of certain ones. Conclusive evidence has not been found regarding the exact daily intake amounts necessary, since some of the actual requirements may be too small to measure; hence the name "trace." Other trace minerals which are still being studied as possibly essential or possibly contaminant include arsenic (true!), boron, cadmium, lithium, strontium, aluminum, barium, and beryllium.

After this, the marketplace takes over and science bows out. People are out there talking about glacial milk, 88-mineral toddies, minerals from ancient lakes, iceberg moss, longevity of 150 years, calcium from pasteurized milk, "normal" doses of lead, eye of newt, etc., making unproven claims about this or that combination, trumpeting anecdotal cures for everything from cancer to hangnails.

The purpose of this section will be to try to sift through the debris and leave behind only the fundamental information which can be verified.

In the past few years, even mainstream medicine is beginning to acknowledge the incontrovertible importance of mineral supplementation. In an article appearing in *JAMA*, the top American medical journal, 24 Dec 1996, a controlled study of **selenium use for cancer patients** was written up. Selenium as you remember, effects powerful antioxidant activity, neutralizing free radicals, which are rampant in the presence of cancer. In this study, 1312 subjects were divided into groups. Some were given selenium; others the placebo. Soon it was noticed that there was a decrease of 63% with prostate cancer, and 46% with lung cancer in the selenium group. The results were so blatant that the designers actually terminated the study early so that everyone could begin to benefit from selenium. This is just one example of the research that is currently being done on mineral supplementation. The problem is, if the results of studies economically threaten a current drug protocol, like chemotherapy, it is unlikely that an inexpensive natural supplement like selenium would be promoted by oncologists as a replacement any time soon.

There are six nutrient groups:

Water
Vitamins
Minerals
Fats
Protein
Carbohydrate

All groups are necessary for complete body function.

The necessity for minerals is a recent historical discovery, only about 150 years old. In the 1850s, Pasteur's contemporary, Claude Bernard, learned about iron. Copper came about 10 years later, and zinc about the turn of the century. With the discovery of Vitamin A in 1912, minerals were downplayed for about 50 years in favor of vitamin research. By 1950, after about 14 vitamins had been discovered, attention returned once more to minerals when it was shown that they were necessary co-factors in order for vitamins to operate. Minerals are catalysts for most biological reactions.

Soon the individual functions of minerals in the body were demonstrated:

Structural: bones, teeth, ligaments
Solutes and electrolytes in the blood
Enzyme actions
Energy production from food breakdown
Nerve transmission
Muscle action

Table of some minerals with the specific functions most commonly agreed upon today

Calcium	Muscle contraction	Bone building		
Chlorine	Digestion	Normal blood pressure		
Chromium	Insulin action	Immune function		
Copper	Immune system	Artery strength	Forms hemoglobin from iron	
Fluorine (NOT Fluoride)	Teeth enamel			
Iodine	Thyroid function			
Iron	Blood formation	Immune function		
Magnesium	Muscle contraction (Relaxation)	Nerve transmission	Calcium metabolism	
Manganese	Enzyme action			
Molybdenum	Enzyme action			
Nickel	Immune regulation	Brain development	DNA synthesis	
Phosphorus	Bone formation	Cell energy		
Potassium	Nerve transmission	Cell Life	Normal blood pressure	Muscle contraction
Selenium	Immune stimulant	Fight free radicals	Activates Vit E	
Silicon	Enzyme action			
Sodium	Cell life	Waste removal		
Sulfur	Protein synthesis			
Tin	Enzyme action			
Vanadium	Circulation	Sugar metabolism		

Larry Berger, PhD

Mineral deficiency means that some of these jobs will not get done. The body is capable of prodigious amounts of adapting, and can operate for long periods of time with deficiencies of many of the above. But someday those checks will have to be cashed. The result: premature aging. Cell breakdown. Without minerals, vitamins may have little or no effect. Minerals are catalysts - triggers for thousands of essential enzyme reactions in the body. No trigger - no reaction. Without enzyme reactions, caloric intake is meaningless, and the same for protein, fat, and carbohydrate intake. Minerals trigger the vitamins and enzymes to act; that means digestion. In general, most discussions about calories are without content.

A virtually undisputed fact is **mineral deficiency**. Observe the titanic output of websites, articles, and supplements visible today. The majority of mineral websites quote a 1936 source

- *Senate Document #264*, as scientific proof that dietary minerals were generally inadequate for optimum health.

> *"...most of us are suffering from certain diet deficiencies which cannot be remedied until deplete soils from which our food comes are brought into proper mineral balance."*
>
> *"The alarming fact is that food...now being raised on millions of acres of land that no longer contain enough...minerals are starving us, no matter how much of them we eat."*
>
> *"Lacking vitamins, the system can make use of minerals, but lacking minerals, vitamins are useless."*
>
> **Senate Document 264**
> **74th Congress, 1936**

The same document went on to quantify the extent of mineral deficiency:

> *"99% of the American people are deficient in minerals, and a marked deficiency in any one of the more important minerals actually results in disease."*

Congressional documents are not generally highly regarded as scientific sources, and other reference texts cite other percentages. The figures quoted by Albion Laboratories, the world leader in patents on supplemental minerals, are somewhat lower, but the idea begins to come across:

DEFICIENCY - U.S. Population

Magnesium	75%
Iron	58%
Copper	81%
Manganese	50%
Chromium	50%
Zinc	67%

The most obvious reasons for mass mineral deficiencies of mineral intake are:

1) **Soil depletion and demineralization.** In 1900, forests covered 40% of the earth. Today, the figure is about 27**%.** (*Relating Land Use and Global Land Cover*, Turner, 1992).Aside from hacking down rainforests in order to raise beef cattle or to build condos, one of the main reasons for the dying forests is mineral depletion. According to a paper read at the 1994 meeting of the International Society for Systems Sciences, this century is the first time ever that "mineral content available to forest and agricultural root systems is down 25%-40%." Less forests means less topsoil. In the past 200 years, the U.S. has lost as much as 75% of its topsoil, according to John Robbins in his Pulitzer-nominated work “Diet for a New America”. To replace one inch of topsoil may take anywhere from 200-1000 years, depending on climate. (Utah Teachers Resource Books)

Demineralization of topsoil translates to loss of productive capacity. Contributing further to this trend is the growing of produce that is harvested and shipped far away.

The standard **NPK** (nitrogen-phosphorus-potassium) fertilizer farmers commonly use is able to restore the soil enough to grow fruits and vegetables which are healthy looking, but may be entirely lacking in trace minerals. The inventor of the entire NPK philosophy, Baron von Leibig, recanted his theories before he died when he saw the deficiencies his methods were fostering as they became the agricultural standard in both Europe and America.

Mineral depletion in topsoil is hardly a controversial issue. The question is not if, but how much. Plants are the primary agents of mineral incorporation into the biosphere. The implication for our position on the food chain is simply: lowered mineral content in produce grown in U.S. topsoil. Not much argument here.

I have not found any source that insists that the mineral content of American topsoil is as good today as it was 50 years ago. Generally, studies talk in terms of how much, if any, minerals are still present.

2) **The second contributor to mineral deficiency within the population is obviously, diet.** Even if our produce did contain abundant minerals, less than 4% of the population eats sufficient fruits and vegetables to account for minimal RDAs. To compound matters further, mass amounts of processed food, excess protein, and refined sugars require most of our mineral stores in order to digest it and remove it. The removal process involves enzymes, which break things down. Enzyme activity, remember, is completely dependent on minerals like zinc and copper and chromium. No minerals - no enzyme action. In addition, milk, dairy products, alcohol and drugs inhibit the absorption of these minerals, further depleting reserves. So it is cyclical: refined foods inhibit mineral absorption, which then are not themselves efficiently digested because of diminished enzyme activity. And then we go looking for bugs as the cause of disease?

3) **The third reason for inadequate minerals in the body is a phenomenon known as secondary deficiency**. It has been proven that an excess of one mineral may directly cause a deficiency of another, because minerals compete for absorption, compete for the same binding sites, like a molecular Musical Chairs. Secondary deficiency means an excess of one mineral may cause a deficiency of another.

For example, iron, copper, and zinc are competitive in this way. Copper is necessary for the conversion of iron to hemoglobin, but if there is excess zinc, less iron will be available for conversion. This may cause a secondary deficiency of iron, which can manifest itself as iron deficiency anemia. All due simply to excess zinc. Researchers have found that these secondary deficiencies caused by excess of one mineral are almost always due to mineral supplements, since the quantities contained in food are so small. Thus the hazards of mega-mineral toddies.

4) **A fourth reason for mineral deficiency in humans is overuse of prescription drugs**. It has been known since the 1950s that antibiotics interfere with uptake of minerals, specifically zinc, chromium, and calcium. (The Plague Makers) Also Tylenol, Advil, Motrin, and aspirin have the same inhibitive effect on mineral absorption. When the body has to try and metabolize these drugs to clear the system, its own mineral stores are heavily drawn upon.

Such a waste of energy is used to metabolize laxatives, diuretics, chemotherapy drugs, and NSAIDs such as Tylenol, Advil and aspirin out of the body. This is one of the most basic mechanisms in **drug induced immunosuppression**: minerals are essential for normal immune function.

Ultimately, the only issue that really counts with minerals is **bioavailability.** It really doesn't matter what we eat; it only matters what makes it to the body's cells. Let's say someone is iron deficient, for example. Can't he just take a bar of iron and file off some iron filings into a teaspoon, and swallow them? Just took in more iron, didn't he? Will this remedy the iron deficiency? Of course not. Here is a major distinction: the difference between elemental minerals and nutrient minerals. Iron filings are in the elemental form; absorption will be 8% or less. Same with most iron pills and most calcium supplements.

Food-bound iron, on the other hand, like that contained in raisins or molasses, will have a much higher rate of absorption, since it is complexed with other living, organic forms, and as such is classed as a nutrient mineral. Minerals are not living, though they are necessary for life. Minerals are necessary for cell life and enzyme reactions and hundreds of other reasons. But they must be in a form that can make it as far as the cells. What is not bioavailable passes right through the body, a waste of time and sometimes money. (Glenn's note: Or the improper form of a mineral may build up to toxic levels)

Bioavailability has a precursor, an opening act. It is called **absorption**. Take a mineral supplement pill. Put it in a glass of water and wait half an hour. If it is unchanged, chances are that the tablet itself would never even dissolve in the stomach or intestine, but pass right out of the body. You would be astounded how many mineral supplements there are in this category.

OK, let's say the tablet or capsule actually does dissolve in the digestive tract. Then what? In order to do us any good, the mineral must be absorbed into the bloodstream, through the intestinal walls. Elemental minerals are absorbed about 1-8% in this manner. The rest is excreted. Elemental means rocks. Elemental minerals are those found in the majority of supplements, because they're very cheap to produce. For the small percentage that actually makes it to the bloodstream, the mineral is available for use by the cells, or as catalysts in thousands of essential enzyme reactions that keep every cell alive every second. Use at the cellular level is what bioavailability is all about.

With this background in mind we can begin to understand that varying amounts of the seven macrominerals and approximately 14 trace minerals, in a bioavailable form are necessary for optimum cell activity, optimum health and would seem to contribute to long lifespan. So besides epidemic mineral deficiency, what's the problem?

In a word, **supplementation**. Mineral deficiency has become such an obvious health concern, causing specific diseases because of a lack of a single mineral, and general immune suppression with a lack of several, that the obvious need for supplementation has spawned an entire industry to the rescue. But in any market-driven industry involving pills, again we find that often the cures are worse than the original problems. Why?

First off, **toxicity**. Remember, even macrominerals are only necessary in **tiny amounts**. Most trace minerals are necessary in amounts too small to be measured, and can only be estimated.

Toxicity is a word that simply means extra stuff. When extra stuff gets put into the body, it's a big deal. All forces are mobilized for removal of the extra stuff, which are called antigens, toxins, poisons, reactants, etc, but you get the idea - it doesn't belong there. Toxicity means taking a nonessential non-nutrient mineral into the body.

Take lead poisoning, for example. If lead gets into the blood, the body will try to remove it. Since the metal atoms are so heavy compared with the body's immune forces, removal may be impossible without the use of a chelating agent. Lead can initiate a chronic inflammatory response and can remain in the body permanently, which is why we don't have lead in paint or gasoline any more.

Most minerals can be toxic if taken to excess. And this excess would not happen from food; only from supplements. (Glenn believes that an excess can happen from food, even though it is uncommon. Think of eating lots of kelp for its health benefits. Kelp is very high in iodine and it is possible to get to much iodine from kelp).

What supplements would be bad?

Well, for starters, any supplement containing more than about 21 minerals, because that's all that have been proven to be necessary for humans. New toxicities are always being discovered. Aluminum linked to Alzheimer's is a recent discovery. Beyond these 21 or so it's simply anybody's guess, no matter what they tell you about the 5 civilizations where people live to be 140 years old. People who show dramatic improvements from taking these 60 and 80 mineral drinks generally were so depleted that they rapidly absorbed the essential minerals in which they were deficient. But the toxicities from the nonessential, unknown minerals may take a long time to show up. Why take in anything extra?

> Glenn's comment: The minerals listed in the paragraph below are in mostly improper forms and are NOT in Ionic form and are NOT angstrom sized. In addition many of them are synthetic versions.

Here's an example of an ingredient list from one of these mega-mineral drinks. I pulled it off the Net: Calcium, Magnesium, Zinc, Vanadium, Manganese, Potassium, Selenium, Chromium, Phosphate, Iron, Sulfur, Carbon, Sodium, Barium, Strontium, Cesium, Thorium, Molybdenum, Nickel, Cerium, Germanium, Copper, Rubidium, Antimony, Gallium, Neodymium, Lanthanum, Bismuth, Zirconium, Thallium, Tungsten, Ruthenium, Boron, Iodine, Chloride, Bromine, Titanium, Cobalt, Dysprosium, Scandium, Samarium, Fluoride, Niobium, Praseodymium, Erbium, Hafnium, Lithium, Ytterbium, Yttrium, Cadmium, Holmium, Rhenium, Palladium, Gold, Thulium, Terbium, Iridium, Tantalum, Europium, Lutetium, Rhodium, Tin, Indium, Silver, Beryllium, Tellurium, and Platinum.

Any questions?

Again, we only need a little. So the mineral supplements we take should be as absorbable and as bioavailable as possible - that way we won't have to take much. Less chance of toxicity.

So the question then becomes: which mineral supplements are the most absorbable and the most usable, and therefore effective in the smallest amounts possible?

Four candidates present themselves, all contending for the title:

Elemental	Least Beneficial and often toxic
Colloidal	*"A colloidal mineral is one that has been so altered that it will no longer pass through cell walls or other organic membranes."* Does that sound like easy absorption? (from later in this article)
Ionic	Need to be in angstrom size particles instead of micron
Chelated	Chelated minerals may be superior to ionic, provided it's the right chelate. Only a specific chelate can resist digestion and maintain its integrity as it is absorbed through the gut. Again, all chelates are not created equal. Inferior chelates, used because they are cheaper to produce are listed later in this article.

Unraveling this puzzle is one area where the internet actually impedes progress. Try it and you'll see why. There's only one answer, but it's buried deep. To find it, we have to review a little basic plumbing.

The digestive tract goes like this: mouth, esophagus, stomach, small intestine, large intestine, and out. Mineral absorption means transferring the mineral from the digestive tract through the wall of the intestine, into the bloodstream. You really have to picture this: the digestive tract is just a long tube, from one end to the other. As long as food and nutrients are inside this tube, they are actually considered to be still outside the body, because they haven't been absorbed into the bloodstream yet. This is an essential concept to understanding mineral absorption. Minerals can't do any good unless they make it into the bloodstream. This is exactly why most minerals bought at the grocery store are almost worthless: they pass right through the body - in one end and out the other. It's also why many nutritionists' and dieticians' advice is valueless; they commonly pretend everything that is eaten is absorbed. When they start talking about calories, look for another speaker.

Two main reasons for lack of mineral supplement absorption:

The pill never dissolved

The mineral was in its elemental form (non-nutrient, e.g., iron filings)

Let's say these problems are overcome. Or let's say the mineral is contained within some food, such as iron in molasses, or potassium in bananas. Food-bound minerals are attached or complexed to organic molecules. Absorption into the blood is vastly increased, made easy. The mineral is not just a foreign metal that has been ingested; it is part of food.

Fruits and vegetables with high mineral content are the best way to provide the body with adequate nutrition. Food-bound minerals are the original mode. As already cited above, however, sufficient mineral content is an increasingly rare occurrence. Foods simply don't have it. How little, what portion of normal depends on what studies one finds. Soon the necessity for supplementation becomes obvious: if the food no longer has it, and we need it, pass the supplements, please. At that point, the marketplace assaults one's awareness and we're almost back to the days of the tonics, brews, toddies, and snake potions of yesteryear.

Let's look at the four types of minerals one by one. Least beneficial are the supplements containing minerals in the elemental form. That means the mineral is just mentioned on the label. It's not ionized, it's not chelated, it's not complexed with an oxide or a carbonate or a sulfate, or with a food, and it's not colloidal. Under "ingredients" it just says "iron" or "copper," or "calcium," etc.

1. Elemental

Elemental minerals are obviously the cheapest to make. A liquid would only have to be poured over some nails to be said to contain iron. Elemental minerals are the most common in grocery store supplements. They may not be toxic, as long as only the minerals mentioned on the label are included in the supplement. The problem is absorption: it's between 1 and 8 percent. The rest passes right through. Not only a waste of money; also a waste of energy: it has to be processed out of the body. This can actually use up available mineral stores.

2. Colloidal

Speaking of overloading, the third type of supplemental minerals is the one we hear the most about: **colloidal.** What does colloidal really mean? Colloidal refers to a solution, a dispersion medium in which mineral particles are so well suspended that they never settle out: you never have to shake the bottle. The other part of the dictionary definition has to do with diffusion through a membrane: "will not diffuse easily through vegetable or animal membrane." Yet this is supposed to be the whole rationale for taking colloidal minerals - their absorbability. Colloidal guru Joel Wallach himself continuously claims that it is precisely the colloidal form of the minerals that allows for easy diffusion and absorption across the intestinal membrane, because the particles are so small. Wallach claims 98% absorption, but cites no studies, experiments, journal articles or research of any kind to back up this figure. Why not? Because there aren't any. The research on colloidal minerals has never been done. It's not out there. Senate Document 264 doesn't really cover it.

In reality, colloidal minerals are actually larger than ionic minerals, as discussed by researcher Max Motyka PhD. Because of the molecular size and suspension in the colloid medium, which Dorland's Medical dictionary describes as "like glue," absorption is inhibited, not enhanced. No less an authority than **Dr. Royal Lee**, the man responsible for pointing out the distinction between whole food vitamins and synthetic vitamins, stated

"A colloidal mineral is one that has been so altered that it will no longer pass through cell walls or other organic membranes."

Does that sound like easy absorption?

For a mineral to be absorbed, it must be either in the ionic state, or else chelated, as explained above. The percentage of colloidal minerals which actually does get absorbed has to be ionized somehow, due to the acidic conditions in the small intestine. Only then is the mineral capable of being taken up by the carrier proteins in the intestinal membrane, as mentioned above. By why create the extra step? Ionic minerals would be superior to colloidal, because they don't have to be dissociated from a suspension medium, which is by definition non-diffusible. All this extra work costs the body in energy and reserves.

Max Motyka further points out the error of Wallach's claims. Wallach states that colloidals are negatively charged, and this enhances intestinal absorption. The problem is his science is 180 backward: Wallach claims the charge of the intestinal mucosa is positive, but all other sources have known for decades that the mucosal charge is negative. This is why ionic minerals are presented to the intestinal surface as cations (positively charged ions). Opposites attract, like repels - remember? Another big minus for colloidals.

Quality control. Consistency of percentages of each mineral from batch to batch. Very simply, there isn't any with the mega mineral supplements, as the manufacturers will themselves admit. The ancient lakes and glaciers apparently have not been very accommodating when it comes to percent composition. Such a range of variation might be acceptable in, say, grenade tossing or blood dilution in seawater necessary to attract a shark, or IQ threshold of terrorists, or other areas where high standards of precision are not crucial. But a nutritional supplement that is supposed to enhance health by drinking it - this is an area in which the details of composition should be fairly visible, verifiable and the same every time. In these 80-trace-mineral toddies, there is no way of testing the presence or absence of many of the individual minerals. Many established essential trace minerals do not even have an agreed-upon recommended daily allowance, for two reasons:

The research has never been done

The amounts are too small to measure

How much less is known about the amounts and toxicities of those unknown minerals which have never been studied, but are claimed to be present in these "miraculous" toddies?

Many essential minerals are toxic in excess, but essential in small amounts. Iron, chlorine, sodium, zinc, and copper are in this category. Toxic levels have been established, and resulting pathologies have been identified: we know what diseases are caused by their excesses. How risky is it to take in 40 or 50 minerals for which no toxicity levels have ever been set?

Doug Grant, a nutritionist, cites several minerals which frequently appear on the ingredient labels of certain mega-mineral products. They actually admit their supplements contain or "may contain" some of the following: (the phrase "may contain" has always been scary for me. If they're not sure, then what else is there that this product "may contain" that they don t know about?)

Aluminum: Documented since the article in *Lancet* 14 Jan 1989 to be associated with Alzheimer's Disease, as well as blocking absorption of essential minerals like calcium, iron, and fluoride.

Silver: questionable as a single-dose antibiotic, consistent intake of silver accumulates in the blood-forming organs - spleen, liver, and bone marrow-, as well as the skin, lungs, and muscles. Serious pathologies have resulted: blood disorders, cirrhosis, pulmonary edema, chronic bronchitis, and a permanent skin condition known as argyria, to name just a few. Silver is better left in the ancient lakes, and in tableware.

Gold: Manufacturers of mega-minerals hawk that "there's more gold in a ton of seawater than there is in a ton of ore." So what? Our blood is not seawater; it evolved from seawater. Gold used to be used to treat rheumatoid arthritis, but has largely been abandoned when they proved that it caused kidney cell destruction, bone marrow suppression, and immune abnormalities.

Lithium: Rarely used as an antipsychotic medication, lithium definitely can cause blackouts, coma, psychosis, kidney damage, and seizures. Outside of that, it should be fine.

The list goes on. The above are just a few examples of mineral toxicities about which we have some idea. But for at least half the minerals in the mega toddies, we know nothing at all.

3. Ionic

Next comes ionic minerals. Usually a step up. Ionic means in the form of ions. Ions are unstable molecules that want to bind with other molecules. An ion is an incomplete molecule. There is a definite pathway for the absorption of ionic minerals through the gut (intestine) into the blood. In fact, any percent of the elemental minerals that actually got absorbed became ions first, by being dissolved in stomach acids.

Ionic minerals are not absorbed through the intestine intact.

The model for mineral ion absorption through the intestine is as follows. Ions are absorbed through the gut by a complicated process involving becoming attached or chelated to some special carrier proteins in the intestinal wall. Active transport is involved; meaning, energy is required to bring the ionic mineral from inside the intestine through the lining, to be deposited in the bloodstream on the other side.

Ionic minerals may be a good source of nutrients for the body, depending upon the type of ions, and on how difficult it is for the ion to get free at the appropriate moment and location. Minerals require an acidic environment for absorption. Remember low pH (less than 7) is acidic; high pH (above 7) is alkaline. As the stomach contents at pH 2 empty into the small intestine, the first few centimeters of the small intestine is the optimum location for mineral absorption. The acidic state is necessary for ionization of the dissolved minerals. If the pH is too alkaline, the ions won't disassociate from whatever they're complexed with, and will simply pass on through to the colon without being absorbed.

As the mineral ions are presented to the lining of the intestine, if all conditions are right, and there are not too much of competing minerals present, the ions will begin to be taken across the intestinal barrier, making their way into the bloodstream. This is a complicated, multi-step process, beyond the scope of this section. Simply, it involves the attachment of the free mineral ion to some carrier proteins within the intestinal membrane, which drag the ion across and free it into the bloodstream. A lot happens during the transfer, and much energy is required for all the steps. Just the right conditions and timing are necessary - proper pH, presence of vitamins for some, and the right section of the small intestine.

Iron, manganese, zinc, copper - these ions are bound to the carrier proteins which are embedded in the intestinal lining. The binding is accomplished by a sort of chelation process, which simply describes the type of binding which holds the ion. The carrier protein or ligand (ligand is usually a molecule which produces a signal by binding to a site on a target protein), hands off the mineral to another larger carrier protein located deeper within the intestinal wall. After several other steps, if all conditions are favorable, the ion is finally deposited on the other side of the intestinal wall: the bloodstream, now usable by the cells.

Ionic mineral supplements do not guarantee absorption by their very nature, although they are certainly more likely to be absorbed than are minerals in the raw, elemental state. However, ionic minerals are in the form required for uptake by the carrier proteins that reside in the intestinal wall.

The uncertainties with ionic minerals include **how many, how much,** and **what else** are the unstable ions likely to become bound to before the carrier proteins pick them up. All ionic supplements are not created equal. Just because it's an ion doesn't mean a supplemental mineral will be absorbed. Too many minerals in a supplement will compete for absorption, crowding out the others. The idea is to offer the body an opportunity for balance; rather than to overload it with the hope that some will make it through somehow.

4. Chelated

The fourth form of supplemental minerals is the chelated variety. Some clarification of this term is immediately necessary. Chelated is a general term that describes a certain chemical configuration, or shape of a compound in which some molecule gets hooked up with some other chemical structures. When a mineral is bound or stuck to certain carrier molecules, which are known as chelating agents, or ligands, and a ring-like molecule is the result, we say that a chelate is formed. Chelate is from the Greek word for claw, suggested by the open v-shape of the two ligands on each side, with the mineral ion in the center.

Chelation occurs in many situations. Many things can be chelated, including minerals, vitamins, and enzymes. Minerals in food may be bound with organic molecules in a chelated state. Many molecules in the body are chelated in normal metabolic processes. The carrier proteins in the intestinal wall discussed above, whose job it is to transport ionic minerals - these chelate the ions. Another sense of the word chelation as exemplified in a mainstream therapy for removing heavy metals from the blood is called chelation therapy. The toxic metals are bound to a therapeutic amino acid ligand called EDTA or to another chelating agent. With a Pac-Man action, the metals are thus removed from the blood.

Molecular weight is measured in units called daltons. The ligands or binding agents may very small (800 daltons) or very large (500,000 daltons) resulting in a many sizes of chelates. Mineral + ligand = chelate. Generally the largest chelates are the most stable, and also the most difficult to absorb. Ionic minerals absorbed through the intestine are chelated to the carrier proteins, at least two separate times.

Using the word chelated with respect to mineral supplements refers a very specific type of chelation. The idea is to bind the mineral ion to ligands that will facilitate absorption of the mineral through the intestine into the bloodstream, bypassing the pathway used for ionic mineral absorption. Sometimes minerals prepared in this way are described as "pre-chelated" since any ionic mineral will be chelated anyway once it is taken up by the intestinal membrane.

After decades of research at Albion Laboratories in Utah, it was learned that small amino acids, especially glycine, are the best ligands for chelating minerals, for three reasons:

1) Bypasses the entire process of chelation by the intestine's own carrier proteins.

2) Facilitates absorption by an entirely different pathway of intestinal absorption, skipping the intermediate steps which ionic minerals go through.

3) The chelate will be the at the most absorbable molecular weight for intestinal transfer: less than 1500 daltons.

It has also been established beyond controversy that certain pairs of amino acids (dipeptides) are the easiest of all chelates to be absorbed, often easier than individual amino acids. Proteins are made of amino acids. Normal digestion presumably breaks down the proteins to its amino acid building blocks so they can be absorbed. But total breakdown is not always necessary. It has long been known that many nutrient chains of two or three or even more amino acids may be absorbed just as easily as single amino acids. Food-bound copper, vitamin C with hemoglobin molecule, animal protein zinc, are some examples of amino acids chelates that are easily absorbed intact.

To take another example, in abnormal digestion it is well known that chains of amino acids - dipeptides, tripeptides, even polypeptide proteins - sometimes become absorbed intact in a pathology known to gastroenterologists as Leaky Gut Syndrome. Obviously it is not healthy and has many adverse consequences, but the point is that amino acids chains are frequently absorbed, for many different reasons. It's not always like it says in the boldface section headings in Guyton's Physiology.

The reason these dipeptide chelates are absorbed faster than ionic minerals is that the chelated mineral was bonded tightly enough so that it did not dissociate in the acidic small intestine and offer itself for capture by the intestinal membranes carrier proteins. That whole process was thus avoided. The chelate is absorbed intact. An easier form. This is a vast oversimplification, and the most concise summary, of why **chelated minerals may be superior to ionic, provided it's the right chelate**. Only a specific chelate can resist digestion and maintain its integrity as it is absorbed through the gut. Again, all chelates are not created equal. Inferior chelates, used because they are cheaper to produce, include the following:

carbonates

citrates

oxides

sulfates

chlorides

phosphates

If the label gives one of these chelates, it means the mineral is bound either too strongly or not tightly enough, and will be released at the wrong time and the wrong place. Chelation of minerals in nutrient supplements is a very precise science, yielding chelates superior to those occurring naturally in foods.

Intact absorption is faster, easier, and requires less metabolic energy, provided the chelate is about 1500 daltons.

To compare chelated and ionic minerals, once the research is presented, there is really not much of a dispute about which is absorbed faster, ionic minerals or dipeptide-like amino acid chelates. Meticulous isotope testing has shown the following increases in percent absorption of chelates, as compared with ionic:

Glenn's comment: Remember, this is only if the right chelate is used. Only a specific chelate can resist digestion and maintain its integrity as it is absorbed through the gut. Again, all chelates are not created equal. How do you know which chelate was used and if it is the right chelate?

Iron	**490% greater**
Copper	**580% greater**
Magnesium	**410% greater**
Calcium	**421% greater**
Manganese	**340% greater**

***Journal of Applied Nutrition* 1970; 22: 42**

Again, this is just the briefest glance at the prodigious amount of research comparing ionic with chelated minerals, but the results are uniform. The winner of the bioavailability contest is: chelated minerals, provided the chelate was maintained as small as possible, generally using glycine as the amino acid ligands, at a total weight of about 1500 daltons.

Food-bound chelated minerals. Often you will hear this or that company claiming that "organic" minerals contained in food are the best, cannot be improved upon, and are superior to all possible types of mineral supplements. This is almost true. The only exception is glycine-chelated minerals, for two reasons:

> The exact amount of minerals in any food is extremely variable and difficult to measure, even if there is high mineral content of the soil. Pesticides destroy root organisms in the soil. These bugs play a major role in selective mineral absorption into the plant.
>
> The ligands that bind the mineral in the food chelate may be too strong or too weak to dissociate at exactly the right time for maximum absorption in the human digestive tract. Glycine chelates are uniform and easily measurable. No question about dosage.

Marketing is a wonderful thing - two different companies are now attributing the longevity of the Hunza tribe in Pakistan to two entirely different properties of their water: one, the minerals; the other, molecular configuration. A classic error in logic is described as "post hoc, ergo propter hoc" - after this, therefore because of this. Maybe it was the weather that made the Hunzas live longer, or their diet, or their grains, or the absence of toothpaste or web servers or... Marketing is the art of persuasion by suspending logic.

The average lifespan of an American is about 75 years. No one has ever proven that taking mineral supplements will extend life. Many old people never took a mineral or a vitamin in their life. It really comes down to quality of life. Incidence of disease during the lifespan. For how many days or months of the total lifespan was the person ill? We are the walking petri dishes of Alexis Carrel, remember? Carrel was the French biochemist, a Nobel prize winner, who did the famous experiment in which he kept chicken heart cells alive in a petri dish for 28 years just by changing the solutes every day. Could've gone longer, but figured he'd proven his point. Mineral content factors largely in the quality of our solutes: the blood - the milieu interior, the biological terrain.

The U.S. has the highest incidence of degenerative diseases of any developed country on earth. In addition, the infectious diseases are coming back; antibiotics are getting less effective every year. Americans' confidence in prescription drugs is weakening. Allow me to disabuse you of unfounded hopes: **cancer and AIDS will never be cured by the discovery of some new drug.** It's not going to happen. There probably will never be another Alexander Fleming - turns out penicillin was just a brief detour anyway. Bacteria have had **50 billion years** to figure out ways to adapt. The only way that anyone recovers from any illness is when the immune system overcomes the problem. Allergy shots never cured an allergy - people who take allergy shots always have allergies.

Our only hope of better health is to do everything possible to build up our natural immune system. One of these preventative measures is nutritional supplementation. It may not be dramatic, but daily deposits to the immune system bank account will pay off down the road. Healthy people don't get sick.

With respect to minerals, then, what are our goals? My opinion is that having once realized the necessity for mineral supplementation, our objectives should be simple:

Take only the minerals we absolutely need

Take the smallest amounts possible

Nothing left over (no metabolic residue)

Some of the above ideas may seem strange and difficult to understand, on first reading. But it is truly a very simplified version of what actually takes place. Most of the technical details were omitted for the sake of clarity and brevity. However, the correctness of the above basic framework is verifiable.

We are living in the age of the **Junk Science Hustle.** Everybody's an expert, often quoting shaky sources, shaky facts, and shaky claims which may have no foundation in physical reality. Seems there's a formula:

Get a product.
Get a marketing company (preferably in Utah or Texas).
Get some university MD endorsements.
Get some miraculous testimonials.
Get a downline.

In a certain way, all this is actually a good sign - a natural consequence of the explosion in holistic nutrition and supplementation. Because in the midst of the quagmire of hype and junk science, some truly superlative items have emerged onto the marketplace which have benefitted indirectly from biomedical advances evolved in the challenged, time-bomb world of mainstream pharmacology. Most of the new holistic supplements are less toxic than standard pharmaceutical drugs, because they're in a category the FDA calls GRAS (Generally Regarded As Safe. That's probably more than we can say for Prozac, fen-phen, and Viagra.) Many of the extraordinary holistic supplements won't be sold in stores, and no one is going to give them away. So welcome to the American marketplace. Very time-consuming and confusing is the screening process one must go through to unearth the treasures that can reward the patient who does resolute search. Caveat emptor.

Above is adapted from < http://www.chiro.org/nutrition/ABSTRACTS/minerals.shtml about 2012 (web site no longer available as of 2016)

I found the article on Sept 24, 2016 at http://www.life-enthusiast.com/minerals-tim-oshea-a-68.html

****

Below is from an audio tape that is no longer available. Excellent information.

Minerals and Enzymes

Calcium Carbonate Is Not Calcium and Chelates

Calcium carbonate consists of one calcium atom attached to one carbon atom, attached to three oxygen atoms. Most people believe they are getting calcium when they take calcium carbonate. They ARE NOT. The body does not have the ability to break this compound down and utilize it.

Calcium Carbonate, Real Calcium, Digestion, Osteoporosis and PH

Because calcium is an alkaline element, the body uses calcium as the main co-enzyme to adjust the PH of digesting foods as it enters the bloodstream. Calcium carbonate does not work properly as a co-enzyme because it does not bind to hydrogen. This would explain why people can take calcium carbonate all day long, but their body continues to rob calcium from their bone structure, causing the condition known as osteoporosis. Calcium carbonate is blackboard chalk. It is the scale that builds up on your shower wall, gums up your swamp cooler or humidifier and it does not mix with water (it is not water soluble). It tends to gum up your bodies circulation system. The beautiful coral reefs are made from calcium carbonate, from the bodies of the tiny ocean creatures. If this calcium were water soluble there would be no barrier reefs. Therefore, calcium carbonate is organic for sea creatures, but inorganic and in the wrong form for man. It is also organic for chickens, but we have no way to discharge it properly. That is why it is in the wrong form for us. It does dissolve in stomach acid. It is used in antacid products. It neutralizes the acid and is then absorbed into the bloodstream, but not in the form that can be used by the tissues. Since the dissolved blackboard chalk migrates out of the blood, it deposits into joints and organs, around the brain and plugs up the vascular system. On the other hand if you consume real calcium that is water soluble, not carbonated, your PH can start rising to correct levels. I have seen many instances where pure calcium has helped remove the flu symptoms in thirty minutes or less by neutralizing acidic crystalline neural toxins produced by the infection. My theory is that the body uses calcium to flush out and neutralize crystalline acidic neural toxins that are created by the infection. This helps to maintain the proper PH levels.

Above is from an audio tape that is no longer available. Excellent information.

Below is from http://articles.mercola.com/sites/articles/archive/2012/07/11/calcium-turmeric-and-resveratrol-benefits.aspx

Calcium: Good From Food, Not From Supplements?

Calcium is one of the most popular dietary supplements on the market, largely because of the widely circulated belief that regular supplemental doses of this mineral are essential for building and maintaining healthy bones. As a result, many people believe that taking a calcium supplement is one of the best - if not an essential - strategy to prevent bone fractures resulting from osteoporosis.

However, it's becoming increasingly clear that while organically-bound calcium from your diet is beneficial, elemental calcium supplements, e.g. calcium carbonate, calcium citrate, etc., may dramatically increase heart attack risk, and other health problems.

A recent study published in the journal "Heart" found that people who took calcium supplements regularly had an *86 percent* greater risk of having a heart attack, which led researchers to suggest such pills should be "taken with caution." *Dietary* calcium, on the other hand, had no such risk! In fact, those who got their calcium exclusively from supplements more than doubled their risk of a heart attack compared to those who took no supplements.

A similar trend has been seen for kidney stones, with people taking calcium supplements at a greater risk, while those who consume a high level of calcium in food are at a *reduced* risk. There have been a number of studies that indicate calcium supplements increase your risk for cardiovascular incidents and other problems, as well as NOT being of much benefit to your bones.

Cardiovascular

- A 2010 meta-analysis showed calcium supplements (without coadministered vitamin D) are associated with a 27% **increased risk for heart attack. Even when calcium was administered with vitamin D, which helps you absorb and utilize calcium,** elemental calcium *still* increased heart attack risk by 24 percent.
- A 2008 study found calcium supplements are associated with a **greater number of heart attacks** in postmenopausal women.
- A 2004 study showed that people with excess calcium in their coronary artery and who take statins have a **17-fold higher risk of heart attacks** than do those with lower arterial calcium levels; researchers concluded that the two most definitive indicators of heart attack were LDL levels *and arterial calcium build-up.*

Osteoporosis and Bone Density

- A 2010 article presented evidence for a total lack of support in the research for calcium supplements reducing fracture risk.
- A 2007 study showed that calcium from dietary sources has more favorable effects on bone health than calcium from supplements in postmenopausal women.
- A 2009 study of postmenopausal women using calcium supplements showed that, although calcium loss from bone was slowed, **bone loss was still occurring.**

What Makes Calcium Supplements Potentially Dangerous?

Your body does not make calcium, and in fact loses this important mineral daily through your skin, nails, hair, sweat and elimination, which is why you must replace it on a regular basis. Historically this has been through dietary sources.

It has been estimated, however, that your body excretes as little as 100 mg a day, making the current recommendations by the National Osteoporosis Foundation for women over 50 to take 1,200 mg a day a bit troubling. When we compare our calcium-rich diet to the traditional calcium-poor Chinese peasant diet, which was free of cow's milk and calcium supplements, approximately 250 mg a day of plant-based calcium was all that was needed to fulfill their bodily needs – and this is a culture with no word for "osteoporosis" in its 3,000+ year old language!

Due to the fact that about 99 percent of your body's calcium is stored in your bones and teeth, if you don't get enough calcium, your body will use the calcium reserves in your bones to perform vital metabolic functions. This is where the idea that supplementing with calcium could prevent calcium loss from your bones comes from - but it is an overly simplified theory that lacks solid evidence to back it up, especially in Western, modernized cultures, which consume unprecedentedly large amounts of dairy-derived, fortification-based and supplemental calcium.

The truth is that taking any calcium in excess or isolation, without complementary nutrients like magnesium, vitamin D and vitamin K2, which help keep your body in balance, can have adverse effects, such as calcium building up in coronary arteries and inducing heart attacks. Even taking calcium *with* vitamin D does not appear to be sufficient to prevent these types of adverse effects.

So when you take a biologically foreign form of calcium (such as limestone, oyster shell, egg shell and bone meal (hydroxylapatite)), or when your body's ability to direct calcium to the right places becomes impaired (as when you are deficient in vitamin K2), calcium may be deposited where it shouldn't be, which can lead to multiple health problems, including heart attacks. It's more likely your body can use calcium correctly if it's food-based calcium.

Above is from http://articles.mercola.com/sites/articles/archive/2012/07/11/calcium-turmeric-and-resveratrol-benefits.aspx

****

Below is from:http://www.mercola.com/nutritionplan/intermediate_proteins.htm

Up the ante to organic butter and eggs.

Ideally you should be consuming as many USDA organic food products as possible, however, if you only get one organic food it should be butter. This is because it is a highly concentrated form of milk. It is not uncommon for non-organic butter to have up to 20 times the level of pesticides of non-organic fruits and vegetables.

Remember eggs?

Now that you've reached the intermediate level, it's time to move up to organic pastured free-range eggs. Compared to official U.S. Department of Agriculture (USDA) nutrient data for commercial eggs, eggs from hens raised on pasture contain:

- 2/3 more vitamin A
- 2 times more omega-3 fatty acids
- 3 times more vitamin E
- 7 times more beta carotene

These dramatically differing nutrient levels are most likely the result of the differences in diet between free-range pastured hens, vs. commercially farmed hens. Organic eggs don't have to be certified by law, so if you are fortunate enough to know someone who grows chickens and controls the feed and conditions, those eggs are typically better than organic store-bought eggs.

How to Find High Quality Eggs

True free-range eggs are from hens that walk about freely outdoors on a pasture where they can forage for their natural diet, which includes seeds, green plants, insects, and worms. A hen that is let outside into a barren lot for a few minutes a day but is fed a diet of corn, soy and cottonseed meal, plus synthetic additives, is NOT an organic free-range hen, and will not produce the same quality eggs as its foraging counterpart. Likewise, a hen that is fed an organic diet, but never gets to go outside is also NOT a true free-range hen, although it may currently slide through as an "organic" one…

A MAJOR part of a hen being truly organic is having free range access to outdoor pasture. It's not just about being fed organic grains. And this is a primary point of contention within the egg industry.

How to Know if You Found High Quality Eggs

The key to getting high quality eggs is to buy them locally, either from an organic farm or farmers market. You can gauge the quality of the egg by the color of its yolk. Organic pastured eggs have deep yellow or orange yolks, whereas commercially-farmed eggs tend to have very light-yellow colored yolks. You will need to be diligent about this as I have found many reliable sources of healthy eggs that invariably wind up cheating and don't put their hens on the grass Fortunately this is easy to tell as the egg yolks from these hens are yellow and not bright orange.

Finding organic eggs locally is far easier than finding raw milk as virtually every rural area has individuals with chickens. To locate a free-range pasture farm, try asking your local health food store, or check out the following web listings:

If you absolutely must purchase your eggs from a commercial grocery store, look for ones that are marked free-range organic. They're still going to originate from a mass-production facility (so you'll want to be careful about eating them raw), but it's about as good as it gets if you can't find a local source. The Cornucopia Institute's report, "Scrambled Eggs: Separating Factory Farm Egg Production from Authentic Organic Agriculture", contains a scorecard that rates nearly 70 different organic egg brands based on 22 organic criteria.

I would strongly encourage you to AVOID ALL omega-3 eggs, as they are some of the least healthy for you. These eggs typically come from chickens that are fed poor-quality sources of omega-3 fats that are already oxidized. Also, omega-3 eggs perish much faster than non-omega-3 eggs.

Above is from:http://www.mercola.com/nutritionplan/intermediate_proteins.htm

****

Below is by the author

Some General Diet Guidelines

There is a strong correlation between the "Metabolic Typing Diet's" "Protein Type" and Blood Type O as well as a strong correlation between the "Metabolic Typing Diet's" "Carbohydrate Type" and Blood Type A. There is a weaker correlation between the "Metabolic Typing Diet's" "Mixed Type" and Blood Types AB and B.

As a general rule Blood Type O ("Protein Type") requires more protein than a Blood Type A ("Carbohydrate Type").

Typical Protein, Carbohydrates and Fats ratios by calorie

Blood Type "A": 20% to 30% protein by calorie with equal amount of good fats by calorie; The rest will be carbohydrates

Blood Type "B": 20% to 40% protein by calorie with equal amount of good fats by calorie; The rest will be carbohydrates

Blood Type "AB": 20% to 40% protein by calorie with equal amount of good fats by calorie; The rest will be carbohydrates

Blood Type "O": 30% to 40% protein by calorie with equal amount of good fats by calorie; The rest will be carbohydrates

Many say that Protein Foods, Carbohydrates and Fats should be combined at each meal and snack

DIET AND FOOD GENERAL NOTES

Vegetable and fruit juices are plain juice as listed **with no other ingredients**.

Soups, dressings etc. require a careful **look at the ingredients**.

Seven major hidden **food allergens** are: dairy, soy, corn, eggs, chocolate (cocoa), gluten (especially wheat) and peanuts.

Gluten containing grains: wheat, rye, barley, oats, millet, Durham, triticale, bulgur, spelt and kamut. The most problematic is wheat. Also these grains in any form including bran, flour, cereals. Eat whole grains only. Acceptable grains should be limited and eaten in moderation by most people.

Nitrites and nitrates are not good for anyone (ham, lunch meats, bacon, and other "cured" foods)

Fruits and Fruit Juice - All fruit juices can cause diarrhea. Prunes, apples and pears are very high in sorbitol which can cause diarrhea and flatulence

Everyone should avoid **artificial sweeteners, msg, food colorings and preservatives**.

Phytates are phosphorus compounds found primarily in cereal grains, legumes, and nuts. They bind with minerals such as iron, calcium, and zinc and interfere with their absorption in the body. Not everyone believes that phytates are a bad thing. Although phytates do bind with minerals, they may actually be preventing the formation of free radicals, thereby keeping the minerals at safe levels in the body. Phytates also have a role to play in cell growth and can move excess minerals out of the body.

Soybeans contain high levels of phytates; more than other beans. Additionally, soy's phytates are so stable that many survive phytate-reducing techniques such as cooking or soaking. (The phytates in whole grains can be deactivated simply by soaking or fermenting). Only long periods of soaking and **fermenting - as used in making miso, natto, shoyu, tamari, and tempeh** (but not tofu, soymilk, texturized soy protein, or soy protein isolate) - significantly reduce the phytate content of soybeans. Also, eating too much unfermented soy may lead to a shortage of crucial minerals, estrogen dominance and will act as an enzyme inhibitor. From my research I feel it may be best to avoid ALL unfermented soy, whether it is GMO or Organic

Oxalic acid combines with other substances to form various salts, called oxalates; usually, those salts are in solution, but if their concentration is high enough some may precipitate out in crystalline form. Such tiny crystals of these salts can be irritating to human tissue, especially to the stomach, the kidneys, and the bladder. It is commonly believed that oxalates contribute to the formation of kidney and bladder stones; one common nutrient with which oxalic acid combines is calcium, making the salt calcium oxalate. Some have argued that by readily combining with calcium, oxalic acid in the diet reduces one's effective intake of dietary calcium.

Purine, High Fructose Corn Syrup and Gout: Gout is an arthritic type of pain in your joints; typically, about 75 percent of people will experience it as an excruciating pain in their big toe. (Hence, if you ever experience sudden, severe pain in your big toe, you may want to go get checked for gout.)

The symptoms of gout - the stiff, swollen and painful joints - are due to excess uric acid forming crystals in your joints, and the pain is caused by your body’s inflammatory response to these crystals.

Besides gout, elevated uric acid is related to a variety of other health conditions, including; Diabetes, High cholesterol, High blood pressure, Kidney disease and Heart disease.

You CAN address the underlying cause of excess uric acid formation via all natural means. Avoid foods high in Purine and High-Fructose Corn Syrup (HFCS). Both can wreck your uric acid levels, putting you at high risk of gout.

Biochemist Russ Bianchi claims that in some processed products, HFCS is either intentionally mislabeled or uses deceptive, legal, non-compliant names, like: Chicory, Glucose-fructose syrup/ glucose syrup/ iso glucose Insulin, Dahlia syrup, Tapioca syrup, Crystalline fructose, Fruit fructose, Agave

Thiocyanate can cause thyroid dysfunction. It inhibits Iodine metabolism and yet is very important to have. It is a chemical found in cigarettes and in some foods. Unless you have an Iodine deficiency or Thyroid problems it probably is fine in food.

Thiocyanate is found in specific foods, common foods indigenous to the African diet as well as some Middle Eastern and Mediterranean diets.
When thiocyanate is present in the diet, it acts as an oxygen carrier and increases the capacity of the blood to transport the life-giving oxygen to every single cell of the body. Thiocyanate is a must have substance if one is dealing with the challenge of sickle cell anemia. Because of the oxygen-enhancing properties of thiocyanate pertaining to the cells of the body, a diet rich in thiocyanate is effective in prevention and healing of sickling of the red blood cells, commonly referred to as or known as sickle cell anemia. According to Andoh, "Just as iron deficiency anemia is corrected with the addition of iron rich foods to the diet, so can sickle cell anemia be corrected with the addition of thiocyanate foods to the diet."
Further, Andoh states: "The painful crisis of sickle cell anemia is infrequent and not as severe in people whose diet is rich in thiocyanate. In fact, many people who grow to adulthood with the traditional diet, often are not aware that they have a blood disorder. Often, when these people migrate to foreign countries and do not eat their traditional diet, they experience a sickle cell crisis for the first time."

LIST OF GOAT CHEESES

France: Bucheron, Chabis, Chavroux, Clochette,Couronne Lochoise, Crottin de Chavignol, Montrachet, Pélardon, Picodon,Pouligny Saint-Pierre, Rocamadour, Sainte-Maure de Touraine, Chabichou du Poitou, Valençay, and Pyramide.

Spain and Portugal: Castelo Branco, Garrotxa

United States: none

United Kingdom: Pantysgawn, CapricornGevrik, Tesyn

Greece: Feta, mizithra, anthotyros are made from a mixture of goat's and sheep's milk.

Norway: Brunost (U.S. name is often Gjetost)

Ireland: Tullyboy

Italy: Caprino

China: Rubing

Australia: Buche Noir

Venezuela: Pasta Firme

Turkey: Tulum cheese

Above is by the author

Chapter 8

Meditation, Exercises and Prayer

Below is by author.

Prayers made up from tool 8 in Two Choices - Divine LOVE or Anything Else

Help me to make it so and keep it so I always breathe in LOVE and breathe out peace with proper deep breaths and practice this consciously for several minutes, several times per day until it becomes automatic.

Help me to make it so and keep it so I always simply sit in the LOVE 'That I AM' and relax into the heart.

Help me to make it so and keep it so I always surrender to the simplicity of living from the 'Heart Space'.

Help me to make it so and keep it so I always receive 'Cosmic LOVE', 'which I AM', and allow it to flow through in a seamless 'State of LOVE'.

Help me to make it so and keep it so I always rest and am nourished in the Simplicity and the peace which surpasses understanding.

Help me to make it so and keep it so I always live and breathe each moment from the Heart with the great LOVE of self and 'All That I AM'.

Help me to make it so and keep it so I always release and let go of all the 'stuff', knowing that I AM omniscient, omnipresent, omnipotent and can retrieve any information that may be needed in any given moment.

Help me to make it so and keep it so I always realize each of us must take responsibility for that which we receive.

Help me to make it so and keep it so I always take time to rest. Help me to soak in, absorb and radiate the pure simple frequencies and LOVE of the cosmic energies continually radiating through the universe.

Help me to make it so and keep it so I always share 'That Which I AM' with LOVE.

Help me to make it so and keep it so I am always ready, willing and open and that the doors open with utter Divine LOVE, Grace, ease and effortlessness to now bring forth, for fair exchange, "All That I AM'; all that I have to share.

Help me to make it so and keep it so I always allow all the programming to simply dissolve and be transmuted in the 'VIOLET FLAME' of God's Infinite Perfection.

Help me to make it so and keep it so I always realize and am aware that past, present and future are all here in the center of the present.

Help me to make it so and keep it so I always know that true prosperity goes hand-in-hand with peace and LOVE.

Help me to make it so and keep it so I always have clarity about whatever the topic may be and am in alignment with 'The Divine Flow', moment to moment.

Help me to make it so and keep it so I always let all the stories go, let all the identities go, let all the strategies go and let all the modalities go. Help me to make it so and keep it so that I only use them when best in the moment, with 'All That I AM' in utter trust as guided.

Help me to make it so and keep it so I always let go, relinquish control, think less and *feel* more.

Help me to make it so and keep it so I always trust 'All That I AM' more.

Help me to make it so and keep it so I always allow all my Helpers of LIGHT and LOVE to bring all of my energies and all of my timelines gathered together in all 'That I AM'.

Help me to make it so and keep it so I always gather all my parts and pieces, 'All That I AM', into the Heart with LOVE.

Help me to make it so and keep it so I always am resting in the Heart, with all the LOVE, with all the feeling, with all the vulnerability; with all the openness, flow and creativity that comes through the heart.

Help me to make it so and keep it so I always let go of all the tensions deeply held through many cycles of time and allow this to trigger a deep, deep, deep relaxation of the physical vehicle. Help me to make it so and keep it so I always refocus in this way so I breathe in Divine LIGHT and LOVE through the heart and breath out peace.

Help me to make it so and keep it so I always bring 'All That I AM' into alignment with Great Spirit, ready to move forward with ease and grace in full alignment with that which I AM here to do at this time.

Help me to make it so and keep it so I always have a deep trust in 'All That I AM', in Creator and in the unfolding of Creation and that I let go of any conceptions of what 'reality' is, of what is going on, of what is happening , of what I need to 'do'.

Help me to make it so and keep it so I always am simply open to LOVE, to the unfoldment of life and creation, as it continues, breath to breath, moment to moment.

Help me to make it so and keep it so I always am in 'The Divine Flow' and am utterly grounded.

Help me to make it so and keep it so I always am in alignment with my infinite chakras, energy centers and centers of consciousness.

Help me to make it so and keep it so I always am in alignment with the 'Heart of Mother' in LOVE.

Help me to make it so and keep it so I always am in alignment through the 'Heart of Mother'.

Help me to make it so and keep it so I always am in alignment with the infinite spirals of chakras, energy centers and centers of consciousness that represent 'All That We Are', in LOVE.

Above is by author.

****

Below is adapted from http://kundalini-teacher.com/guidance/testgui.php

Testing Your Guides

An appeaser is one who feeds a crocodile, hoping it will eat him last.
Winston Churchill

A parasite cannot live alone.
African (Ovambo) Proverb

A half-truth is a whole lie.
Jewish Proverb

If you get side tracked listening to entities it will slow your progress. The oldest and wisest sages say to pay no attention to the phenomena along the path. This is sage, safe advice, but often difficult for westerners to take. We are too curious. If you choose to pay attention to the entities, results could be embarrassing at the least, and disastrous at the worst. How many times have you heard of the homicidal psycho who says, the 'voices' or 'God' told them to do it? Yikes, don't go there.

I sometimes observe a funny sort of one-up-man-ship among some new agers. Who has the most guides, and whose guides have the fanciest names and titles - this is all very silly. Illusion. When it comes to guides, quality is essential, and quantity does not mean a thing! What the boasters are really saying, is how many different critters have persuaded them to hand their internal, essential Divine power of free will over. How gullible they are, and how widely they are enslaved...

Many types of critters who may appear claiming to be guides, are simply not worth the energy of your attention. They are self centered entities who will use fear, flattery, fancy titles and prophecies of doom, to persuade you to direct your power towards their own agendas.

This is how people sometimes find themselves on a mountain top, having given away all their possessions, waiting for the Lightships to come save them from Armageddon. Most entities feed on emotional energy (fear, anger, guilt, shame). They stay away from LOVE. The more they can get you riled up, the bigger the buffet - and of course they will often want you to start some sort of cult or movement so you will bring more people for them to feast on. That way they can impress their buddies by inviting them to a human energy smorgasbord.

Your emotional energy is their food. Without it they cannot continue to exist. They are parasites, and they may use flattery, predictions, warnings, or pranks to provoke your emotional reactions. Some entities may go on and on about how unique and special you are.

Yes, we are all special and unique in Great Spirit's eyes, regardless of who we are and what we do! Infinite manifestation creates uniqueness, and all of creation is special, loved and cherished - from the smallest pebble to the greatest leader.

Integrating that, actually leads to humility, not self aggrandizement. When you really begin to feel how much you are loved by the Divine, unconditionally, no matter what you say or do, there is no need to build yourself up with stories of your specialness. Simply Being, is enough. More blissful and radiant than self esteem via any other method could ever be.

Entities, (and some professional psychics who channel entities!) may give you fancy titles or famous past lives so you will pay attention to them. Where your attention goes your energy goes, so flattering you that you are Napoleon or Cleopatra reincarnated is a way for them to feed on your energy if you believe the flattery.

Funny, too how the entities tend to stick with what works. I've lost track of how many people have told me their guides said they had been "Keeper of the temple in Atlantis"... It means they were the janitor, I think! The Atlantis temple must have needed a lot of staff to do the cleaning up, like Disneyland...

Beware of guides, human or discarnate, who want to give you a fancy title or special name, and tell you that you have some special mission to save the world. Believing it is the path to Kundalini psychosis. They may use flattery to get your attention and persuade you to invest your time and energy into their personal agendas. Usually a closer look into their preaching reveals a decidedly fear based paradigm, or limits that do not truly exist.

Appearances can be deceiving. Just because an entity or guide looks pretty, all glowy and nice, does not mean they have your highest good in mind. There is an old story of a spiritual teacher: a lovely radiant female spirit, crowned and clothed in light appeared to him and said "you can have success or happiness, but not both. Which will you choose?" The teacher said "you're WRONG!" and banished the entity... and went on to have happiness ***and*** success!

On the other hand, sometimes entities that appear very dark and scary at first, turn into angels if you can love them unconditionally. **The scary appearance is to give you the option to exercise your free will choice to love or fear.** They are a reflection of your own fears, and loving them releases the fear blockage within you.

There is a place for compassion, certainly but much of what is called compassion is more about projections of what someone else needs! Sometimes the fear may be hard to discern; "The road to hell is paved with Good Intentions." If the mission you are given is about what someone else needs, that is one clue.

On the higher chakra levels of perception, All is One and there is no one else. All that you see, is yourself reflected. What you think someone else needs is more about what you think you need.

The genuine guides know, "Change the world by changing inside yourself."

The even wiser ones know, that the world does not need changing, everything is unfolding as it should. True spiritual beings know that the world is perfect in Great Spirit's eyes, and all is Great Spirit, so what needs to be "saved?"

If the entities are giving you predictions of the future, chuck them into the Light. Truly Divine beings know that the power is in the Now, and predictions that take you out of the moment, do not serve. Occasionally the Heart may offer some clues about the future, but rarely.

If the entities are very judgmental, boot them into the Light. If they are telling you that someone is evil, boot them into the Light. Unconditional love does not judge. It sees with eyes of compassion, and finds something loveable or at least sympathetic, about everyone, even history's most notorious villains.

Sending entities into the light is very easy, I have dozens of methods. Simply asking your Guardian Angels to take the entities into the light works very well. On the chakra level universes of duality, there are boundaries and individuality. Every animal has its territory and home, and the right and power to defend its space. You have a Divine Right to be sovereign in yourself, and Angels will be the enforcers of that, if you ask them.

(Glenn's comment: Make sure you ask for Angels of Love and Light. My way is, "Great Spirit and Great Spirit helpers as are best....")

Glenn's prayer for sending entities into the light is:

"Great Spirit, show this entity's spirit, soul and being Your Pure Divine Love and Light.

Help it recognize, get used to, accept and embrace Your Pure Divine Love and Light.

Bring it home to You as soon as it is ready and it is time.

Do what is best with it and for it. *Thank You."*

This prayer can be said for deceased animals and people too.)

I have encountered entities, especially ghosts, that try to convince me that they are not supposed to go into the light yet, that there are still things they must do. Don't believe a word of it. Send them all into the light and let Great Spirit sort them out. Great Spirit has it handled. The truly worthy beings will not resist, and will not be offended at your caution. They can take a trip into the light and enjoy it, and come right back to thank you.

It is important to test the guidance and the 'voices' that you hear. The still small voice within will never ask you to do anything that would hurt anyone, or cause them harm... including yourself. It is a voice of love. It will never give you scary warnings. It will never lie to you. It may sometimes give you predictions of the future, but generally not, because it knows that staying "in the moment" is more important. If you ever get questionable advice from your heart voice do not hesitate to do an entity clearing on yourself as many times as you need to.

It is very important that you be grounded when you are talking to the still small voice of the heart, otherwise you may very well hear instead the fearful voice of your own ego. You've already been listening to your ego for most of your life, probably you are tired of hearing it. Tired of the hamster wheel of your own thoughts going round and round, and that wheel motivates you to seek the peace that is to be found in stillness.

Sometimes the advice of the heart voice can be confusing, sometimes it may say things that will unground you, because you react emotionally, but usually if you can stay grounded and ask enough questions you will get to a place of clarity and insights.

For example, the heart voice may tell you that you are Christ... This very typically happens, at a certain phase of awakening, and it can be very destabilizing for some people who invent their own interpretation instead of asking the Heart for more clarity.

Quite a few psychos have heard this and gone off on some disastrous messiah mission, resulting in events like Waco. If you stay grounded and ask for more information, you may learn that Jesus was an embodiment of heart chakra unconditional love, and he himself said, that the same potential he manifested, is within us all. The heart is the center of the Christ-consciousness, which is the light of compassion and unconditional love. The "second coming", is all of us, growing into greater love and understanding.

You are All that Is, Christ and Hitler, both... but which will you choose to manifest? Hitler probably heard it too, he believed himself to be the "German messiah." Certainly at the beginning of his leadership, Hitler did some good things for Germany, like inventing the Volkswagen... he got much crazier, later, although the insane beginnings were present, potential in his book, "Mein Kamph."

On that subject, one needs to be careful of human guides, too. Kundalini awakening is not always a clear road to enlightenment. There are many casualties along the way. Sadly, many fall into the trap of psychosis, typically believing that they are somehow specially chosen to lead some great mission.

Because of the amazing charisma that is part of awakening, some psychotics may drag quite a few others along with them. Hitler was awakened, and his charisma could make women faint and grown men weep, when he spoke... he dragged a whole country along with him, and after the war many Germans snapped out of the trance and felt like they were waking from a long, bad dream. He is a human embodiment of my previous warnings about entities, with all his noise about the superior, special Aryans and their right to rule the world, for the good of the world, and at any cost.

The heart voice will never lie, and can always be trusted, but first you have to make certain that what you are hearing, really is the genuine Heart voice. I have cleared more entities and ghosts of people's heart chakras then I care to count. Most often, it is ghosts who took up residence there by invitation, when you were a child. Sometimes, a heart full of entities will choose to be silent, instead of allowing the unworthy to speak. Better no guidance, than bad guidance that lies.

Test your guidance by sending it into the light. If it is the true heart voice then it will remain, you cannot remove it, it is a part of you. If you are hearing a ghost or an entity, it is very easy to clear. I can only think of one occasion where a voice could not be removed easily. One out of thousands, and even that one eventually came around to be transmuted, when it was loved enough.

Love is all that is. Sadly, beings that are polluted with fear sometimes do not know that they are love. Probably you are not entirely convinced that you are love either, so it is easy to see how other beings might share the same confusion.

Above is adapted from http://kundalini-teacher.com/guidance/testgui.php

****

Below is adapted from *Going Within* by Shirley MacLaine

In This Section

Mirroring As A Catalyst

...With each personal drama I began to see that stress wasn't necessary if I chose not to allow myself to experience it. The script changed if I changed my perspective on the "scenes" around me. The *reality* of the scenes themselves shifted as I shifted my outlook on what I was observing. I found that no matter what unpleasantness I found myself involved with, if I stopped and asked myself, "Why have I created this? What am I learning from this?" - the circumstance became not a tragedy but an enlightening experience.

This was not easy when a mugger lunged at me on First Avenue with the clear intention of doing whatever he deemed necessary to get my handbag. I remember my flash reaction that I, by God, did not like playing the part of a victim. Instinctively I changed my "part" and lunged back at him, shrieking like the Wicked Witch of the North until the mugger thought *my* insanity was something he didn't want to tangle with. I changed the script.

I began then to view almost anything negative as a question of *my* point of view, which I could alter. I watched myself as closely as though I were a character in my own play. Then I'd ask myself, "What am I learning about me?" When a producer would renege on a promise, or a director would humiliate me or someone else in front of the crew, or when an airline would lose my luggage, or a cabdriver was rude, or a friend or a lover did something that really hurt my feelings, I would ask myself what I was learning from it and wonder if I needed to learn about myself in *that* fashion any longer. I found that when I took the responsibility for what happened to me and claimed the power to have created such a circumstance in the first place, I could then give it up. To continue to blame someone whom I considered to be a culprit was to abdicate my own power. I was, on some level, drawing the unpleasantness to me, participating fully in the throes of the conflict, and, more than anything else, creating the environment for it to happen so that I could learn more about myself.

When I began to experiment with this shift in perception, a new world of positive attitudes began for me. It was as though I was constantly opening up windows onto new landscapes.

I first noticed the phenomenon with a friend of mine who was sick. I felt helpless in trying to help her. I didn't approve of the drugs she was taking. I felt she was giving up and had adopted a negative attitude toward life and her situation. I became despondent about her future. Then it occurred to me that maybe I had created her in my life for a reason. What was I learning from that then? Why did I need her to play such a part in my play? Was she a mirror for me? Was she going through an experience that I did not want to go through myself? Was I observing her as though I were observing myself?

Suddenly the depth of such a new perspective hit me, and as I absorbed the truth of it, I began to work into a system of thought in which I pictured myself releasing her from her pain because I didn't want it anymore. In one month, she was better and off the painkilling drugs.

Maybe it was coincidence. Maybe not. I do know that as soon as I allowed myself to take responsibility for my depression about her, *she* began to take responsibility for her healing. I'm still not sure how it works, but I believe it does.

Another time I was involved in a lawsuit with a person who was unreasonably demanding money from me. I became very self-righteous and decided to fight it all the way to the Supreme Court. I was outraged. My lawyers recommended that I settle. I refused, saying the whole thing was grossly unfair. They agreed but said I should pay the money and forget about it. I lay awake nights, fuming, running endless dialogues in which I justifiably devastated this person, playing out scenes in courtrooms with the whole world watching while I reduced him to ruins, which I thought was fair under the circumstances. Internal anger doing its ugly thing to *me.* Then one afternoon in the court chambers I stood off from myself and tried to use my "new perspective" technique. I consciously decided to perceive this man who was demanding money from me as a "teacher." I thought, "This person is serving as a catalyst for *my* growth. I am being afforded the opportunity here to look at my own anger and study why it is so intense."

Almost involuntarily I dissolved into tears. Slowly the frustration subsided and I realized that it had been there a long, long time. It was not just the result of this immediate situation. Then I *really* cried, relieved that the conflict was gone, grateful that this man had acted as a teacher and a motivator for my evolvement. As a matter of fact, I went even further. I *decided* to see him as a person who had interrupted his own growth to serve as a catalyst for mine. The effect of such a shift in perspective was immediate.

First, when I stopped crying, I instructed my attorneys to pay what he had demanded. To my astonishment, they came back later and said they couldn't understand why, but he had withdrawn his gargantuan claim and now wanted a modest sum. I had never spoken directly to him, but the shift in my attitude somehow neutralized the energy creating the conflict between us. In giving up the battle, or "surrendering my anger," the fundamental energy in the polarity between us shifted until tugging and war were not possible. In the most personal way I realized it does indeed take two to tango, and when I checked out of the dance, the music stopped too.

Again, I don't know how it works, but when sincerely undertaken, this attitude in perspective becomes very powerful. If there is a tug-of-war and one side ceases to pull, the other side collapses because the game depends upon the polarity of opposites. I was learning that to assure a positive and fresh outlook, it was necessary to release the feelings that gave me pain. Not to control those feelings, but actually to let them go. But first came the need to recognize that *it was my choice* to have had those feelings in the first place.

To express with anger and hostility is to receive the same. To express with Love is to receive Love.

> Glenn's Note: Is the following also valid?
>
> To think with anger and hostility is to receive the same. To think with Love is to receive Love.
>
> Glenn's Note: Is it possible that you are the one who is sick, broke, depressed, in pain, etc. because someone else does not want to go through it or experience it? Have they given you 'stuff' that you are going through for them? Is it always an individual doing the mirroring or can it even be a group, organization, government agency or 'the government'? Have you given them "stuff" to go through for you?

<Above from pages 32-34 and 36>

Releasing Emotions And Excessive Concern For Others

Third Chakra

The third chakra is located in the solar plexus. Its glandular externalization manifests in the pancreas and it governs the action of the liver, stomach, gallbladder, spleen, and certain aspects of the nervous system. This chakra is the clearinghouse for emotional sensitivities and issues of personal power.

Sensitives often comment that they see most people who have unhealthy emotional attachments to children and loved ones "leaking" from the third chakra. Energy spills out of its center and depletes the energy of the individual experiencing concern, possessiveness, and proprietary interest in the lives of those they love. This does not mean one should not be concerned, for instance, about one's children and those they care about. But the concern should be in terms of the child's or loved one's well-being, not for the relief of one's own possessive anxiety.

This third chakra gives almost all of us more problems than any other because it is essentially the "seat of emotional living." Out of unbalanced emotions come ulcers, digestive problems, and liver, spleen, and pancreatic troubles. The positive and negative energy polarities are located in the solar plexus (third) chakra, which, when balanced, is bi-polar, meaning that the positive (masculine - yang) and negative (feminine - yin) are perfectly harmonious. When a person crosses his arms in front of his solar plexus, he is blocking off the energy of that potential balance by adopting a defensive posture; or to put it another way, he is protecting his feelings by crossing his arms.

When a person is overwhelmed with emotion there is an automatic triggering of an almost involuntary act called crying. When tears well up, if allowed to proceed, they often lead to sobbing. The physical act of sobbing produces a gentle - or sometimes not so gentle - massage of the solar plexus. The deep and heavy sob caresses the solar plexus, which can then relax, releasing the pent-up emotion that it was unable to process in the first place. "Having a good cry" enables the third, yellow, chakra at the solar plexus center to reestablish its balance and release itself from emotional overload.

If the sobbing doesn't bring this about, sometimes a person will vomit. The act of vomiting activates the diaphragm muscles. The diaphragm itself is a dome-shaped muscle that separates the lower three chakras from the upper four chakras. Vomiting actually clears out the physical manifestation of what is causing the emotional overload. That is why we often feel so "spacey" and mellow after a good cry or a purging vomit! It is the body's defense mechanism against feeling more of an emotional overload than it is able to handle.

<Above adapted by from pages 79 and 80>

If I had created the pain and the healing in my body, was I also creating the pain and the healing in every area of my life?

Anyone who is intensely involved with the physicality of performance knows that the body does not perform well if the spirit is gloomy. Therefore, the connection between the two needs improvement and the access to "interior light" is necessary.

One night, after dancing two shows on fifty-odd-year-old legs, Vita-Bath therapy and massage were not enough. In the stillness of my bedroom, I sat cross-legged on the floor and shut my eyes. I got up and put a cassette of music on the tape recorder, sat down, and shut my eyes again. I listened to a quiet tinkle of harp music and tried to allow my mind to have no thoughts at all. This wasn't easy. It required trust and a kind of passive discipline that I was not used to because I am an overachiever who is motivated by will and by thought: but thoughts were what were causing the emotional glitches that in turn manifested as pain and tension in my body.

Then I tried directing my thoughts to my body, beginning with my feet, to relax. Slowly and with care and attention, I told each area of my body to drop its tensions: "Knees, thighs, abdomen, chest, neck, and head, drop your tension!" I knew that each area carried tension for its own reasons. I concentrated on each muscle, flexed and relaxed it, waiting between each new relaxation to make sure the tension was not returning. I allowed the tensions to drift away. And waited, consciously enjoying the growing relaxation. Then slowly I allowed myself to drift away. I drifted and floated . . . drifted and floated. If a thought bothered me, I told it to go away or evaded it by concentrating on a small muscle in a toe or finger. Slowly I realized that my body was completely relaxed. Then I shifted my focus to my interior center.

It was easier than I had suspected. I found a ball of light that I'd heard was always there. It was small. I don't know whether I "found" it or whether I visualized it. It was irrelevant. It was there. At first it was barely recognizable in the "darkness" within. So I visualized it until it became larger. Now it glowed. Again I wasn't certain whether it was actually there or whether it was my creation. Again it didn't matter. Slowly I visualized the light growing, becoming a larger and larger ball of pulsating brilliance. Then, when I felt ready, I directed the light to the pain in my back. It was as though I could feel, on another level of reality, the warmth of the light. I held it as long as I could, and my back pain subsided somewhat. I moved on to my legs, particularly my knees, which took a pounding from the high heels I danced in. I visualized the ball of light splitting into two balls, one for each knee. I bathed my knees in the light. I *literally* felt warmth, because I believed in my visualization. I held the two balls of light firmly in my mind. They were real to me because I wanted them to be real. I *perceived* them as real. It was my choice, my power to hold such a reality. I went with it even further. I decided to make the balls of light blue-a brilliant royal blue. I had read that blue was a healing color. Not only did the balls of light become royal blue; they seemed to be speaking to me as though grateful to be recognized at last! The blue lights melted into my knees. It was as though I was listening to the internal language of color and light, which had a meaning all its own. Yet, I was listening to something I had created. Or had I? Had it always been there inside me, waiting to be recognized as a healing device had I only been conscious of it?

I answered my own question: I had created everything myself. I had created the pain. And I had created the healing. I was in control of it all. The pain *and* the healing were inventions of mine. On some level I didn't understand yet, my knees felt healed. So did my back. I had read about people using visualizations in hospitals (with the aid of doctors) to help heal cancer, tumors, and so on. One boy had apparently healed a hole in his heart by visualizing golden threads sewing it shut. Using some unseen talent and understanding from some other dimensional truth, I had used my own unrecognized power to heal my tired, tense body. **If I had created the pain and the healing in my body, was I also creating the pain and the healing in every area of my life?** And was that light inside me a tool with which I could create my reality to be whatever I desired?

Any change externally begins with a change internally.

<Above from pages 39, 40 and 57>

Yin (Feminine) And Yang (Masculine) Balance

In the Indian, Middle Eastern and Oriental cultures the feminine represents the yin energy, the masculine the yang energy. These two energies are basically complementary, the two energies operating in the universe that make a whole, the yang being external and manifesting and the yin internal and creative.

Looking at the sexual drive from this perspective - i.e., the need to complement or unite yin and yang - it was interesting for me to investigate the emotional issues surrounding sexual needs relating to the human chakra system.

I learned that in the aforementioned cultures the three lower chakras, in men *and women,* operate basically with yang energy, the energy of those issues that relate predominantly to the physical, Earth plane of existence. The three higher chakras, in women *and men,* operate basically with yin energy, which relates predominantly to issues of the spirit.

The heart chakra, which is located in the center, is androgynous. It is the seat and home of the soul, or Higher Self, and it is perfectly balanced in its yin and yang expressions. The Higher Self is connected and interfaced with God energy, which also is perfect in its balance of creating and manifesting, the yin and the yang.

Therefore, the more we each resonate to the perfection of the Higher Self, the more we are reflecting perfect balance in ourselves, the more androgynous we are. This does not mean bisexual. It simply means perfectly balanced recognition of the feminine and masculine aspects in each of us.

When we carefully examine our problems and conflicts relating to life, liberty, and the pursuit of happiness, it becomes quite clear that many revolve around our perceptions of masculine and feminine issues, relating not only to sex but also to how we express ourselves vis-a-vis creativity and manifestation. Do we need to be assertive because we fear annihilation from passivity and gentleness? Do we need to control for fear of being controlled? Do we dare listen to the whispers of intuition rather than the loud demands of the intellect?

<Above from page 124>

Tipping Point (Critical Mass) Of Mankind's Consciousness

Talbot's masterly work *Beyond the Quantum* is a particularly clear and fascinating presentation of complex theories and experiments of several New Age scientists. Some of their conclusions have given rise to speculation about the "realness" of reality and highly controversial views (in scientific circles at least) on what can only be described as mysticism. Science and spirituality seem to be converging. Alain Aspect, for instance, in his 1982 experiment, proved that at least one of two conclusions had to be true - either reality as we define it does not exist, i.e., *we* create reality to be what we think it is, *or* communication with the past *and with our future* does exist.

Rupert Sheldrake, a biochemist, has postulated a superimposed *field* (web of information) which he calls a "morphogenetic field," or M-field, to account for the conveyance of information within like species. He calls this informational movement "morphic resonance." On an experimental basis his theory gains support from a thirty-four-year study (about 1905 to about 1938)by William McDougall in which rats from totally different, widely separated genetic lines, nevertheless learned the new useful habits that only one group was working with-except that "learn" is slightly misleading as this information appears to have become universally available once a certain number of rats had acquired it. In other words, the information had entered the rat M-field.

Again, there is the famous "hundredth monkey effect" - not really a controlled experiment, but an observed event that occurred in the 1950's on the island of Koshima. Researchers performing various studies of the local population of monkeys dumped sweet potatoes on the beach. This particular species of monkey had never encountered sweet potatoes before, and while they liked the vegetable they clearly did not like its sandy coating. Then one monkey genius discovered she could clean the potatoes by washing them in the sea. First a few other monkeys, observing this, did the same, later followed by several more busy potato washers. Then quite suddenly, all at once, the entire troop took to washing their potatoes. At this point, other researchers, *on islands far removed from the original,* reported that all *their* monkeys started to *utilize the same washing technique!*

The conclusion is that **information acquired by a certain number of any given species acts like a flashpoint** - from that point forward the species as a whole is equipped with that information.

The new knowledge has entered their M-field via morphic resonance. Moreover, since the species can be widely separated geographically and all its descendants everywhere will also be born with that information, when Sheldrake talks about an M-field he is talking about a subatomic informational web that operates across both space and time. In addition, the M-field may well be connected to the subatomic particle behavior that always expresses itself as a movement toward *wholeness,* a movement that is true for all forms and species, including crystals.

<Above from pages 64 and 65>

Glenn's Questions:

If enough people practice and learn LOVE, will it somehow become a tipping point for all mankind and will the world be a LOVING place? Will earth be heaven? Will the people who choose LOVE be transported to another more LOVING dimension of reality?

If enough people practice and learn fear, judgment, anger and hate will it somehow become a tipping point for all mankind and will we destroy ourselves and our planet?

Skeptics Effects On Sensitives

When we are each in tune with ourselves, we Significantly affect the attunement of others. When we are seriously out of "sync" with ourselves, we also disrupt, disturb, and distress others. This is why someone who is aggressively skeptical *can* affect or even distort the effectiveness of "sensitives."

I remember the first day in Ojai; Alex Orbito (a psychic surgeon from Manila) had set up a clinic room in the vestibule of a Unity church. Thirty people wanted to see someone else operated on before they would allow any healing on their own bodies. I volunteered, since so many were there because of me.

They quietly filed into the room. I lay on a table fully clothed. Alex was behind the table with his head in his hands, bowed in prayer. He prayed for a long time. I supposed it was because of the diversity of energies in the room (psychics and sensitives tune in to everyone else's energy patterns, which sometimes has a negative impact on them).

Alex didn't raise his head. Finally, with his head still bowed, whispered to me. "Shirley," he said hesitantly. "There is man in blue sweater against the wall who is negative, very negative. He doesn't like me or what I do. Very difficult. You can ask him to leave please?"

I turned my head from the lying position and spotted the man Alexwas talking about. It was the friend of a journalist whom I had invited. Rather than single him out, I said, "There is evidently someone here exuding a lot of skeptical negative energy. You know who you are. It would be better if you came back later when you felt more positive." The man in the blue sweater, along with two other people, quietly left. No one blamed them. Alex prayed again and went into a slight trance. His expression changed and the "operation" on me proceeded.

I felt deep pressure inside my abdomen and I had to admit this time there was slight pain. I knew it was coming from the disbelief in the room, so I closed my eyes and put my own mind into a consciousness of complete trust. The pain subsided.

It was then that I realized so clearly the importance of trust when working with spiritual healing, or anything spiritual for that matter. At the same time I flashed on the times in my life when I believed I would get well as opposed to believing the illness would last longer. I remembered regular doctors I had had. If I trusted them, I fared better. It seemed to be as much up to me as it was to the doctor. The healer and the healed working together. On reflection, my body always reacted to my expectations. Physicality follows mind.

<Above from pages 118, 181 and 182>

Primary Mission Of Spiritual Healing

Alex Orbito (a psychic surgeon from Manila) said that he was only an instrument. "I am a human being like anyone else, but when I'm doing my healing, I am an instrument of God . . . without the aid of the Divine province, I cannot do anything."

The most important thing I heard Alex say was, "The primary mission of spiritual healing is not the elimination of physical ailments, but to promote inner awareness, a sense of spiritual attachment, and a personal fellowship with God."

<Above from page 186>

Alex warned someone he had done psychic surgery on and relieved the pain she had been suffering, " ...that if the pain stemmed from a karmic cause she would have to work that out herself by aligning herself with the God energy more faithfully than she had up till then."

<Above from page 172>

Need For Physical Proof

As for the accusations that Filipino surgeons use blood capsules and animal innards to create what appears to be physical proof of extraction, the evidence is confusing.

When tested in a laboratory, the blood is sometimes human blood and sometimes more of a watery plasma. The healers themselves say they don't understand why. They explain only that it isn't really necessary to break the skin and produce real blood or physical extractions to effect healing. They say that many patients need physical proof that they are being healed in order to become better. So they materialize and manifest blood for that purpose. They say that if a patient "sees" he was operated upon, the healing is more profound. So just as they "dematerialize" the epidermis in order to enter the body, they "materialize" blood and clots to effect healing. They say the body is only an illusion anyway, the *physical* being only the manifestation of one's thought. I found the issue of physical "reality" to be the central question, not whether Alex Orbito (a psychic surgeon from Manila) was a fraud or not.

There was no doubt in my mind that his hands had entered my body

<above from page 179>

Self Healing

In my reading on the relationship between mysticism and quantum physics, I was fascinated to learn that each organ of the human body has a harmonious energy pattern that science can now identify. The organs are matter within an electromagnetic energy field, which William Burr described as "the blueprint for life." In the spatial relationship between the molecules in that energy field the molecules are, relatively speaking, farther apart than the planets in our perceived universe are to each other. The universe within, then, is more vast than the universe without! Furthermore, according to science the solidity of matter is actually an illusion. The grand illusion, as a matter of fact, is that our physical world is solid. It is not. It is a molecular structure of subatomic particles that *appears* to be solid. Is this science or is this mysticism?

Science says there are three basic components to the event of an experience: time, space, and matter. When there is a consensus that each of those component parts exists, we have what we term reality. So it only takes an agreement of perception for anything to exist as real. According to science, the physical dimension becomes real only through the consciousness of our intentions. Reality is then actually an intention that becomes an illusion of consciousness.

The molecules that create the illusion of physical reality are organized by electromagnetic fields of energy. If through our "intentional consciousness" we alter the frequency of those electromagnetic fields, we "defy" (or alter) reality. Examples of that are feats by yogis who stop their heartbeats by will (i.e., intention of consciousness), fire-walking, levitation (reversing the polarities of the body relating to gravity), and so on.

So each of us is a living, walking electrical field of energy. Our field of energy organizes the molecular structure that we *perceive,* both within and without, as physical reality.

One of the most extraordinary and beautiful truths about subatomic worlds is that they tend to "move" toward order. Each of us is an amalgamation of frequencies that *needs* to be harmonious and compatible, whose natural order is to move toward harmony. This harmony, this order, is impeded and distorted by feelings of fear, anger, hatred, et cetera. Here, right here, is the interface between who we think we are and the subatomic world from which we have created ourselves.

Conscious awareness of these dynamics within can help to bring our frequencies into balance. When that occurs, "reality" itself goes beyond our customary comprehension of it - the form of reality takes on a dimension we do not normally perceive.

Highly self-realized and disciplined people with total self-awareness can create antibodies that cure disease. Of course, that is a contradiction in itself because totally self-realized people rarely become dis-eased. They are in total "easement" within themselves. They will be more, or less, disease free depending on the degree of their spiritual awareness. Disease in the body, as I have learned from experience, begins first with a blockage of energy in the spirit. For me, *all* of my physical problems begin in my *consciousness.* **And when I stop to meditate, when I go within and literally "ask" my Higher Self why I am manifesting a particular physical problem, I usually get an answer and always it relates to some fear, rejection, or feeling of "nonworthiness."** I try to reconnect with spiritual harmony and God. If I'm successful, I get well. This particular aspect of New Age thinking - self healing - is a highly developed stage, obviously a long way down the road to full self-awareness.

It requires patience and a full confrontation of one's own consciousness, which can sometimes be extremely painful, because it involves the most difficult of all human feelings: *self* forgiveness. I have found that I first have to *admit* that I am afraid, or angry, or rejected, or feeling undeserving. *Then* I can forgive myself for allowing myself such disharmony. When I forgive myself, healing begins.

So, since both scientists *and* mystics claim that harmony is the natural order of life, I try continually to remind myself that I have the right and indeed the Divine inheritance to reflect that harmony in myself. It's not always easy in a world full of suffering and anger and anguish, but **I am learning that if I work on myself to attempt to achieve an internal reality of harmony, it alters my physical reality.**

It is now possible to monitor and correlate how a change of consciousness affects physical reality. An individual capable of this is manipulating his or her physical reality by manipulating his own electromagnetic fields of energy. And he does that by consciously orchestrating his patterns of thought. The resulting manifestation of the thought patterns alters the physical reality. Thus, we begin to see how it is possible to create one's own physical reality with the use of thought and higher conscious awareness.

<Above from page 67 and 68>

One's Responsibility In Exposing Others to Spiritual Concepts

In the below section Alex is a psychic surgeon from Manila and Ted Bennett (an alias) is a traditional western doctor invited by Shirley MacLaine to observe.

Alex claimed that whenever he sat down to meditate in order to operate and heal, he could feel the Divine force descend upon him, causing a cold sensation in his arms and fingers. They become energized with this magnetic force, which enables him to separate molecules of the flesh without using incising instruments. Sometimes he uses no "surgery," but rather heals only by touching.

Whatever was going on in Ted Bennett's mind was as interesting to me as the phenomenon itself. "This makes me feel that the body itself is a trick," he said. "A physical trick that we play on ourselves in order to experience life, or something. Or, is Alex the trick?"

I could feel Ted's confusion. Had I suggested he come to New Mexico to witness a sophisticated sleight-of-hand act? Had we both been fooled?

After a few days with Alex, Bennett didn't say much. We'd have meals together but I could feel him deliberately avoiding the subject. He seemed not only to be sifting the information he was witnessing, but somehow he was evaluating what he thought of me for placing him in such an untenable position. Was he embarrassed, perhaps, because he felt *I* was deluded? I found that I didn't know what to say. I felt Ted back away from discussing anything with me. He took walks alone in the desert. He had seen Alex's hands in people's bodies. He had smelled and seen the blood. He had stood behind, in front of, and closely beside this "spiritual surgeon" from the Philippines. He had studied Alex's work with expert eyes, yet he could find nothing that evidenced fraud or fakery. In fact, Bennett had said that the human body, not the surgery, seemed to be the illusion.

"I'm very uncomfortable with what I'm seeing," he said. "I can't understand. I have spent my life training in medical science, yet what I am seeing seems to make a mockery of that."

As a result of Bennett's genuine philosophical quandary, I realized the significance of what I had done. I had invited him here and he had trusted me enough to come. Yet, I had called into play and exposed him, almost as a metaphysical lark, to invisible truths and forces of nature hich, by their very existence, defied scientific explanation. I had almost playfully knocked the traditional pins out from under his support system. Confronted with something inexplicable in terms of present empirical knowledge, such an intelligent, caring, and rational person required a personal patience in the face of his Own confusion, to say nothing of the required appreciation of wider and deeper truths - truths that science might somehow suspect existed but couldn't countenance yet in a responsible manner. The challenge for Ted, then, was to respect that there were finer perspectives in everything within which a more subtle science of understanding would someday be acknowledged. On top of all that, I had forced him to take responsibility for what he had seen. This, I believe, was the most stressful aspect of all. If the psychic surgery wasn't a trick, then what was it?

By the time Bennett left New Mexico, he hadn't reached a solution in his own mind or within his own system of truth. I have not discussed it with him since. More than anything, *I* began to take more seriously my responsibility in exposing people to phenomena that completely upset their personal sense of reality. Spiritual technology is not a game. It isn't a parlor adventure to entertain, or a diversion. It is a serious and profound recognition that there are energies and forces at work in the universe that lie waiting to be accessed so that the human race can heal itself into a more spiritual state of truth and being.

<Above from page 189>

Above is adapted from MacLaine, Shirley. (1989). *Going Within.* New York: Bantam Books

Remember

We are much more than this body.

We, as our body, are limited only by our own belief in limitation.

In The Following Tables

In the following tables you may also want to ask for "My Unihipil" as you are guided. Unihipili is the Hawaiian name for the sub conscious.

Questions You May Want To Ask Yourself (Self)

Tables below are by the author. Some questions are Shirley MacLaine's and some are his.

I was taught to make all questions into statements because the universe only understands yes or no. I recently realized if the statement is a negative, saying it as a statement can sometimes energize the negative. I have reworded these negative statements into questions with *yes* or *no* answers to avoid inadvertently energizing a negative.

Caused by your judgment towards or fear for someone you know.

If you have a friend or loved one who is sick, depressed, etc., do you feel helpless in trying to help them? Do you disapprove of their choices and life style? Do you feel they are giving up and adopting a negative attitude toward life and their situation? Are you despondent about their future? Then it occurred to me that maybe I had created them in my life for a reason.

Question (Be specific if you wish.)	Answer Before Clearing	Answer After Clearing
Person's Name if someone specific in mind. (__________)		
Do I feel helpless in trying to help a friend or loved one? (name)		
Do I disapprove of their choices and life style?		
Do I feel they are giving up and adopting a negative attitude toward life and their situation?		
Am I despondent about their future?		
Is this a mirror for me?		
Have I decided to perceive this person or situation as a 'teacher'?		
Do I realize that the person(s) or organizations involved have interrupted their own growth and have I thanked them?		
Do I need to learn in this unpleasant manner any longer?		
Am I still learning in this unpleasant manner?		

Why have I created this and brought them into my life?	
What am I learning from this?	
What am I learning about me?	
Why am I drawing this unpleasantness to me?	
Why have I drawn this person into my life?	

<u>Caused by someone you know</u> who is judging you in some way or is fearful for you.

In some way that I am unable to explain in words you are responsible for energizing or accepting this.

Do I have a friend or loved one who feels helpless in trying to help me? Do they disapprove of my choices and life style? Do they feel I am giving up and adopting a negative attitude toward life and my situation? Are they despondent about my future? Have they created this version of me in their life for a reason.

Question (Be specific if you wish.)	Answer Before Clearing	Answer After Clearing
Person's Name if someone specific in mind. (____________)		
Do I have a friend (name) who disapproves of my choices and life style?		
Do I have a friend (name) or loved one who feels helpless in trying to help me?		
Do I have a friend (name) who feels I am giving up and adopting a negative attitude toward life and my situation?		
Do I have a friend (name) who is despondent about my future?		
Have they created this version of me in their life for a reason.		
Is this a mirror for me?		
Have I decided to perceive this person or situation as a 'teacher'?		
Do I realize that the person(s) or organizations involved have interrupted their own growth and have I thanked them?		
Do I need to learn or teach in this unpleasant manner any longer?		
Am I still learning in this unpleasant manner?		

What am I learning from this?	
What am I learning about me?	
Why am I drawing this unpleasantness to me?	
Why have I drawn this person_into my life?	

Releasing Emotions And Excessive Concern For Others

Third Chakra

Questions	Answer Before Clearing	Answer After Clearing
Person's Name if someone specific in mind. (____________)		
Am I overly concerned for (name) to the point of possessiveness or trying to help too much?		
Am I overly concerned because of *my* fear?		
Am I overly concerned because I think I know better?		
Do I feel helpless in trying to help him or her.?		
Is there something I disapprove of in their life or the choices they make?		
Do I feel they have adopted a negative attitude toward life and their situation?		
Am I despondent about their future?		
Have I released (name) from his/her pain or life's challenge by releasing my fear, judgment, need to 'fix' and allowed them their own path?		
Have I turned the person's (name) challenge over to Great Spirit and (same name) as is best?		
Am I assisting as is best?		
Have I released the need to 'fix it'/them?		
Have I released all excessive concern for the person (name)?		
Am I allowing the person (name) their own path and their own opportunity for their soul's growth?		
Are my emotions in relation to (name) balanced as best?		

If I had created the pain and the healing in my body, was I also creating the pain and the healing in every area of my life?

Question	Answer Before Clearing	Answer After Clearing
Do I know and accept that I have created my own pain. (physical, emotional or mental)?		
Have I created my own pain?		
Do I know and accept that I create the pain and healing in every area of my life?		
Do I know that I created the pain in every area of my life?		
Am I ready to heal the pain in my life?		
Am I ready to let go of the pain in my life?		

Yin (Feminine) And Yang (Masculine) Balance

Question	Answer Before Clearing	Answer After Clearing
Do I allow my lower three chakras to operate basically with yang (masculine)energy, the energy of those issues that relate predominantly to the physical, Earth plane of existence?		
Do I allow my higher three chakras to operate basically with yin (feminine) energy, which relates predominantly to issues of the spirit?		
Is my fourth (heart) chakra open and fully balanced with masculine and feminine energy so the energy is androgynous and allows all the other chakras to work together in harmony and balance?		
Do I allow the masculine and feminine energies to be complimentary to each other in perfect balance?		
Do I need to be assertive because I fear annihilation from passivity and gentleness?		
Do I need to control for fear of being controlled?		
Do I allow others to control me in order to avoid taking responsibility for myself?		
Do I dare listen to the whispers of intuition rather than the loud demands of the intellect?		

Tipping Point (Critical Mass) Of Mankind's Consciousness

Question	Answer Before Clearing	Answer After Clearing
Do I know and accept that information acquired by and beliefs accepted by a certain number of any given species acts like a flash point and tipping point?		
Do I know and accept that if enough people practice and learn LOVE, LOVE will somehow become a tipping point for all mankind and the world be a LOVING place?		
Do I know and accept that if enough people practice and learn fear, judgment, anger and hate, the negative thoughts, words and actions will somehow become a tipping point for all mankind and famine, earthquakes, tsunamis, global warming etc. will be more severe. We may even destroy ourselves and our planet?		
Do I all too often go into fear and judgment?		
Have I chosen LOVE and almost always or always practice LOVE?		

Skeptics Effects On Sensitives

Question	Answer Before Clearing	Answer After Clearing
Do I know and accept that we are each in tune with ourselves, and we significantly affect the attunement of others?		
Do I know and accept that when we are seriously out of "sync" with ourselves, we also disrupt, disturb, and distress others, even at a distance?		
Do I know and accept that someone who is aggressively skeptical *can* affect or even distort the effectiveness of "sensitives"?		
Do I know that I can, with the assistance of Great Spirit, be immune to people who are aggressively skeptical?		
Do I know that if my work is being negatively impacted or made difficult by someone who is aggressively skeptical it is ok to leave or ask them to leave?		
Do I fear and judge skeptics and energies I perceive as negative or dangerous?		
Do I know that I am fully protected by and with LOVE?		

Primary Mission Of Spiritual Healing

Question	Answer Before Clearing	Answer After Clearing
Do I know the primary mission of spiritual healing is not the elimination of physical ailments, instead, it is to promote inner awareness, a sense of spiritual attachment, and a personal fellowship with Great Spirit/God?		
Do I know and accept that it is ok to 'cure' physical, emotional, mental and life's ailments as long as the 'cure' is in harmony with the primary mission of spiritual healing?		
If the pain or ailment stems from a karmic cause or serves another purpose, I know that I can work that out myself by aligning with the God energy more fully during and after surgery or other forms of intervention?		
Do I know and accept that sometimes "curing" someone will interfere with thier souls growth and highest good?		

Need For Physical Proof

Some say the body is only an illusion; the *physical* being only the manifestation of one's thought.

Question	Answer Before Clearing	Answer After Clearing
Is it necessary to understand why miracles and healing happens to affect a healing?		
Is it ok if a patient needs to "see" he was operated upon, for the healing to be more profound?		
Do I know and accept that the body is only an illusion when perceived from a higher perspective and the *physical* is only the manifestation of one's thought?		
Do I believe that if I let go of the need to see physical proof and accept that true healing is energized at some un-namable upper realm I can be healed without physical proof?		
Have I let go of the need for physical proof?		

Self Healing

According to both science and many new age thinkers, the physical dimension becomes real only through the consciousness of our thoughts and intentions. Many of these thoughts and intentions come from our Subconscious and Superconscious minds.

Question	Answer Before Clearing	Answer After Clearing
Do I know and accept that disharmony, dis-ease and life's unpleasant challenges are caused by feelings of fear, anger, unworthiness, hatred, self hatred, etc?		
Do I know and accept that harmony, health and a joyful life are somehow energized by LOVE, as well as feelings of love, self worth, inner peace and a strong connection to Divinity/Great Spirit?		
Have I admitted to myself that I am afraid or angry, or *feel* rejected, undeserving or unworthy?		
Have I forgiven myself for being afraid or angry, or *feeling* rejected, undeserving or unworthy?		
Have I reconnected with spiritual harmony and God as is best at this time?		
Does reconnecting with spiritual harmony and God benefit my physical reality and body for the best in some way beyond words ?		
Am I doing what is best as a human being here on earth in order to fulfill my life's purpose and soul's growth and to heal physically in harmony with LOVE?		

Go within and literally 'ask' your Higher Self,

"Why I am manifesting (a particular physical or life problem)?

The answer almost always, or always, relates to some fear, rejection, or feeling of "unworthiness."

One's Responsibility In Exposing Others to Spiritual Concepts

If you expose a person to invisible truths and forces of nature which, by their very existence, defy scientific explanation or the person's existing beliefs, it is possible to unintentionally knock the traditional pins out from under his or her support system. Confronted with something inexplicable in terms of present empirical knowledge, even an intelligent, caring, and rational person can be forced to take responsibility for more than they can handle and you may just confuse them.

Question	Answer Before Clearing	Answer After Clearing
Do I want to share because of my ego?		
Is the person ready for what I have to share?		
Am I willing to learn from them?		
Will sharing with them assist them on their souls journey?		
Will sharing with them interfere with their soul's journey or life's purpose?		
Will what I want to share make the person uncomfortable?		
Is it best they are made uncomfortable?		
Will what I want to share confuse the person?		
Will what I want to share put the person in a genuine philosophical quandary that will interfere with their path?		
Will what I want to share force the person to take responsibly beyond their wisdom and ability?		
Will exposing the person to phenomena that is foreign to them upset their personal sense of reality to their detriment?		

Tables above are by the author. Some questions are Shirley MacLaine's and some are his.

****

Below is by author

WAYS OF HEALING -- IS THIS A PROMPT?

Keep in mind that the undesired issue can be physical, emotional or mental and includes habits and obsessions/compulsions.

Questions to ask yourself and Great Spirit. Set the ego aside. Let go of all expectations and desires as to the answer. Clear them as guided.

First question: "Is this a prompt?" What I am asking is if I need to do some healing, releasing and transmuting at the spiritual level using my conscious mind.

If the answer is no, you need to 'work' at the physical, emotional/feeling and mental levels here in 3D. There is always 'work' to do at the Spiritual and energetic levels, however, sometimes the physical, emotional/feeling and mental levels need to be addressed more directly.

If the answer is yes, the most important 'work' is at the Spiritual level. You may also want to ask, "What are you trying to tell me?" Without healing at the Spiritual/Energetic level the symptom or problem may come back as the same problem or even a new one. Also work in the 3D.

3D explanation and Levels of healing:

First Level Diet Therapy, Exercise, Osteopathy & Chiropractic, Surgery, Physical Therapy, Drugs & Herbs, Orthomolecular Medicine, Aromatherapy, Healthy Life Style

Second Level: Micro current Therapies, Acupuncture, BodyWork/Touch, Breath Therapy, Yoga, Qigong, Meditation, Radiation Therapy

Third Level: Mental Field Therapy, Psychotherapy, TFT (Thought Field Therapy), EMDR (Eye movement desensitization and reprocessing), Homeopathy

Forth Level: Systemic Family Constellation, Color and Sound Therapies, Shamanism, Hypnotherapy, Jungian Psychotherapy, Radlonics, Rituals

Fifth Level: Is beyond 3D. It is between the individual and Great Spirit/God/Divinity. It includes Self Healing, Prayer, Awareness, LOVE and True Meditation

Infinite Levels of Healing. There may be infinite levels. The conscious mind needs to know the five above.

Five main methods of healing I use are described and summarized in my book *Awareness, A Path To Spiritual And Physical Health and Well-Being.*

Prayer

Affirmations

Self-Identity Ho'oponopono based on Ihaleakala Hew Len's teachings

Releasing trapped emotions/feelings based on Bradley Nelson's *Emotion Code*

Witnessing by "Entering The Witness" based on John Ruskan's *Emotional Clearing Process*

Another way to heal that may be helpful.

Meditation for Cellular Healing (later in this book)

Examples of Questions to assist in pinpointing a prompt and 'work' needed follow.

I was taught to make all questions into statements because the universe only understands yes or no. I recently realized if the statement is a negative, saying it as a statement can sometimes energize the negative. I have reworded these negative statements into questions with yes or no answers to avoid inadvertently energizing a negative.

In The Following Tables

In the following tables any place you see (Other Name) can be changed to (My Unihipili) as you are guided. Unihipili is the Hawaiian name for the sub conscious.

Illness Or Pain (can also be used for habits/ obsessions/ compulsions)

Name of what you want to heal/let go of. Can be physical, mental or emotional.

Name the problem/challenge: (   )

Question / Statement (replace the word 'illness with the appropriate word)	Answer needs to be	Answer before clearing	Answer after clearing
This illness, discomfort or habit is a prompt.			
Do I seek attention through my illness(s)?	NO		
Does (Full birth name) seek attention through his/her illness(s)?			
Does (Other Name) seek attention through his/her illness(s)?			
Am I invested in my illness(s)?	NO		
Is (Full birth name) invested in his/her illness(s)?			
Is (Other Name) invested in his/her illness(s)?			
Would I feel lost without my illness(s)?	NO		
Would (Full birth name) feel lost without his/her illness(s)?			
Would (Other Name) feel lost without his/her illness(s)?			
Am I punishing myself through this illness?	NO		
Is (Full birth name) punishing himself/herself through this illness?			
Is (Other Name) punishing himself/herself through this illness?			
Do I truly want to be healed?	YES		
Does (Full birth name) truly want to be healed?			
Does (Other Name) truly want to be healed?			
Do I truly want to be cured?	YES		
Does (Full birth name) truly want to be cured?			
Does (Other Name) truly want to be cured?			
Is my intention set to heal?	YES		
Is (Full birth name) intention set to heal?			
Is (Other Name) intention set to heal?			

Question / Statement	Answer needs to be	Answer before clearing	Answer after clearing
Is my intention to heal pure and clear?	YES		
Is (Full birth name) intention to heal pure and clear?			
Is (Other Name) intention to heal pure and clear?			
Is my intention to heal completely?	Most effective if Yes		
Is (Full birth name) intention to heal completely?			
Is (Other Name) intention to heal completely?			
Do I truly want to stay here on earth in this physical body for a while? (specify time if desired)			
Does (Full birth name) truly want to stay here on earth in this physical body for a while? (specify time if desired)			
Does (Other Name) truly want to stay here on earth in this physical body for a while? (specify time if desired)			

Finances, Abundance and Prosperity

Question / Statement	Answer needs to be	Answer before clearing	Answer after clearing
My financial woes is a prompt.	N/A		
Do I seek attention through my financial woes?	NO		
Does (Full birth name) seek attention through his/her financial woes?			
Does (Other Name) seek attention through his/her financial woes?			
Am I invested in my financial woes?	NO		
Is (Full birth name) invested in his/her financial woes?			
Is (Other Name) invested in his/her financial woes?			
Would I feel lost without my financial woes?	NO		
Would (Full birth name) feel lost without his/her financial woes?			
Would (Other Name) feel lost without his/her financial woes?			
Am I punishing myself with my financial woes?	NO		
Is (Full birth name) punishing himself/herself with his or her financial woes?			
Is (Other Name) punishing himself/herself with his or her financial woes.			
Do I feel, believe and know it is possible to be financially independent, self sufficient and wealthy and still be in harmony with LOVE and the highest good, and to fulfill my soul's purpose in this lifetime?	YES		
Does (Full birth name) feel and know it is possible to be financially independent, self sufficient and wealthy and still be in harmony with LOVE and the highest good, and to fulfill his/her soul's purpose in this lifetime?			
Does (Other Name) feel and know it is possible to be financially independent, self-sufficient and wealthy and still be in harmony with LOVE and the highest good, and to fulfill his/her soul's purpose in this lifetime?			

Question / Statement	Answer needs to be	Answer before clearing	Answer after clearing
Do I truly want to be financially independent and wealthy?	YES		
Does (Full birth name) truly want to be financially independent, self sufficient and wealthy?			
Does (Other Name) truly want to be financially independent, self sufficient and wealthy			
Is my intention set to be financially independent, self sufficient and wealthy?	YES		
Is (Full birth name) intention set to be financially independent, self sufficient and wealthy?			
Is (Other Name) intention set to be financially independent, self sufficient and wealthy			
Is my intention to be financially independent, self sufficient and relatively wealthy pure and clear?	YES		
Is (Full birth name) intention to be financially independent, self sufficient and relatively wealthy pure and clear?			
Is (Other Name) intention to be financially independent, self sufficient and relatively wealthy pure and clear?			
Do I feel and believe I am deserving of financial independence and wealth?	YES		
Does (Full birth name) feel and believe he/she is deserving of financial independence and wealth?			
Does (Other Name) feel and believe he/she is deserving of financial independence and wealth?			
AFFIRMATION: I will use my wealth wisely and with LOVE.	YES		
AFFIRMATION: (Full birth name) will use his/her wealth wisely and with LOVE.			
AFFIRMATION: (Other Name) will use his/her wealth wisely and with LOVE.			

Smoking and Other Habits/Addictions

Question / Statement	Answer needs to be	Answer before clearing	Answer after clearing
My smoking (or other habit/addiction)is a prompt.			
Do I seek attention through my smoking?	NO		
Does (Full birth name) seek attention through his/her smoking?			
Does (Other Name) seek attention through his/her smoking?			
Am I invested in my smoking?	NO		
Is (Full birth name) invested in his/her smoking?			
Is (Other Name) invested in his/her smoking?			
Am I punishing myself by my smoking?	NO		
Is (Full birth name) punishing himself or herself by smoking?			
Is (Other Name) punishing himself or herself by smoking?			
Do I smoke to keep any romantic interest/life partner at bay?	NO		
Does (Full birth name) smoke to keep any romantic interest/life partner at bay?			
Does (Other Name) smoke to keep any romantic interest/life partner at bay?			
Do I smoke as a form of suicide?	NO		
Does (Full birth name) smoke as a form of suicide?			
Does (Other Name) smoke as a form of suicide?			
Would I feel lost without my smoking?	NO		
Would (Full birth name) feel lost without his/her smoking?			
Would (Other Name) feel lost without his/her smoking?			

CAUTION: The following three questions may be better to leave as YES, if that is the answer, until you have learned to quiet your mind in other ways.			
Question / Statement	Answer needs to be	Answer before clearing	Answer after clearing
Do I Smoke to quiet, calm, slow down, and/or numb my mind and thoughts?	NO		
Does (Full birth name) smoke to quiet, calm, slow down, and/or numb his/her mind and thoughts?			
Does (Other Name) smoke to quiet, calm, slow down, and/or numb his/her mind and thoughts?			
Do I Smoke to block or filter out unwanted thoughts and energies?	NO		
Does (Full birth name) smoke to block or filter out unwanted thoughts and energies?			
Does (Other Name) smoke to block or filter out unwanted thoughts and energies?			
Do I Smoke to tone down my intuition and awareness?	NO		
Does (Full birth name) smoke to tone down my intuition and awareness?			
Does (Other Name) smoke to tone down my intuition and awareness?			

Question / Statement	Answer needs to be	Answer before clearing	Answer after clearing
Do I know how to quiet my mind and keep unwanted and/or intrusive thoughts and energies out with healthy/positive FLOW?	YES		
Does (Full birth name) know how to quiet his/her mind and keep unwanted and/or intrusive thoughts and energies out with healthy/positive FLOW?			
Does (Other Name) know how to quiet his/her mind and keep unwanted and/or intrusive thoughts and energies out with healthy/positive FLOW?			

Question / Statement	Answer needs to be	Answer before clearing	Answer after clearing
Am I ready, willing and able to quiet my mind and keep unwanted and/or intrusive thoughts and energies out with healthy/positive FLOW?	YES		
Is (Full birth name) ready, willing and able to quiet his/her mind and keep unwanted and/or intrusive thoughts and energies out with healthy/positive FLOW?			
Is (Other Name) ready, willing and able to quiet his/her mind and keep unwanted and/or intrusive thoughts and energies out with healthy/positive FLOW?			
Am I ready to have the world see me as I AM?	YES		
Is (Full birth name) ready to have the world see him/her as he/she IS?			
Is (Other Name) ready to have the world see him/her as he/she IS?			
Is my intention set to have healthy/positive FLOW?	YES		
Is (Full birth name) intention set to have healthy/positive FLOW?			
Is (Other Name) intention set to have healthy/positive FLOW?			
Is my intention set to have healthy/positive FLOW pure and clear?	YES		
Is (Full birth name) intention set to have healthy/positive FLOW pure and clear?			
Is (Other Name) intention set to have healthy/positive FLOW pure and clear?			
Do I truly want to have healthy/positive FLOW?	YES		
Does (Full birth name) truly want to have healthy/positive FLOW?			
Does (Other Name) truly want to have healthy/positive FLOW?			
Is there a frequency (flower essence, essential oil, Zeolite, Celandine, etc.) that will assist in letting go of and releasing the undesired habit/addiction?			

Question / Statement	Answer needs to be	Answer before clearing	Answer after clearing
Do I truly want to stay here on earth in this physical body for a while? (specify time if desired)			
Does (Full birth name) truly want to stay here on earth in this physical body for a while? (specify time if desired)			
Does (Other Name) truly want to stay here on earth in this physical body for a while? (specify time if desired)			

Physical Heart

Question / Statement	Answer needs to be	Answer before clearing	Answer after clearing
This heart problem is a prompt.			
Do I seek attention through my heart problem(s)?	NO		
Does (Full birth name) seek attention through his/her heart problem(s)?			
Does (Other Name) seek attention through his/her heart problem(s)?			
Am I invested in my heart problem(s)?	NO		
Is (Full birth name) invested in his/her heart problem(s)?			
Is (Other Name) invested in his/her heart problem(s)?			
Would I feel lost without my heart problem(s)?	NO		
Would (Full birth name) feel lost without his/her heart problem(s)?			
Would (Other Name) feel lost without his/her heart problem(s)?			
Am I punishing myself with my heart problems?:	NO		
Is (Full birth name) punishing himself/herself with their heart problems?			
Is (Other Name) punishing himself/herself with their heart problems?			
Do I truly want my heart to heal?	YES		
Does (Full birth name) truly want his/her heart to heal?			
Does (Other Name) truly want his/her heart to heal?			
Is my intention set to heal my heart?	YES		
Is (Full birth name) intention set to heal his/her heart?			
Is (Other Name) intention set to heal his/her heart?			
Is my intention to heal my heart pure and clear?	YES		
Is (Full birth name) intention to heal his/her heart pure and clear?			
Is (Other Name) intention to heal his/her heart pure and clear?			

Question / Statement	Answer needs to be	Answer before clearing	Answer after clearing
Is my intention to heal my heart completely?	YES		
Is (Full birth name) intention to heal his/her heart completely?			
Is (Other Name) intention to heal his/her heart completely?			
Do I truly want to stay here on earth in this physical body for a while? (specify time if desired)			
Does (Full birth name) truly want to stay here on earth in this physical body for a while? (specify time if desired)			
Does (Other Name) truly want to stay here on earth in this physical body for a while? (specify time if desired)			

Digestion and Digestive System Problems

Question / Statement	Answer needs to be	Answer before clearing	Answer after clearing
My digestive system problem(s) is a prompt.			
Do I seek attention through my digestive system problems?	NO		
Does (Full birth name) seek attention through his/her digestive system problems?			
Does (Other Name) seek attention through his/her digestive system problems?			
Am I invested in my digestive system problems?	NO		
Is (Full birth name) invested in his/her digestive system problems?			
Is (Other Name) invested in his/her digestive system problems?			
Would I feel lost without my digestive system problems?	NO		
Would (Full birth name) feel lost without his/her digestive system problems?			
Would (Other Name) feel lost without his/her digestive system problems?			
Am I punishing myself with my digestive system problems?	NO		
Is (Full birth name) punishing himself/herself with their digestive system problems?			
Is (Other Name) punishing himself/herself with their digestive system problems?			
Do I truly want my digestive system to heal?	YES		
Does (Full birth name) truly want his/her digestive system to heal?			
Does (Other Name) truly want his/her digestive system to heal?			

Question / Statement	Answer needs to be	Answer before clearing	Answer after clearing
Is my intention set to heal my digestive system?	YES		
Is (Full birth name) intention set to heal his/her digestive system?			
Is (Other Name) intention set to heal his/her digestive system?			
Is my intention to heal my digestive system pure and clear?	YES		
(Full birth name) intention to heal his/her digestive system pure and clear?			
(Other Name) intention to heal his/her digestive system pure and clear?			
Is my intention to heal my digestive system completely?	YES		
Is (Full birth name) intention to heal his/her digestive system completely?			
Is (Other Name) intention to heal his/her digestive system completely?			
Do I truly want to stay here on earth in this physical body for a while? (specify time if desired)			
Does (Full birth name) truly want to stay here on earth in this physical body for a while? (specify time if desired)			
Does (Other Name) truly want to stay here on earth in this physical body for a while? (specify time if desired)			

Life Too Hectic

Question / Statement	Answer needs to be	Answer before clearing	Answer after clearing
My hectic lifestyle is a prompt.			
Do I avoid looking at things and feeling too much through my hectic life?	NO		
Does (Full birth name) avoid looking at things and feeling too much through his/her hectic life?			
Does (Other Name) avoid looking at things and feeling too much through his/her hectic life			
Am I invested in my hectic life style?	NO		
Is (Full birth name) invested in his/her hectic life style?			
Is (Other Name) invested in his/her hectic life style?			
Would I feel lost without my hectic life style?	NO		
Would (Full birth name) feel lost without his/her hectic life style?			
Would (Other Name) feel lost without his/her hectic life style?			
Am I punishing myself with my hectic life style?	NO		
Is (Full birth name) punishing himself/herself with their hectic life style?			
Is (Other Name) punishing himself/herself with their hectic life style?			
Do I truly want to have a less hectic life?	YES		
Does (Full birth name) truly want to have a less hectic life?			
Does (Other Name) truly want to have a less hectic life?			
Is my intention set to heal my hectic life style and have a more balanced and joyful life?	YES		
Is (Full birth name) intention set to heal his/her hectic life style and have a more balanced and joyful life?			
Is (Other Name) intention set to heal his/her hectic life style and have a more balanced and joyful life?			

Question / Statement	Answer needs to be	Answer before clearing	Answer after clearing
Is my intention to heal my hectic life style pure and clear?	YES		
Does (Full birth name) intention to heal his/her hectic life style pure and clear?			
Does (Other Name) intention to heal his/her hectic life style pure and clear?			
Is my intention to heal my hectic life style completely?	YES		
Is (Full birth name) intention to heal his/her hectic life style completely?			
Is (Other Name) intention to heal his/her hectic life style completely?			
Do I truly want to stay here on earth in this physical body for a while? (specify time if desired)			
Does (Full birth name) truly want to stay here on earth in this physical body for a while? (specify time if desired)			
Does (Other Name) truly want to stay here on earth in this physical body for a while? (specify time if desired)			

Too Much Drama In Life

Question / Statement	Answer needs to be	Answer before clearing	Answer after clearing
The drama in my life is a prompt.			
Do I feel a need for drama in my life?	NO		
Does (Full birth name) feel they have a need for drama in their life?			
Does (Other Name) feel they have a need for drama in their life?			
Am I invested in the drama in my life?	NO		
Is (Full birth name) invested in the drama in his/her life?			
Is (Other Name) invested in the drama in his/her life?			
Would I feel lost without drama in my life?	NO		
Would (Full birth name) feel lost without drama in his/her life?			
Would (Other Name) feel lost without drama in his/her life?			
Am I punishing myself with the drama in my life?	NO		
Is (Full birth name) punishing himself/herself with the drama in their life?			
Is (Other Name) punishing himself/herself with the drama in their life?			
Do I truly want to have less drama in my life?	YES		
Does (Full birth name) truly want to have less drama in his/her life?			
Does (Other Name) truly want to have less drama in his/her life?			
Is my intention set to heal and do away with the drama in my life and have a more balanced and joyful life?	YES		
Is (Full birth name) intention set to heal and do away with the drama in his/her life and have a more balanced and joyful life?			
Is (Other Name) intention set to heal and do away with the drama in his/her life and have a more balanced and joyful life?			

Question / Statement	Answer needs to be	Answer before clearing	Answer after clearing
Is my intention to heal and do away with the drama in my life pure and clear?	YES		
Is (Full birth name) intention to heal and do away with the drama in his/her life pure and clear?			
Is (Other Name) intention to heal and do away with the drama in his/her life pure and clear?			
Is my intention to heal and do away with the excess drama in my life completely?	YES		
Is (Full birth name) intention to heal and do away with the excess drama in his/her life completely?			
Is (Other Name) intention to heal and do away with the excess drama in his/her life completely?			
Do I truly want to stay here on earth in this physical body for a while? (specify time if desired)			
Does (Full birth name) truly want to stay here on earth in this physical body for a while? (specify time if desired)			
Does (Other Name) truly want to stay here on earth in this physical body for a while? (specify time if desired)			

Overly Concerned And Overly Anxious For Others

Question / Statement	Answer needs to be	Answer before clearing	Answer after clearing
My Over Concern And Worry For Others is a prompt.			
Am I overly concerned or overly anxious for others?______ (name if someone specific in mind)	NO		
Is (Full birth name) overly concerned for others? (name if someone specific in mind)			
Is (Other Name) overly concerned for others? (name if someone specific in mind)			
Am I overly fearful that something wrong may happen to those I care about?	NO		
Is (Full birth name) overly fearful that something wrong may happen to those he/she cares about?			
Is (Other Name) is overly fearful that something wrong may happen to those he/she cares about?			
Do I blame myself for the mistakes and hard-times of others?	NO		
Does (Full birth name) blame himself/herself for the mistakes and hard-times of others?			
Does (Other Name) blame himself/herself for the mistakes and hard-times of others?			
Do I allow others what I perceive as mistakes, faults and imperfect actions without judgment?	YES		
Does (Full birth name) allow others what he/she perceives as mistakes, faults and imperfect actions without judgment?			
Does (Other Name) allow others what he/she perceives as mistakes, faults and imperfect actions without judgment?			
Do I forgive others their imperfect actions?	YES		
Does (Full birth name) forgive others their imperfect actions?			
Does (Other Name) forgive others their imperfect actions?			

Self Forgiveness

Question / Statement	Answer needs to be	Answer before clearing	Answer after clearing
Do I forgive my imperfect thoughts?	YES		
Does (Full birth name) forgive himself/herself for their imperfect thoughts?			
Does (Other Name) forgive himself/herself for their imperfect thoughts?			
Do I forgive my imperfect actions?	YES		
Does (Full birth name) forgive himself/herself for their imperfect actions?			
Does (Other Name) forgive himself/herself for their imperfect actions?			
Do I love myself even with my perceived imperfections?	YES		
Does (Full birth name) love himself/herself even with his/her perceived imperfections?			
Does (Other Name) love himself/herself even with his/her perceived imperfections?			

Above is by the author

****

Explanation of What Makes Up "All The Aspects" Of DNA to make the following meditations even more effective.

Scientists use the term "double helix" to describe DNA's winding, two-stranded chemical structure. If untwisted, DNA looks like two parallel strands. One strand is complementary to the other. The images below may help you to visualize while doing the menitations.

The structure of DNA is illustrated by a right handed double helix.

Two images of how it is often depicted are below.

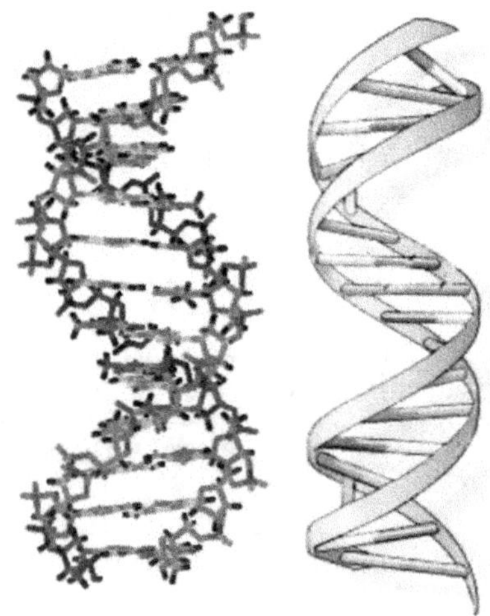

Glenn's thoughts are on the next several pages and the Actual Exercise is after the explanation.

What if our genes were merely building blocks, and a greater intelligence was in charge of the physical as well as the unseen?

There is more to this 'Greater Intelligence' than mentioned here. The following will give you a good basic idea why the meditation can be so effective.

DNA (Deoxyribonucleic acid) provides the genetic information necessary for the development and reproduction of all living organisms and is often described as a genetic blueprint. Harmful mutations cause gene-based diseases. All of the cells within a complex multicellular organism such as a human being contain the same DNA; however, the body of such an organism is clearly composed of many different types of cells. What, then, makes a liver cell different from a skin or muscle cell and what affects the DNA?

What causes one part of the body to be healthy and another part to be diseased? What causes emotional and mental instability? It can be a chemical or nutritional imbalance or a physical injury. It can also be energetic.

In the following meditations "DNA **<u>and all its aspects"</u>** refers to the physical DNA, RNA, Soul Echoes and Epigentics as explained below, as well as everything that effects gene expression, emotions and even more that is beyond words.

"Soul Echoes"

The distortions, mutations and all lower vibration (dense) disharmonic thought forms from what we perceive as past moments can be thought of as *miasms, 'cellular memory', 'Imprints On The Luminous Energy Field', memories replaying, beliefs, vows, oaths, covenants, promises, agreements*, *concepts, attitudes, 'truths'*, and *contracts* that are no longer in harmony with our highest good and well being. Some of these are personal, some are between you and another person or soul and some are between you and God. All of these, and more, can be thought of as "***Soul Echoes***" to be released. There is no need to forget them. Keep the information and release/desolve the patterns and assosiated energies.

Transmuting "***Soul Echoes***" and embodying higher identity levels allows healing of the DNA and activation of higher DNA strands **and all its aspects**. The activation of higher strands initiates a realignment in a person's life direction and physical health towards a more harmonious and joyful path.

"**Soul Echoes**" in your conscious and unconscious fields or awareness that you are living by affect all aspects of your being. Some are over thousands of years old. These "***Soul Echoes***" create and magnetize lower frequency events and experiences in our current incarnate reality and cause the mutations in our physical DNA. Physical toxins and impurities from our environment and diet can also cause disease and damage to the DNA.

Our current life situations are not only created through our past and present choices. We inherit "***Soul Echoes***" from our other lives, parents and ancestors at conception through the DNA and EpiGenetics. We also inherit them from Mother Earth and the collective. Since we have simultaneous incarnations in different time/space zones which are all connected to one DNA template, we also have karmic bleed through from our soul extensions (parallel selves) who are still in incarnation. An example of this is that karmic bleed through can manifest as physical symptoms being experienced that are not in truth your own. If another soul extension (parallel self) is experiencing something, you can be experiencing this same 'thing' through your physical body.

When we clear the DNA template we clear the time line and destiny of all our selves.

Allow the highest priority '**Soul Echoes**' to clear as Spirit chooses.

The clearing of the DNA template progressively purges ancient distortions and mutations within the gene codes.

Emotions and '**Soul Echoes**' can trigger the expression of DNA strands.

Clearing '**Soul Echoes**' can also clear and resolve phobias, and blocks to your mental, emotional and spiritual health as well as limitations and 'lack'.

You can even affect you car, computer and other inanimate 'things' with '**Soul Echoes**'. Just ask someone who believes their computer will crash when mercury is in retrograde.

Once this negative 'data' is removed any resulting voids need to be filled.

Epi-Genetics as well as '**Soul Echoes**' affects the DNA **and all its aspects** .

Epigentics is a scientific field of study. Two good sources of information are mercola.com and the University of Massachusetts.

"Soul Echoes", diet, quality of our physical environment, exercise or lack thereof all affect Epi-Genetics.

Epigenetics literally means "above" or "on top of" genetics. It refers to external modifications to DNA that turn genes "on" or "off." These modifications do not change the DNA sequence, but instead, they affect how cells "read" genes.

Epigenetics is the study of potentially heritable changes in gene expression (active versus inactive genes) that does not involve changes to the underlying DNA sequence — a change in phenotype without a change in genotype — which in turn affects how cells read the genes.

The epigenome is a multitude of chemical compounds that can tell the genome what to do. The human genome is the complete assembly of DNA

What makes up the epigenome?

The epigenome is the set of chemical modifications to the DNA and DNA-associated proteins in the cell, which alter gene expression. The modifications can be altered in response to environmental exposures, disease, thoughts, beliefs and emotions.

There are different types of epigenetic marks, and each one tells the proteins in the cell to process those parts of the DNA in certain ways.

There is no doubt there are many marks we don't even know about yet.

You actually have a tremendous amount of control over how your genetic traits are expressed, by changing your thoughts and altering your diet and your environment.

The work of Dr. Bruce Lipton and other epigenetic researchers shows that the "environmental signals" also include thoughts and emotions—both of which have been shown to directly affect DNA expression.

Quantum physics shows us that the invisible, immaterial realm is actually far more important than the material realm.

This new science reveals that your perceptions control your biology. If you can change your perceptions, you can shape and direct your own genetic readout.

You are in control of your genes … You can alter them on a regular basis, depending on the foods you eat, the air you breathe, the thoughts you think and your emotions. It's your environment and lifestyle that dictates your tendency to express disease or health. In fact, your thoughts may shape your environment far more than physical matter.

It's interesting to note that the word 'spirit' by spiritualists, and the word 'field' by physicists, use the same definition for those two words.

Epigenetics Controls Genes. Certain circumstances in life can cause genes to be silenced or expressed over time. In other words, they can be turned off (becoming dormant) or turned on (becoming active).

Epigenetics Is Everywhere. What you eat, where you live, who you interact with, when you sleep, how you exercise and even your conscious and unconscious thoughts – all of these can eventually cause chemical modifications around the genes that will turn those genes on or off over time. In certain diseases, various genes are switched into the opposite state, away from the normal/healthy state.

Epigenetics Is Reversible. We can reverse the gene's state to keep the good while eliminating the bad…

"**Soul Echoes**" affect EpiGenetics. "**Soul Echoes**" and Epigenetics affect RNA, DNA and Gene Expression. Thus, they also affect health and emotions.

Questions you may want to ask yourself before doing the actual meditations.

You need to be clear for the meditation to be as effective as possible. Set the ego aside. Let go of all expectations and desires as to the answer. Clear them as guided.

If you are unable to get answers from Great Spirit, you may want to make them into prayers.

> An example is: "Great Spirit and Great Spirit helpers as are best,
> Help me to make it so and keep it so I let go of any need or inclination to get attention through illness or discomfort. *Thank You.*"

I was taught to make all questions into statements because the universe only understands yes or no. I recently realized if the statement is a negative, saying it as a statement can sometimes energize the negative. I have reworded these negative statements into questions with ***yes*** or ***no*** answers to avoid inadvertently energizing a negative.

In the following table any place you see (Other Name) can be changed to (My Unihipili) as you are guided

Unihipili is the Hawaiian name for the sub conscious>

Question / Statement	Answer needs to be	Answer before clearing	Answer after clearing
Do I seek attention through my illness(s)?			
Does (Full birth name) seek attention through his/her illness(s)?	NO		
Does (Other Name) seek attention through his/her illness(s)?			
Am I invested in my illness(s)?			
Is (Full birth name) invested in his/her illness(s)?	NO		
Is (Other Name) invested in his/her illness(s)?			
Would I feel lost without my illness(s)?			
Would (Full birth name) feel lost without his/her illness(s)?	NO		
Would (Other Name) feel lost without his/her illness(s)?			

Question / Statement	Answer needs to be	Answer before clearing	Answer after clearing
Am I willing to recreate myself and my SELF as a healthy individual?			
Is (Full birth name) willing to recreate his/her self and his/her SELF as a healthy individual?	YES		
Is (Other Name) willing to recreate his/her self and his/her SELF as a healthy individual?			
Do I truly want to be healed?	YES		
Does (Full birth name) truly want to be healed?			
Does (Other Name) truly want to be healed?			
Is my intention set to heal?			
Is (Full birth name) intention set to heal?	YES		
Is (Other Name) intention set to heal?			
Is my intention to heal pure and clear?			
Is (Full birth name) intention to heal pure and clear?	YES		
Is (Other Name) intention to heal pure and clear?			
Do I know what I will do with myself and my life without any illness?			
Does (Full birth name) know what he/she will do with his/her self and his/her life without any illness?	YES		
Does (Other Name) know what he/she will do with his/her self and his/her life without any illness?			
I would ( )			
Is my intention to heal completely?	Most effect ive if YES		
Is (Full birth name) intention to heal completely?			
Is (Other Name) intention to heal completely?			
Do I truly want to stay here on earth in this physical body for a while? (specify time frame if desired)			
Does (Full birth name) truly want to stay here on earth in this physical body for a while? (specify time frame if desired)			
Does (Other Name) truly want to stay here on earth in this physical body for a while? (specify time frame if desired)			

Even if you get no visuals when doing the following meditations, just read the meditations with Love, have faith, and allow the Divine Flow. Healing has taken place, even if the conscious mind is unaware of it. Conscious awareness will come.

Metatron's Introduction to The Meditation For Cellular Healing

Below was given to me in March 2015 by a medical professional and shared with her permission.

Metatron's Introduction to the Meditation For Cellular Healing as she received it from Spirit.

I wish to bring you a message of healing; an exercise which you may do to improve your overall health and well-being.

This exercise was initially devised to work with those on the Earth plane suffering from autoimmune dysfunctions. It also heals more than can be put into words. The immune system in many humans at this time is functioning poorly, secondary to stress. This stress can take the form of illness. This stress might also cause emotional or spiritual, rather than physical problems. The result on the immune system can be just as devastating.

Ones with autoimmune illnesses often find themselves easily fatigued, feeling weak, unable to think clearly as if in a mental fog and often in pain. There are more specific symptoms related to each individual type of disorder.

The exercise I am offering is quite simple and can be done by anyone. For the exercise to work one must truly want to be healed. It is a common fault of humans to seek attention through their illness. The illness often serves as a large part of that person's identity. Those people would feel lost without their illness. For someone invested in their illness, the continued attention to the illness feeds it, deeply ingraining it into the cells of the body, thus making it more and more difficult for healing to occur. A shift in consciousness is necessary for them to be healed. The intention must be set to heal.

If your intention is to be healed, then you are a ripe candidate for this healing exercise. This powerful meditation utilizes the Star Tetrahedron, Healing Light, and Vortex Energies.

Once is often enough for this most powerful Visualization exercise. Your intention must be to heal completely. If you find yourself wavering, you may repeat the exercise. Also, if multiple body systems are involved, you may extract cells from these other areas, one at a time.

Allow at least two weeks before repeating this exercise. Give the vitalized cell(s) the opportunity to do their work. Repeating this process too soon may confuse the body.

To make optimal use of this exercise, attention must be given to your diet, exercise and rest. Drink copious amounts of pure, fresh water. It is beneficial to eat very little grain and lots of vegetables and fruit. Protein should be found in vegetables, fish, and poultry. Take care to use natural foods without chemical additives (organic, non-GMO is best). Fresh air is important every day. Sunshine is optimal. A brisk walk, if you are able, can accomplish this. Other daily exercise is recommended as tolerated. Sleep is essential and restorative. It is the time when the regenerating cells are hard at work. Get at least eight hours of sleep nightly with naps during the day as needed. As a daily practice, close your eyes and listen to your body. Let it tell you what it needs.

As you are entering this new time of clarity, creativity and a heightened sense of Being, I wish you to be healthy in body, mind and spirit. My hope is that this meditation exercise will be a valuable tool for you on your journey.

With Blessings and Radiant Love

Metatron

Personal Notes

Actual Meditation

Metatron's Meditation For Cellular Healing as given to Glenn

If you have not already read pages 294-298 for an explanation of what influences the DNA and what "all its aspects" means, I suggest you read it now.

Before beginning the exercise, it is optimal to be clean and dressed in comfortable clothing as you would be for meditation. Next, please ground yourself. You may also want to enter your 'sacred space.'

> Glenn's note: I have slightly modified this and written it for the plural. Sometimes more than one cell comes to awareness.
>
> Two ways to ground that may be helpful.
>
> 1) "Great Spirit and Great Spirit Helpers, as are best, help me stay grounded and fully connected to EARTH and all of Her Selves through CENTRAL SUN and YOUR LOVE and help me keep EARTH and all Her Selves connected to CENTRAL SUN through me, so we heal each other with and through YOUR LOVE and LIGHT. *Thank You.*"
>
> 2) "Great Spirit and Great Spirit Helpers, as are best, keep me grounded to Mother Earth and all Her selves and fully connected to you as I do this meditation. *Thank you.*"
>
> You may also visualize the grounding links.

During this meditation if you choose a body part and cell to heal, choose only one. If Spirit spontaneously guides you to more than one, follow that guidance. This is written for the plural.

If at any time during this meditation, you have any doubts, ask Spirit to lead. Also, if at any time you need more time, say "pause", and when you are ready to continue, say "go."

At this point, enter into your meditative state.

Ask yourself and Spirit what parts of your body are most out of harmony and/or balance. Send attention to those places, focusing on the individual cells of that area. As you are looking at the individual cells, choose which ones to work with. Bring the cells out of your body and place them in front of you. Turn them around, examining them closely, looking at them from all angles. Next, turn these chosen cells on their side, the flatter side down, so that from the side they look a little like oblong dinner plates. Place them horizontally out from your body in front of your heart chakra.

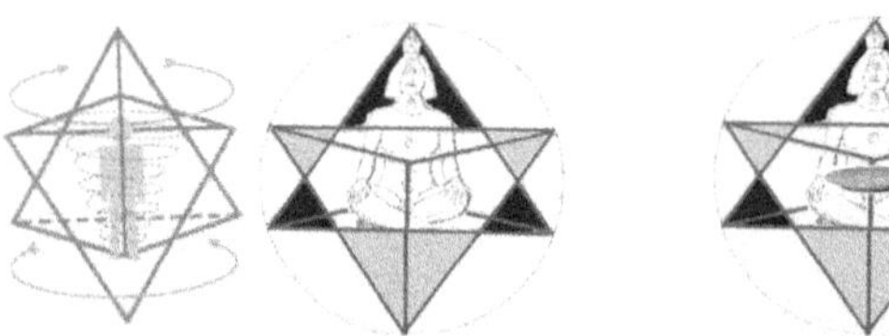
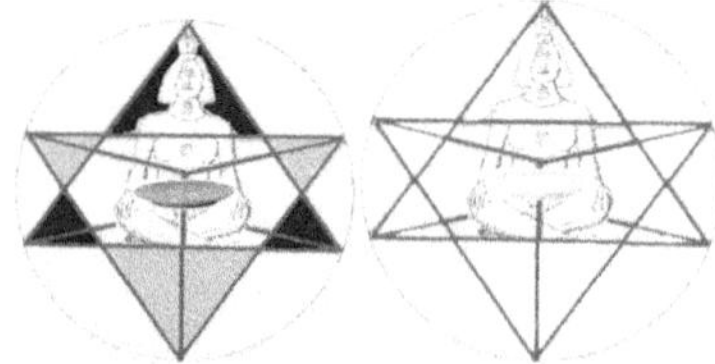

Next, allow the cells to be stationary in space as you visualize a three sided, upward pointing pyramid floating down from above and sliding over the cells, so that the cells are completely enclosed within the center of the pyramid. Allow this upward pointing pyramid to remain stationary around the cells, as you visualize a second pyramid with its point facing down, rising up over the cells, again enclosing them.

> If you were looking at this figure in two dimensions, straight on from the side, it would look like a Star of David, with the cell floating horizontally in the center. In three dimensions, however, as you are doing this exercise now, you see that you have created a Star Tetrahedron, with the cells floating horizontally in its center.

Now bring a beautiful healing blue light down from above to fill and completely saturate the first (upward pointing) pyramid and your cells floating in its center.

After that, bring up from below, a beautiful healing green light to fill the second (downward pointing) pyramid and enclosed cells.

As these beautiful blue and green lights meet in the overlapping pyramids, they fuse into a brilliant white light. This light begins to swirl in a clockwise direction. It becomes a vortex of healing energy in, through and around the cells. The contents of the cells, including the DNA **and all its aspects**, are cleaned and cleared. The white light and vortex energies within the Star Tetrahedron clean and clear the cells much like a high efficiency washing machine.

As the healing of the cells is completing, allow the spinning to slow to a halt. Now allow the white light to dissipate, leaving you with healthy, renewed, fully viable cells with their DNA **and all its aspects** vitalized to a higher vibratory level.

In your meditation, take these healthy cells out of the Star Tetrahedron by sliding them toward you.

Place these healthy, vibrant cells into your Third Eye (brow chakra).

Then move the cells back into their original body part(s).

> These cells are used as a template model, regenerating and repatterning all of the other cells in the affected body part(s) and additionally for the body as a whole.

Metatron

When you are ready, open your eyes. Thank yourself and Great Spirit for the healing/clearing and let it go.

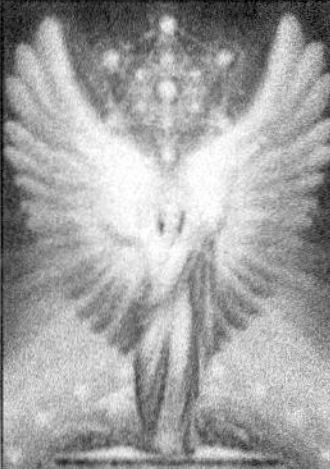

Metatron

Graphic by Marius Michael-George

Web site: http://mariusfineart.com/

Above was given to me in March 2015 by a medical professional and shared with her permission.

Below is adapted from *Metatron's Meditation For Cellular Healing* on the previous pages.

Explanation of Metatron's Meditation As Adapted by Glenn For Healing The Non Physical/Energetic

This meditation can be used for clearing, healing, releasing and deenergizing The Non Physical/Energetic that is adversely affecting you and your well-being. It, in some way, also assists in eliminating toxins and impurities.

If you have not already read pages 294-298 for an explanation, I suggest you read it now.

A brief explanation of the meditation is given below.

This meditation can be used for healing what can be thought of as non-physical/energetic aspects **of DNA**. Let go of the names and the need to analyze. This 'non-physical affects the mental, emotional and spiritual levels and bodies. This in turn affects the physical body, and all aspects of your life as a physical being. It works similarly to 'cellular healing', however healing the non-physical/energetic may be more effective than 'cellular healing' when dealing with emotional or mental issues as well as with Soul Echoes. It may also be more effective in releasing unconscious and conscious beliefs that energize self limiting or destructive behavior and habits.

Allow a thought or image of something that is bothering you, you hold judgment on or you would like to change. Ask yourself what you want to heal or ask Great Spirit to bring forward what is to be healed at this time. Instead of working with a cell as in *Metatron's Meditation For Cellular Healing* to heal the physical DNA, you will be working with what can be called "energy balls". When you have the thought of what you want to heal, let go of the thought and allow these energy balls to appear in your conscious awareness without any attempt to analyze, count or name them (may be one or many).

You may be guided to do this exercise separately for each of the following:
miasms, ***'cellular memory'***, ***'Imprints On The Luminous Energy Field'***, ***memories replaying***, ***beliefs***, ***vows***, ***oaths***, ***covenants***, ***promises***, ***agreements***, ***concepts***, ***attitudes***, ***'truths'***, and ***contracts*** that are no longer in harmony with our highest good and well being

All of these, and more, can be thought of as "***<u>Soul Echoes</u>***" to be released.

I suggest a prayer or meditation similar to the following before and after the exercise.

"Great Spirit and Great Spirit Helpers as are best,
Help me to always fill all voids and emptiness with 100% Pure Divine LOVE and LIGHT as is best. *Thank You.*"

Personal Notes

Actual Meditation

Metatron's Meditation For Healing The 'Non-Physical'

Healing Beyond The DNA

(Metatron's Meditation adapted by Glenn) Before beginning the exercise, it is optimal to be clean and dressed in comfortable clothing as you would be for meditation.

If you have not already read pages 294-298 for an explanation, I suggest you read it now.

Next, please ground yourself. You may also want to enter your 'sacred space.'

> Glenn's note: Two ways to ground that may be helpful.
>
> 1) "Great Spirit and Great Spirit Helpers, as are best, help me stay grounded and fully connected to EARTH and all of Her Selves through CENTRAL SUN and YOUR LOVE and help me keep EARTH and all Her Selves connected to CENTRAL SUN through me, so we heal each other with and through YOUR LOVE and LIGHT. *Thank You.*"
>
> 2) "Great Spirit and Great Spirit Helpers, as are best, keep me grounded to Mother Earth and all Her selves and fully connected to you as I do this meditation. *Thank you.*" You may also visualize the grounding links.

During this meditation you may see one or several 'energy balls'. Either is fine. This is written for the plural.

If at any time during this meditation, you have any doubts, ask Spirit to lead. Also, if at any time you need more time, say "pause", and when you are ready to continue, say "go."

At this point, enter into your meditative state.

Ask yourself what you want to heal, or ask Great Spirit to bring forward what is to be healed at this time. Let go of intent or analysis, and just allow.

Allow 'energy balls', representing the **<u>Soul Echoes</u>** and anything else which are interfering with and adversely affecting you, to come into awareness.

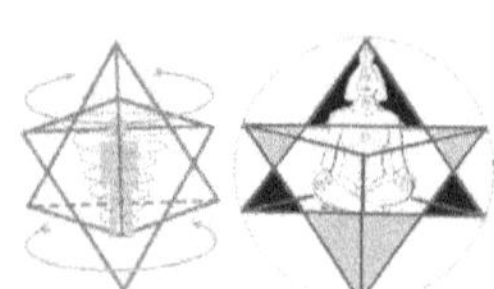

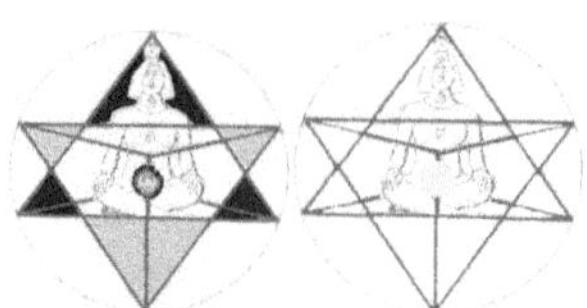

They are stationary in space as you visualize a three sided, upward pointing pyramid floating down from above and sliding over the 'energy balls', so that the 'energy balls' are completely enclosed within the center of the pyramid. Allow this upward pointing pyramid to remain stationary around the 'energy balls', as you visualize a second pyramid with its point facing down, rising up over the 'energy balls', again enclosing them.

> If you were looking at this figure in two dimensions, straight on from the side, it would look like a Star of David, with the 'energy balls' floating in the center. In three dimensions, however, as you are doing this exercise now, you see that you have created a Star Tetrahedron, with the 'energy balls' floating in its center.

Now bring a beautiful healing blue light down from above to fill and completely saturate the first (upward pointing) pyramid and your 'energy balls' floating in its center.

After that, bring up from below, a beautiful healing green light to fill the second (downward pointing) pyramid and enclosed 'energy balls'.

As these beautiful blue and green lights meet in the overlapping pyramids, they fuse into a brilliant white light. Let this light begin to swirl in a clockwise direction. It becomes a vortex of healing energy in, through and around the 'energy balls'. The 'energy balls' and all they represent are cleaned and cleared as Great Spirit sees best. The white light and vortex energies within the Star Tetrahedron clean and clear the 'energy balls' much like a high efficiency washing machine.

As the healing of the 'energy balls' is completing, allow the spinning to slow to a halt. Now allow the white light and the 'energy balls' to dissipate and dissolve. Realize that the energy balls dissipate and dissolve without conscious thought or any attempt to analyze. The energy has been vitalized to a higher vibratory level.

When you are ready, open your eyes. Thank yourself and Great Spirit for the healing/clearing and let it go.

Above is adapted by Glenn from *Metatron's Meditation For Cellular Healing*.

DNA Activation And Re-Patterning described

The actual exercise follows these thoughts.

If you have not already read pages 294-298 for an explanation of what influences the DNA and what "all its aspects" means, I suggest you read it now.

What if our genes were merely building blocks, and a greater intelligence was in charge of the physical as well as the unseen?

Once this negative 'data' is removed any resulting voids need to be filled.

Before beginning the exercise, it is optimal to be clean and dressed in comfortable clothing as you would for meditation. Next, please ground yourself. You may also want to enter your 'sacred space.'

> Glenn's note: I have slightly modified this and written it for the plural. Sometimes more than one DNA strand is ready to heal.

Before beginning the exercise, it is optimal to be clean and dressed in comfortable clothing as you would be for meditation. Next, please ground yourself. You may also want to enter your 'sacred space.'

> One way to ground that may be helpful.
>
> "Great Spirit and Great Spirit Helpers, as are best, keep me grounded to Mother Earth and all Her selves and fully connected to you as I do this meditation. *Thank you.*"
>
> You may also visualize the grounding links.

DNA Activation And Re-Patterning - The Actual Exercise

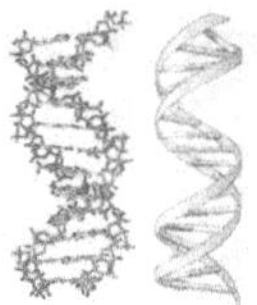

If at any time during this meditation, you have any doubts, ask Spirit to lead. Also, if at any time you need more time, say "pause", and when you are ready to continue, say "go."

As described above, recognize that there is more to DNA than just the physical DNA.

This re-patterning is to bring your DNA **and all its aspects** back to the 'Divine Plan' (often called the Original Blueprint) and 'Divine Manifestation' (often called the Original Weaving)

First find a quiet place and relax. Enter your Sacred Space.

At this point, enter into your meditative state.

Visualize your DNA strands. You may see one pair (two strands) or several pairs.

Use a finger and thumb to pull down the willing DNA strands from the top.

If no DNA strand is willing, try again later.

Place your other hand at the bottom and use a finger and thumb from that hand to pull up the willing strands (or the strings or cords) from the bottom.

Bring the two ends together and allow them to touch.

This allows the DNA **and all its aspects** to heal on the strands that were willing; all the way back to the "Original Blueprint" and "The Original Weaving.

When you are ready, open your eyes. Thank yourself and Great Spirit for the healing/clearing and let it go.

When you are ready, open your eyes. Thank yourself and Great Spirit for the healing/clearing and let it go.

Beyond DNA - Soul Activation And Re-Patterning described

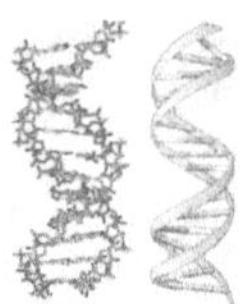

Recognize that there is more to DNA than just the physical DNA.

If you have not already read pages 294-298 for an explanation, I suggest you read it now.

You may be guided to do this exercise separately for each of the following:

miasms, ***'cellular memory'***, ***'Imprints On The Luminous Energy Field'***, ***memories replaying***, ***beliefs***, ***vows***, ***oaths***, ***covenants***, ***promises***, ***agreements***, ***concepts***, ***attitudes***, ***'truths'***, and ***contracts*** that are no longer in harmony with our highest good and well being

All of these, and more, can be thought of as "***Soul Echoes***" to be released

This re-patterning is to bring your Being back to the 'Divine Plan' (often called the Original Blueprint) and 'Divine Manifestation'(often called the Original Weaving)

Glenn's note: I have slightly modified this and written it for the plural. Sometimes more than one strand is ready to heal.

Before beginning the exercise, it is optimal to be clean and dressed in comfortable clothing as you would be for meditation. Next, please ground yourself. You may also want to enter your 'sacred space.'

One way to ground that may be helpful.

"Great Spirit and Great Spirit Helpers, as are best, keep me grounded to Mother Earth and all Her selves and fully connected to you as I do this meditation. *Thank you."*

You may also visualize the grounding links.

The Actual Exercise

Beyond DNA - Soul Activation And Re-Patterning

If at any time during this meditation, you have any doubts, ask Spirit to lead. Also, if at any time you need more time, say "pause", and when you are ready to continue, say "go."

At this point, enter into your meditative state.

First find a quiet place and relax. Enter your Sacred Space.

Visualize strands (or strings or cords) that look like DNA strands. You may see one pair or several pairs.

Use a finger and thumb to pull down the willing strands (or the strings or cords) from the top.

If no strand (or string or cord) is willing, try again later.

Place your other hand at the bottom and use a finger and thumb from that hand to pull up the willing strands (or the strings or cords) from the bottom.

Bring the two ends together and allow them to touch.

This allows the '**Soul Echoes**' and energetic disturbances to heal on the willing strands back towards the "Original Blueprint" and "The Original Weaving"

When you are ready, open your eyes. Thank yourself and Great Spirit for the healing/clearing and let it go.

****

Acupressure

(one hand and then the other)

Thumb (Blood pressure, heart and tension.
Next three fingers
Pinky finger (finances)
Rub palm with thumb from other hand (general wellbeing and energy)
Place palms together.

To Heal the Stomach and Heart and bring them and their chakras into balance.

Use your finger and rub the abdomen in the vicinity of the stomach and 3rd chakra in a clockwise motion.

Above was given to me by Duane Redwolf Miles. His website is http://artoffrequency.com.
****

Below is adapted from *The Dark Side Of The Light Chasers* by Debbie Ford

Bus Trip Adapted by Glenn

A simple way to integrate your other Selfs

Sub-Personalities, Aspects, Soul Fragments and Shadow Selves are different names for essentially the same thing. If they are unrecognized, unloved and yet to be embraced, they are in shadow and thus unintegrated into your Being. They can be what we perceive as 'Light' or ''dark'.

The reason we do 'Shadow Work' is to become whole. Unconceal, own, Love and embrace your shadow as well as your light. This allows the negative energies to be released and retains the positive components and lessons.

If you are ruled by fear you must go within and find your courage. It is your birthright to be whole: to have it all. It only takes a shift in your perception, an opening of your heart. When you can say, "I am that", to the deepest, darkest aspect of yourself and to the Lightest aspect of yourself, then you can reach true enlightenment. It's not until we fully embrace the dark that we can embrace the light. I've heard it said that shadow work is the path of the heart warrior. It takes us to a new place in our consciousness where we have to open our hearts to all of our-selves, and to all of humanity.

Every aspect of ourselves has a gift. Every emotion and every trait we possess helps show us the way to enlightenment, to oneness. Our shadow is here to point out where we are incomplete.

Every single sub-personality has a gift for you. Every aspect of you, whether you like it or not, can benefit your life. To think there is only darkness or only light is to deceive yourself. There is light in every part of us and every part of the universe. To not find our gifts is to reject the extraordinary design of life. Our souls long to learn these valuable lessons. We need to stop judging our souls' journey and trust in the design of our humanity and eternal goodness. There is an ancient saying, "All things must grow, or they die." Our highest purpose is to learn and grow from our experiences and then move on. Once we receive the benefit of our traits we are free to choose the experiences we desire.

Preparation For The Bus Trip Exercise

This is an exercise that requires you to surrender to yourself, so make sure you have created a safe environment for the process and that you are relaxed. You are going to meet your inner voices, so you want to have your mind as quiet as possible.

You may want to open sacred space and surround yourself with LOVE, LIGHT and VIOLET FLAME.

Use your own way or you may say a prayer similar to the following.

Great Spirit and Great Spirit Helpers, as are best,
Help me stay fully connected to YOU and YOUR LOVE and LIGHT. *Thank You.*

Great Spirit and Great Spirit Helpers, as are best,
Help me stay standing fully in YOUR LOVE, LIGHT and VIOLET FLAME. *Thank You.*

Great Spirit and Great Spirit Helpers, as are best,
Keep me completely surrounded by YOUR LOVE, LIGHT and VIOLET FLAME. *Thank You.*

Great Spirit and Great Spirit Helpers, as are best,
Help me stay filled with Your LOVE, LIGHT and VIOLET FLAME as is best. *Thank You.*

Great Spirit and Great Spirit Helpers, as are best,
Help me keep it so only energies and beings of Pure Divine LOVE and LIGHT surround me, influence me and share and communicate through me. *Thank You.*

Great Spirit and Great Spirit Helpers, as are best,
Help me to Open Your Sacred Space of LOVE as is best, keep me in Our Sacred Space and close our sacred space as is best when I have finished this exercise . *Thank You.*

Exercise on next two pages.

Actual Bus Trip Exercise Starts Here

As you are learning this exercise you can open your eyes after each step and read the next to continue. Just remain calm and present.

Close your eyes and start following your breath. Take long, slow, deep breaths, retaining the breath for five or more seconds, and then slowly exhale. Do this a few times until your mind is quiet.

Now imagine stepping onto a large, yellow bus. Take a seat in the middle of the bus. You're feeling excited about taking a long awaited trip. Imagine riding down the street on a clear, beautiful day. You're sitting there minding your own business when someone taps you on your shoulder. You look up and this person says, "Hello, I'm one of your sub-personalities and all the other people on this bus are also your sub-personalities. Why don't you get up now and walk around and see who's on your bus."You get up from your seat and you walk through the entire bus looking at all the different people in their seats.

You see before you every kind of person - tall people, short people, teenagers, and old people. There might be circus people, animals, and homeless people. There may even be some, who look or feel otherworldly. With you on the bus are people of every race, color, and creed. Some of them are waving to get your attention, others may be hiding quietly in the corner. Continue to walk through the aisles, slowly visualizing all the characters on the bus.

Now the bus driver directs you to allow one of your sub personalities to take you for a walk off the bus in a nearby park. The sub-personality may seem angry, sad, lost, or hesitant. It may even seem 'dark'. There should be an underlying *feeling* of LOVE and anticipation.

1) Take your time and allow one of your sub-personalities to come and take your hand, and escort you off the bus into the park. If no sub-personality comes to take your hand be patient and ask again some other time.

Ask that person to tell you what trait he or she represents along with a name. (*For example, if you meet someone angry you could name this person Angry Alfred or Angry Ann. If you don't hear a name you give that person one).* Take all the time you need. Notice how this person is dressed and looks. What does this person smell like? Notice his or her mood and body language.

Take another deep breath and ask this person/Being:

> **"What is your gift to me?"** Be open to the gift and after you have received the gift, ask,
> **"What is the gift of ________; What does it bring to me?"** Then ask,
> **"What do you need to be whole?"**
> **"What do you need to integrate into my psyche with LOVE?"**

After you have heard every answer ask this person,:

> **"Is there anything else you need to say to me?"** When you are finished make sure you acknowledge them, thank them and walk them back to the bus.

Now that you are back on the bus return to **1)** and ask, **"Is there another sub-personality ready for integration with me at this time."**

If the answer is “YES” repeat the exercise.

If the answer is “NO” open your eyes when you are ready and give thanks.

Don't worry if you did not get all the answers you needed from your sub-personalities. It takes time and practice to hear all of their messages. Make a date with yourself to do it again.

Explanation Of Trigger Words

We're taught never to say negative things about ourselves. If I wake up feeling worthless, I'm supposed to pretend that I don't feel that way. I'm supposed to say to myself that I'm worthy and hope I will come to feel worthy later in the day. I have to go to work pretending I feel worthy because feeling worthless is not okay. I have to hide behind my mask of worthiness all day, hoping no one will see through it. But, inside, I'll feel a quiet despair knowing I'm not being myself, all because I'm unable to embrace being worthless. We resist this aspect of ourselves and pass judgments on the kind of person we perceive as worthless.

We are told affirmations will make us okay, however, if we put ice cream on top of poop after a few spoonfuls, we will taste the poop again. When we integrate negative traits into our selves, we no longer need affirmations because we'll know that we're both worthless and worthy, ugly and beautiful, lazy and conscientious. When we believe we can only be one or the other, we continue our internal struggle to only be the right things. When we believe that we are only weak, nasty, and selfish - traits that we believe our friends and families don't possess - we feel shame. When we believe or pretend we are only worthy, conscientious, caring, loving, etc. we are denying and repressing the part we believe to be ‘dark’, thus denying ourselves wholeness. When you own all of the traits in the universe, you'll understand that every aspect within you has something to teach you. These teachers will give you access to all the wisdom in the world.

Using The Words List

Take a moment to quiet your mind. Take several slow, deep breaths and slowly read through the list below. After looking at every word, say to yourself, "I am _________," for every word. If you can say it clearly without any emotional charge, then move on to the next word. Write down any word that you're uncomfortable with or dislike on a sheet of paper. Include words that represent things that you admire in someone else but don't embrace in yourself.

If you are not sure that the word has any charge for you, close your eyes for a minute and meditate on the word. Repeat it to yourself a few times out loud and ask yourself how you'd really feel if someone you respected called you this word. If you'd be angry or upset, write it down. If you would feel flattered and superior, write it down.

Also spend some time thinking about words that are not on this list that run your life or cause you pain.

You possess all these qualities. All you have to do to integrate them is unconceal, own, and embrace each one.

List Of Positive Words

POSITIVE	POSITIVE	POSITIVE	POSITIVE
accepting	Credible	healthy	responsible
acknowledged	Decisive	holy	rich
active	Dedicated	honored	romantic
adored	Delicious	humorous	safe
adorned	Desirable	innovative	Satisfied
affluent	Disciplined	inspiring	secure
alive	Divine	intelligent	self-assured
articulate	deserving	irresistible	sensitive
artistic	easygoing	joyful	sensual
assertive	embracing	juicy	sexy
attractive	empowering	knowledgeable	simple
balanced	energetic	leader	soft
beautiful	enlightened	loved/loving	solid
blissful	enthusiastic	loyal	spiritual
bold	extravagant	lucky	spontaneous
brilliant	fair	magnificent	strong
calm	faithful / faith	mature	successful
capable	famous	non-judgmental	superstar
carefree	fearless	nurturing	talented
centered	flexible	open	tender
champion	focused	optimistic	thankful
cheerful	forgiving	organized	thoughtful
cherished	fortunate	passionate	timely
choice-maker	forward	patient	understanding
clean	free	peaceful	vivacious
compassionate	fruitful	playful	vulnerable
complete	fulfilled	powerful	wanted
confident	full	precious	warm
connected	fun	pretty	warm-hearted
conscious	funny	productive	whole
content	generous	prolific	willing
cool	gentle	punctual	wise
cosmic	genuine	quiet	wonderful
courageous	giving	radiant	worthy
creative	glamorous	realized	
	happy		

List Of Negative Words

NEGATIVE	NEGATIVE	NEGATIVE	NEGATIVE
abuser	condescending	floozy	insensitive
addict	confrontational	foolish	insipid
aggressive	conniving	frail	intrusive
alcoholic	controlling	freak	irresponsible
anal	coward	frigid	jealous
angry	critical	frugal	jerk
anorexic	cruel	full	judgmental
anxious	dangerous	gambler	know-it-all
arrogant	**DARK**	geek	lame
ass	dead	gold	late
asshole	deceitful	good	lazy
ass-kisser	defensive	goofy	liar
bad	delinquent	gossip	lifeless
ball	depressed	Greedy	loser
been	desperate	groupie	loud
beggar	destructive	grudge	love
betrayer	devious	has	lush
better	diabolical	hateful	malicious
big	digger	heartless	mama's
bigot	dirty	hopeless	man-hater
bitchy	disgusting	hormonal	manipulator
bitter	disturber	hot	martyr
black	dominating	hungry	masochistic
bossy	druggy	hyper	mean
boy	dumb	hypocrite	middle
bulimic	dyke	idiot	miser
buster	egocentric	idiot	mouth
buyer	elitist	ignorant	nasty
cagey	emotional	immature	needy
carrier	empty	impatient	neglectful
castrated	energy	imperious	nervous
cheap	enough	imposter	nose
cheater	envious	impotent	nosy
childish	**EVIL**	inappropriate	not
class	explosive	inauthentic	offensive
classless	faggot	incompetent	old
codependent	failure	inferior	opportunist
cold	fat	inflexible	overbearing
competitive	fearful	insane	oversensitive
compulsive	flabby	insecure	

NEGATIVE	NEGATIVE	NEGATIVE	NEGATIVE
pain	secretive	superficial	victimizer
pansy	self-destructive	tasteless	vindictive
passive	shameful	than	violent
perfectionist	shameless	thick-headed	wasteful
perverted	shit	thief	weak
possessive	shot	thoughtless	weasel
POWERLESS	shrew	tight	whiney
predator	shyster	traitor	white
prudish	sick	trash	whore
psychotic	sinister	trashy	wild
pushy	sleazy	unconscious	wimp
racist	sloppy	**UNDESERVING**	withdrawn
resentful	slut	unfair	withholding
resistant	smelly	ugly	woman-hater
ridiculous	sneak	unimportant	womanizer
righteous	snippy	uninteresting	worthless
rigid	snob	**UNLOVABLE**	wretched
ruthless	soulless	unqualified	zombie
sad	spinster	**UNVALUABE**	
sadistic	stingy	**UNWORTHY**	
scammer	stuck	unenlightened	
scared	stupid	useless	
scary	sucker	victim	

Above is adapted from *The Dark Side Of The Light Chasers* by Debbie Ford
****

Below is by the author.

A good prayer to say before any healing or journeying

This is to help you to surrender to yourself. Make sure you have created a safe environment for the process and that you are relaxed. Quiet your mind and open to Sources Love and guidance. You may want to turn off your phone and other devices.

You may want to open sacred space for yourself and the area you are in. Surround yourself with LOVE, LIGHT and VIOLET FLAME.

Use your own way or you may say a prayer similar to the following.

Great Spirit and Great Spirit Helpers, as are best,
Help me stay fully connected to YOU and YOUR LOVE and LIGHT. *Thank You.*

Great Spirit and Great Spirit Helpers, as are best,
Help me stay standing fully in YOUR LOVE, LIGHT and VIOLET FLAME. *Thank You.*

Great Spirit and Great Spirit Helpers, as are best,
Keep me completely surrounded by YOUR LOVE, LIGHT and VIOLET FLAME. *Thank You.*

Great Spirit and Great Spirit Helpers, as are best,
Help me stay filled with Your LOVE, LIGHT and VIOLET FLAME as is best. *Thank You.*

Great Spirit and Great Spirit Helpers, as are best,
Help me keep it so only energies and beings of Pure Divine LOVE and LIGHT surround me, influence me and share and communicate through me. *Thank You.*

Great Spirit and Great Spirit Helpers, as are best,
Help me to Open Your Sacred Space of LOVE as is best, keep me in Our Sacred Space and close our sacred space as is best when I have finished this exercise. *Thank You.*

Great Spirit and Great Spirit Helpers, as are best,
Help me to set aside my conscious mind and all expectations as to the answers to any questions. Help (________your name________) to step aside and allow my higher aspects and "I AM" presence to receive the questions and answers, and bring any healing to me as is best. I ask my Unihipili (sub-conscious mind) to lovingly be my interpreter and gatekeeper as is best. *Thank You.*

Great Spirit and Great Spirit Helpers, as are best,
Do this as is best for all those participating in this healing. *Thank You.*

Above is by the author.
****

Three Versions of The Lord's Prayer and a Native American Prayer

Notice the difference in energy of these prayers.

Christian Version of The Lord's Prayer

The Christian version has slight variations in wording.

Our Father who art in Heaven,
Hallowed be thy name;
Thy kingdom come
Thy will be done
On earth as it is in heaven.
Give us this day our daily bread;
And forgive us our trespasses
As we forgive those who trespass against us;
And lead us not into temptation,
But deliver us from evil.
For thine is the kingdom,
The power, and the glory,
For ever and ever.
Amen.

Below is from http://www.thenazareneway.com/lords_prayer.htm

The Lord's Prayer In the original Aramaic

Abwûn
"Oh Thou, from whom the breath of life comes,

d'bwaschmâja
who fills all realms of sound, light and vibration.

Nethkâdasch schmach
May Your light be experienced in my utmost holiest.

Têtê malkuthach.
Your Heavenly Domain approaches.

Nehwê tzevjânach aikâna d'bwaschmâja af b'arha.
Let Your will come true - in the universe (all that vibrates)
just as on earth (that is material and dense).

Hawvlân lachma d'sûnkanân jaomâna.
Give us wisdom (understanding, assistance) for our daily need,

Waschboklân chaubên wachtahên aikâna
daf chnân schwoken l'chaijabên.

detach the fetters of faults that bind us, (karma)
like we let go the guilt of others.

Wela tachlân l'nesjuna
Let us not be lost in superficial things (materialism, common temptations),

ela patzân min bischa.
but let us be freed from that what keeps us off from our true purpose.

Metol dilachie malkutha wahaila wateschbuchta l'ahlâm almîn.
From You comes the all-working will, the lively strength to act,
the song that beautifies all and renews itself from age to age.

Amên.

Sealed in trust, faith and truth.
(I confirm with my entire being)

Above is from http://www.thenazareneway.com/lords_prayer.htm

Below is adapted from *Co-creation* by Vladimir Megre

Anastasia's Version of The Lord's Prayer

The way she spoke these words was not the way we say prayers. She spoke them the way anyone might talk to a close friend, a loved one, a relative. Her speech contained all the intonations of a live conversation. Passion, joy, fervent ecstasy - as though the One Anastasia was talking to was right there beside her:

"Then why doesn't anyone understand His words?"

"Words? The peoples of the Earth have so many words with different meanings. There are so many diverse languages and dialects. And yet there is one language for all. One language for all Divine callings. It is woven together out of the rustlings of the leaves, the songs of the birds and the roar of the waves. The Divine language has fragrance and color. Through this language God responds to each one's request and gives a prayerful response to prayer."

"Could you translate, or express in words, what He says to us?"

"I could give you an approximation."

"Why just an approximation?"

"Because our language is much too poor to be compatible with the language God speaks to us in."

My father, You are present everywhere!
For the light of life I gladly thank You,
For Your bright kingdom visible here and now,
And for Your loving will. Long live the good!
For daily bread and daily food with joy I thank You!
And for Your loving patience,
And for Your giving of forgiveness of sins on Your Earth fair.
My Father, You are present everywhere!
I am Your daughter here midst Your creations.
Weakness and sin — I shall not let them in,
But prove myself worthy of Your consummations.
My Father, You are present everywhere!
I am Your daughter, Your joy I declare.
My entire self shall magnify Your glory,
In Your bright dream the coming ages all will live and share.
It shall be so! I wish it so! I am a daughter of Yours.
My Father, You are present everywhere.

Above is adapted from *Co-creation* by Vladimir Megre

Below is from http://www.NativeHistoryMagazine.com

Native American prayer

Similar to the Christian version of The Lord's Prayer

Oh, Great Spirit
Whose voice I hear in the winds,
And whose breath gives life to all the world,
hear me, I am small and weak,
I need your strength and wisdom.
Let me walk in beauty and make my eyes ever behold,
the red and purple sunset.
Make my hands respect the things you have
made and my ears sharp to hear your voice.
Make me wise so that I may understand the things
you have taught my people.
Let me learn the lessons you have
hidden in every leaf and rock.
I seek strength, not to be greater than my brother,
but to fight my greatest enemy - myself.
Make me always ready to come to you
with clean hands and straight eyes.
So when life fades, as the fading sunset,
my Spirit may come to you without shame.

Translated by Lakota Sioux Chief Yellow Lark in 1887

Above is from http://www.NativeHistoryMagazine.com

****

Appendix

Concurrent Healing Techniques

1) **Other Styles Of Prayer.**

2) **Inner Child Healing**: Healing of the feeling, emotional and mental wounds of the inner child,

including changed perceptions and integration of the dark side, with forgiveness and LOVE, rather than blame.

3) **Soul Retrieval:** Retrieval of soul pieces ready to integrate. Treatment of fragmented and lost

(or stolen) soul parts that keep one from being Spiritually whole. Missing soul fragments create openings in the manifest and unmanifest bodies.

4) **Personal Empowerment Techniques**: Personal empowerment provided by a Spiritual

reconnection with one's Highest Self and with The All-Powerful, All-Knowing Creator of the Universe. Feelings of aloneness and separation are replaced with compassion, forgiveness and LOVE.

5) **Meditation and Contemplation**

6) **Nutrition and Eating Habits**

7) **Physical Fitness and Exercise**

8) **Minimizing Damaging Habits**: Smoke less or become a non smoker, limit caffeine, limit carbonated beverages, limit alcoholic beverages, limit refined/processed foods, limit other non-nutritious foods.

9) **Acupuncture**

10) **Hypnosis**

11) **Shamanic Healing**

12) **Energy Healing**

13) **Chiropractic**

14) **Massage and 'Bodywork'**

15) **Training**: Train yourself to recognize your State of Being and your health.

16) **Supplements and Medicines**

17) **Holistic Doctors and Practitioners**

18) **Traditional Western Medicine**

Suggested Reading and Web Sites

My First Two Books and Web Site

Two Choices - Divine LOVE Or Anything Else by Glenn Molinari

Awareness - A Path To Spiritual and Physical Health and Well-Being by Glenn Molinari

http://twochoices.net for additional information and FREE PDFs

Reincarnation And Past Lives

Childrens Past Lives by Carol Bowman

Return From Heaven by Carol Bowman

Many Lives Many Masters by Brian L. Weiss, M.D.

Dental And Mouth

Elements of Danger: Protect Yourself Against the Hazards of Modern Dentistry by Morton Walker, D.P.M. (can be overwhelming)

<http://www.hugginsappliedhealing.com/>

<http://www.talkinternational.com/toothchart.html> (for interactive tooth to organ chart)

<http://www.flcv.com/indexa.html>

<http://www.secretofthieves.com/tooth-chart/> (an even more detailed tooth to organ chart)

Nutrition

No one nutritional and eating plan is right for everyone. When looked at with a critical eye the following three plans combine for a good basis.

Eat Right For Your Type by Dr. Peter J. D'Adamo
<http://dadamo.com/>

Enter The Zone by Barry Sears, PhD
<http://zonediet.com/zone-diet-overview>

The Metabolic Typing Diet by William Wolcott and Trish Fahey
<http://www.healthexcel.com/>

<http:/FindaSpring.com> (can help you find a natural spring close to you)

Affirmations

You Can Heal Your Life by Louise L. Hay

Memories Replaying

Zero Limits by Ihaleakala Hew Len, PhD and Joe Vitale

A very good introduction to healing and releasing 'Memories Replaying' by practicing Self Identity Ho'oponopono as developed and taught by Morrnah Nalamaku Simeona and Ihaleakala Hew Len. I have been unable to find a web site that is Ihaleakala Hew Lens'. His teachings are very powerful, however many people have commercialized them.

<http://top411.tripod.com/zero-limits-with-hooponopono/dr_ihaleakala_hew_len.html>

(A web page with links to video interviews with Ihaleakala Hew Len)

Trapped/Hidden Feelings, Emotions and Aspects

The Emotion Code by Dr. Bradley Nelson

<http://www.drbradleynelson.com/filters/the-emotion-code/>

Emotional Clearing Process by John Ruskan

<http://www.emclear.com/index.html>\

The Dark Side Of The Light Chasers by Debbie Ford

<http://store.debbieford.com/product_info.php?products_id=9>

Magnets for Healing

<https://www.lyonlegacy.com/learn/behind_science_magnetics.aspx>

The Ringing Cedars Series by Vladimir Megre

This series of books tells of Vladimir's learning from a Siberian recluse named Anastasia.

Some people believe Vladimir Megre has met Anastasia and the book is based on actual events. Some people say it is a work of fiction. Some people even say that there is no such person as Vladimir Megre.

I just found a web site <http://archive.org/advancedsearch.php> that has all 9 books in the series available as FREE downloads in EPUB, MOBI for Kindle and PDF formats. The PDF with text is searchable for words and phrases.

Book 1 *Anastasia* by Vladimir Megre
Book 2 *The Ringing Cedars of Russia* by Vladimir Megre
Book 3 *The Space of Love* by Vladimir Megre
Book 4 *Co-Creation* by Vladimir Megre
Book 5 *Who Are We?* by Vladimir Megre
Book 6 *The Book Of Kin* by Vladimir Megre
Book 7 *The Energy of Life* by Vladimir Megre
Book 8.1 *The New Civilization* by Vladimir Megre
Book 8.2 *Rites of Love* by Vladimir Megre

<http://www.vladimirmegre.com/vladimir_megre_story.php>
<http://www.anastasia.ca/>

Excellent Practice (modify for yourself)

Everyday Enlightenment - The Twelve Gateways to Personal Growth by Dan Millman

References

In Person

Miles, Duane Redwolf. In person 2015 and 2016. See his website at <artoffrequeny.com>

Books

Bowman, Carol. *(1998). Children's Past Lives.* New York. Bantam Books.

Calhoun, Marcy. (1987). *Are You Really Too Sensitive.* Nevada City, Ca. Blue Dolphin Publishing.

Ford, Debbie. *(1998)The Dark Side Of The Light Chasers*. New York. Berkley Publishing Group.

MacLaine, Shirley. (1989). *Going Within.* New York: Bantam Books.

Megre, Vladimir. (2000). *Co-Creation*. Ed. Leonid Sharashkin. Trans. John Woodsworth. The Ringing Cedars Series. Book 4. Kahului, HI. Ringing Cedars Press.

Weiss, Brian L., M.D. (1988). *Many Lives, Many Masters.* New York. Simon & Schuster.

Web Sites

Burney, Robert. *Emotional Incest - Emotionally devastating child abuse*. 2009 Recovered 2016. <http://www.woundedsouls.com/index.php/emotional-incest> (Originally found in 2014 at http://www.suite101.com/article.cfm/codependency_recovery/50739 which is no longer available)

Burney, Robert. *Inner Child Healing - How To Begin*. 2013. Retrieved 2014. <http://www.healyourinnerchild.com/Book-Content/inner-child-healing-how-to-begin>

Chong, Daniel H. ND. *Real or Synthetic: The Truth Behind Whole-Food Supplements*. 19 Jan 2005. Retrieved about 2008. <http://articles.mercola.com/sites/articles/archive/2005/01/19/whole-food-supplements.aspx>

Hornecker, John. *Soul And Oversoul*. 2010. Retrieved 1 June 2016. <http://www.earthscape.net/soul_oversoul.htm>

Institute of Health Sciences, 819 N. L.L.C. *Lemon (Citrus) - a miraculous product to kill cancer cell"*. 9 July 2011. Retrieved 2014 <http://csn.cancer.org/node/222132>

Kaplan, Teresa M. *Growing Towards Wholeness Through Grief: The Journey of the Wounded Child Within*. No date. Retrieved 2010. <http://www.creativegrowth.com/teresa.htm>

Kardos, Geza. *Habits That Block Creativity*. No Date. Retrieved 2016. <http://pt.slideshare.net/olivianightowl/habits-that-block-creativity>

Klinghardt, Dietrich MD, PhD. *Autonomic Response Testing Laws.* 2010. Retrieved 2014 <http://www.klinghardtacademy.com/Articles/ART-Laws.html >

Klinghardt, Dietrich MD, PhD. *The 5 Levels of Healing*. Retrieved 27 Dec 2014. <http://www.klinghardtacademy.com/images/stories/5_levels_of_healing/Klinghardt_Article_5_Levels_of_Healing.pdf> (originally retrieved as an html about 2005))

Klinghardt, Dietrich MD, PhD. *Applied Psycho-Neurobiology*. No date. Retrieved 2007 <http://www.mercola.com/article/applied_psycho_neurobiology/apn.htm>

Mercola, Joseph, Dr. *Experts Warn Vitamin E Can Trigger Cancer.* 18 Nov 2011. Retrieved 2012 <http://articles.mercola.com/sites/articles/archive/2011/11/18/dangers-of-vitamins.aspx>

Mercola, Joseph, Dr. *How Your Oral Health Contributes to Your General Health and Wellbeing.* 30 Nov 2014. Retrieved 2015. <http://articles.mercola.com/sites/articles/archive/2014/11/30/importance-oral-microbiome.aspx>

Mercola, Joseph, Dr. *Meet Dr. Mercola*. No date. Retrieved 2016 <http://www.mercola.com/forms/background.htm>

Mercola, Joseph, Dr. *New Studies on 3 Important Nutrients.* 11 July 2012. Retrieved 2012. <http://articles.mercola.com/sites/articles/archive/2012/07/11/calcium-turmeric-and-resveratrol-benefits.aspx>

Mercola, Joseph, Dr. *Oil Pulling Craze: All-Purpose Remedy?* 5 May 2014. Retrieved 2015 <http://articles.mercola.com/sites/articles/archive/2014/05/05/oil-pulling-coconut-oil.aspx>

Mercola, Joseph, Dr. *Proteins: Be Selective of Your Protein Sources*. No Date. Retrieved 2016. <http://www.mercola.com/nutritionplan/intermediate_proteins.htm>

Mercola, Joseph, Dr. *Should Parents Be Allowed to Decide About Vaccines?* 29 April 2014. Retrieved 2014. <http://articles.mercola.com/sites/articles/archive/2014/04/29/children-vaccines.aspx?e_cid=20140429-remainder-z1_DNL_art_1&utm_source=dnl&utm_medium=email&utm_content=art1&utm_campaign=20140429-remainder-z1&et_cid=DM45200&et_rid=503112330>

Myers Dennis L., M.D. *A "New" Biology*. No date. Retrieved about 2013 <http://members.iimetro.com.au/~hubbca/dr_dennis_myers.htm>

Myers, Dennis. *Cause of degenerative disease*. 19 Dec 2012. Retrieved in 2013. <http://www.life-enthusiast.com/cause-of-degenerative-disease-a-3526.html>

No author listed. *Bions, Protocells, Biogenesis, Pleomorphism, Live-Blood Microscopy and Genetics*. No date. Retrieved 2015. <http://www.orgonelab.org/cart/xbions.htm>

No author listed. *Darkfield Microscopy or Live Blood Analysis*. No Date. Retrieved about 2005 <http://altered-states.net/barry/darkfield/index.htm>

No author listed. *Discernment*. 15 Jan 2008. Retrieved 2010. <http://kundalini-

teacher.com/guidance/discern.php>

No author listed. *Kinesiology: The Tool for Testing*. No date. Retrieved 2014. <http://www.holistichealthtools.com/muscle.html>

No author listed. *Salts that Heal and Salts that Kill.* No date. Retrieved 2005. <http://curezone.org/foods/saltcure.asp>

No author listed. *Testing your Guides.* 15 Jan 2008. Retrieved 2010. <http://kundalini-teacher.com/guidance/testgui.php>

No author listed. *The Prayer To Our Father(translated into first century Aramaic)*. No date. Retrieved 2015 <http://www.thenazareneway.com/lords_prayer.htm>

No Author listed. *The Shadow Self.* 15 Jan 2008. Retrieved 2010. <http://kundalini-teacher.com/guidance/shadow.php>

No author listed. *Types of Dreams. No Date.* Retrieved 2012 <http://types-of-dreams.info/>

O'Shea, Tim. *Minerals*. 12 Oct 2012. Retrieved 2013 <http://www.life-enthusiast.com/minerals-tim-oshea-a-68.html>

Poehlman Karl Horst. *Dr. Enderlein, Bechamps and other Pleomorphic Researchers*. 1997. Retrieved 2009. <http://curezone.com/forums/fm.asp?i=919966>

Schweitzer, Sophia. *A Beginner's Guide to Craniosacral Therapy*. No date. Retrieved 2016. <http://www.cranialtherapycentre.com/a-beginners-guide-to-craniosacral-therapy/>

Sills, Franklyn. *Cranial Rhythmic Impulse*. 2013. Retrieved 2016 <http://www.craniosacral-biodynamics.org/cranialrhythmic-impulse.html>

Vander Stoep Carol, RDH, BSDH, OMT. *Safer and Healthier Alternatives to Root Canals and Other Common, Yet Harmful, Tooth Restoration Techniques.* 3 May 2014. Retrieved 2015. <http://articles.mercola.com/sites/articles/archive/2014/05/03/root-canal-alternative.aspx?e_cid=20140503Z1_DNL_art_1&utm_source=dnl&utm_medium=email&utm_content=art1&utm_campaign=20140503Z1&et_cid=DM45438&et_rid=508895019>

Velanthas. *[Ascension Information] More On The Galactic Oversoul Merges*. 9 Dec 2008. Retrieved 2014 <https://lightworkers.org/page/58696/ascension-information-more-on-the-galactic-oversoul-merges>

Viadro Claire I., MPH, PhD. *Sulfate, Sleep and Sunlight: The Disruptive and Destructive Effects of Heavy Metals and Glyphosate.* 8 May 2014. Retrieved 2015. <http://articles.mercola.com/sites/articles/archive/2014/05/08/heavy-metals-glyphosate-health-effects.aspx?e_cid=20140508Z1_DNL_art_1&utm_source=dnl&utm_medium=email&utm_content=art1&utm_campaign=20140508Z1&et_cid=DM45823&et_rid=514705428>

Whitaker, Kay Cordell. *Healing On All Levels*. 29 March 2012. Retrieved 2013 <http://www.katasee.com/2012/03/29/healing-on-all-levels/>

Web pages no longer available

Author unknown. <http://http-server.carleton.ca/~gkardos/88403/CREAT/Block4.htm>

Author unknown.<http://www.healwithhope.com/#!muscle-testingapplied-kinesiology/c20dx >

Van Auken, John. *The Body - Temple Of God.* 12 Nov 2007. Retrieved 2009 <http://edgarcayce.org/ps2/body_temple_of_god_J_Van_Auken.html>

About The Author

At the conscious level, my journey that has led to this book began in 1997. I first saw a doctor who used several alternate forms of testing and treating that were outside the usual western medicine 'norm'. Before then I was a follower of traditional Western medicine. As he and other doctors, practitioners and healers retired or moved too far away, I was led to the next; each one being further away from what is considered traditional/normal healing practices. Traditional medicine still has its role to play (surgery saved my life on at least two occasions), as do other modalities, some of which are listed in appendix B. Nutrition, exercise, proper sleep and common sense are also important parts of the whole.

Glenn Molinari was born in Wilmington, Delaware on April 17, 1948. Until 1954, his family lived in Southern New Jersey, at which time the family moved to the suburbs just outside Wilmington. Glenn served our Country in the Air Force from 1968 to 1972. After having been honorably discharged, he moved back to Delaware and in 1996 moved in with his father on the Eastern Shore of Maryland.

While Glenn was learning about alternative therapies and the Body/Mind/Spirit connections, he remained at his father's side as caregiver until 2007. He moved to Cornville, Arizona in 2008, where he resides today.

Glenn continues his interest in choosing Divine LOVE, practicing awareness and alternative healing modalities. He continues to share with those interested.

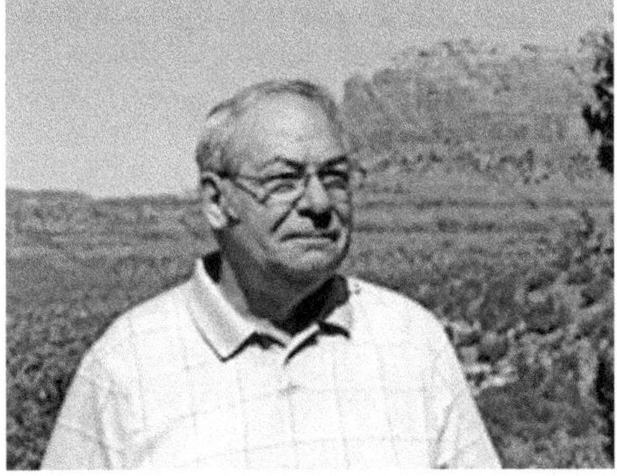

I hope you have found this helpful.

If you wish, you may contact Glenn Molinari

telephone: 1 (928) 300-6202

email: glenn@twoChoices.net

Web Site: http://twoChoices.net

www.ingramcontent.com/pod-product-compliance
Lightning Source LLC
LaVergne TN
LVHW081352060426
835510LV00013B/1784
* 9 7 8 0 9 8 5 4 7 8 4 7 6 *